PREVENTION AND TREATMENT OF HIV INFECTION IN INFANTS AND CHILDREN

ANNALS OF THE NEW YORK ACADEMY OF SCIENCES
Volume 918

PREVENTION AND TREATMENT OF HIV INFECTION IN INFANTS AND CHILDREN

Edited by Arthur J. Ammann and Arye Rubinstein

The New York Academy of Sciences
New York, New York
2000

Library of Congress Cataloging-in-Publication Data

Prevention and treatment of HIV infection in infants and children/ editors, Arthur J. Ammann, Arye Rubinstein.
    p. cm. — (Annals of the New York Academy of Sciences   ;v.918)
    Includes bibliographical references and indexes.
    ISBN 1-57331-267-3 (cloth : alk. paper) . — ISB N1-57331-268-1(pbk. : alk. paper)
    1. AIDS (Disease) in infants. 2. AIDS (Disease) in children. 3. HIV infections. 4. Infants—Health and hygiene. 5. Children—Health and hygiene. I. Ammann, Arthur J., 1936– II. Rubinstein, Arye. III. Series.

Q11.N5 vol. 918
[RJ387.A25]
500 s—dc21
[618.92'9792]   00-061301

GYAT / PCP
Printed in the United States of America
ISBN 1-57331-267-3 (cloth)
ISBN 1-57331-268-1 (paper)
ISSN 0077-8923

ANNALS OF THE NEW YORK ACADEMY OF SCIENCES

Volume 918
November 2000

PREVENTION AND TREATMENT OF HIV INFECTION IN INFANTS AND CHILDREN

Editors
ARTHUR J. AMMANN AND ARYE RUBINSTEIN

This volume is the result of a conference entitled **Second Conference on Global Strategies for the Prevention of HIV Transmission from Mothers to Infants**, sponsored by the International AIDS Society and the American Foundation for AIDS Research (amfAR) in collaboration with the Office of AIDS Research, National Institutes of Health, and the Canadian Association for HIV Research, and held on September 1–6, 1999, in Montreal, Canada. Also included is the **Satellite Conference on Advances in Pediatric AIDS**, which was sponsored by the New York Academy of Sciences and held on September 5–6, 1999, in Montreal, Canada.

CONTENTS

GLOBAL STRATEGIES FOR THE PREVENTION OF HIV TRANSMISSION FROM MOTHERS TO INFANTS

ADVANCES IN PEDIATRIC AIDS

Financial assistance was received from:

GLOBAL STRATEGIES CONFERENCE ON THE PREVENTION OF HIV TRANSMISSION FROM MOTHERS TO INFANTS

Co-sponsors
- CENTERS FOR DISEASE CONTROL AND PREVENTION
- ELIZABETH GLASER PEDIATRIC AIDS FOUNDATION
- FOGARTY INTERNATIONAL CENTER, NIH
- FRANÇOIS-XAVIER BAGNOUD FOUNDATION
- GLOBAL STRATEGIES FOR HIV PREVENTION
- HARVARD AIDS INSTITUTE
- JOSIAH MACY, JR. FOUNDATION
- MARCH OF DIMES
- NATIONAL INSTITUTE OF ALLERGY AND INFECTIOUS DISEASE (NIAID)
- NATIONAL INSTITUTE OF CHILD HEALTH AND HUMAN DEVELOPMENT (NICHD)
- NATIONAL INSTITUTE OF MENTAL HEALTH (NIMH)
- NEW YORK ACADEMY OF SCIENCES
- JOINT UNITED NATIONS PROGRAM ON HIV/AIDS

Corporate sponsor
- GLAXO WELLCOME

Corporate co-sponsors
- AGOURON
- BOEHRINGER INGELHEIM / ROXANE LABORATORIES
- BRISTOL-MYERS SQUIBB COMPANY
- MERCK FROSST (CANADA)

SATELLITE CONFERENCE ON ADVANCES IN PEDIATRIC AIDS

Major corporate funding
- GLAXO WELLCOME

Supporters
- DUPONT PHARMACEUTICALS COMPANY
- JOSIAH MACY, JR. FOUNDATION
- OFFICE OF AIDS RESEARCH, NIH
- PEPSI-COLA COMPANY
- AMERICAN FOUNDATION FOR AIDS RESEARCH (AmfAR)

Contributor
- MERCK & COMPANY

GLOBAL STRATEGIES FOR THE PREVENTION AND TREATMENT OF HIV TRANSMISSION FROM MOTHERS TO INFANTS

Introduction to the Second Conference on Global Strategies for the Prevention of HIV Transmission from Mothers to Infants

ARTHUR J. AMMANN[a]

Global Strategies for HIV Prevention, San Francisco, California, USA

Pediatric AIDS Research Institute, University of California, San Francisco, California, USA

The Second International Conference on Global Strategies for the Prevention of HIV Transmission from Mothers to Infants and the Satellite Conference on Advances in Pediatric AIDS focus on those who suffer as a result of some of the greatest disparities found in this epidemic. Women and children now comprise almost 50% of those who are infected with HIV. We know that they are more easily infected, have little or no contol over the circumstances under which they become infected, progress to disease more rapidly, have poorer health care, benefit from treatment more slowly, and suffer some of the severest consequences of discrimination. A diagnosis of HIV infection often means ostracism, poverty, neglect, loss of family, abuse, or orphan status.

During this conference we asked ourselves why the number of HIV-infected women and children continues to increase when for over a decade we have known how to prevent HIV infection. Are we too slow to act or too timid to apply what we already know? HIV counseling and testing, condoms, delay in first sexual intercourse, monogamy, prevention of pregnancy in HIV-infected women, elective cesarean section, treatment of sexually transmitted diseases, AZT during pregnancy, and alternatives to breastfeeding—the list of methods to prevent HIV infection is long. Since the last Global Strategies Conference in Washington, D.C. in September 1997, we now know that shorter and more economical courses of nevirapine or AZT may be as effective in preventing perinatal HIV transmission as ACTG 076. These are all effective prevention methods. And yet HIV infection continues to increase. We must remember that no amount of funding for research and no economical method of prevention will be effective unless implemented and that implementation requires accountability—accountability from individuals, accountability from health care professionals, and accountability from political and religious leaders.

This volume emphasizes subjects that are becoming increasingly important in preventing HIV infection. Some of these are scientific issues. Others are social, economic, political, and ethical issues. Some, such as breastfeeding, have become increasingly important because we have made advances that now demand that we reexamine previous assumptions. Throughout the conference, issues were highlight-

[a]Address for correspondence: 104 Dominican Drive, San Rafael, CA 94901. Voice: 415-451-1814; fax: 415-456-2622.
Ammanndoc@aol.com

ed in areas where our knowledge is insufficient, not to discourage, but rather to call attention to new areas that require emphasis, resources, or research. Some subjects address more practical and economical methods for preventing HIV infection, which are desperately needed for resource-poor countries. This year's conference will also address the growing number of HIV-infected and -uninfected children who now constitute "the orphan crisis." The satellite conference on pediatric HIV/AIDS emphasized advances that have been made in the treatment of HIV infection and asked how these can be transferred into developing countries.

It is to be hoped that each person who attended the conference left with both a sense of urgency and a clear understanding of his or her role in contributing to the prevention of HIV infection. The meeting can only be called successful if change occurs—in individuals, communities, organizations, governments and policies—change that results in HIV prevention.

Human Immunodeficiency Virus:
An Epidemic without Precedent

ARTHUR J. AMMANN[a]

Global Strategies for HIV Prevention, San Francisco, California, USA

Pediatric AIDS Research Institute, University of California, San Francisco, California, USA

In spite of the now estimated 40 million persons infected with the human immunodeficiency virus (HIV) worldwide, there is no historical precedent to predict the full biologic impact of the epidemic.[1] Compared to the much-feared epidemics of the past that adapted to predictable patterns of dissemination over centuries of time, HIV began an estimated 40 years ago.[2] Thus, HIV is a new virus, and we are just now beginning to understand its origin, variation, and adaptation to its human host. HIV results in an infection in which protective immunity never develops, resulting in a state of chronic immunodeficiency.[3,4] This secondary immunodeficiency promotes the global proliferation of new infectious agents and resurgence of old ones.[5,6] The unique biologic consequences of HIV infection suggest that there will be an ongoing evolution of the epidemic with continued infection of millions of persons at a constant rate. Further, in spite of highly successful combination antiretroviral therapy with suppression of viral levels to almost undetectable levels, recent studies have cast doubt on our ability to eradicate the virus.[7] As we move forward in a prevention agenda, it is clear that the epidemiology and biology of HIV infection provide some sobering thoughts about our ability to bring the epidemic under control before additional massive numbers of persons become infected.

Even though there is universal agreement that ultimate control of HIV infection cannot occur until there is an effective preventative vaccine, there are few scientific advances in HIV vaccinology that bring substantial hope that this will be possible in the near future. Results from studies of subunit vaccines, such as those produced by recombinant DNA technology and, more recently, DNA vaccines, have not resulted in broad-based neutralizing immunity of long duration.[8,9] Viral envelope antigens, obtained directly from patients, have been under evaluation for several decades, are poorly immunogenic, and stimulate low levels of antibody that neutralize laboratory strains of HIV but fail to neutralize broad ranges of HIV.[10] The use of a variety of adjuvants has improved the immune response including cytotoxic T-cell immunity, but it is clear that HIV is capable of "escaping" immunologic control.[11] Entirely new approaches to developing a vaccine, such as DNA immunization or unique methods of antigen presentation, are likely to be required; but while these novel approaches are under evaluation, tens of millions more persons will become infected with HIV.[12]

[a]Address for correspondence: 104 Dominican Drive, San Rafael, CA 94901. Voice: 415-451-1814; fax: 415-456-2622.
Ammanndoc@aol.com

The frustration of not having a vaccine to prevent HIV resulted in the brief embrace of the concept that a live attenuated vaccine might be the solution to the global epidemics. In reality, this was a result of a failure to appreciate the extraordinary ability of HIV to defeat the immune system. The flirtation with a live attenuated vaccine was based on the observation that several patients, infected with a mutated HIV strain that contained a *nef* deletion, failed to develop immunodeficiency.[13] Animal studies were designed using *nef*-deleted attenuated strains of SIV to test the hypothesis that an HIV *nef*-deleted vaccine might be safe to test in humans. However, *nef*-deleted SIV-immunized animals developed disease when challenged with SIV and patients with *nef*-deleted HIV infection went on to disease progression.[14] It is likely that we have a long way to go before we will have an effective vaccine, and it is possible that we have yet to make the critical discovery that will allow for the development of a protective vaccine for HIV.

Therapeutic strategies to control HIV replication and disease progression are increasingly meeting with failure primarily due to drug resistance.[15,16] While this is not a surprise to some, the rapidity with which this has occurred has resulted in rethinking different therapeutic approaches such as delaying therapy or saving the "best" therapy until more advanced disease occurs.[17] In reality, none of these are likely to be effective as long-term strategies for controlling the global epidemic and represent "fall-back" positions rather than true treatment advances.

The demonstration that drug resistance emerges more rapidly under circumstances of monotherapy, simple two-drug combinations, or intermittent treatment raises skepticism about the ability to achieve long-term control of the HIV epidemic in developing countries by means of antiretroviral therapy.[18,19] With 90% of the world's population of HIV-infected persons in developing countries with the least potential for affording combination drug treatment, monotherapy and interrupted therapy are the more likely scenarios, leading to the development and transmission of multidrug-resistant HIV.[20] Like tuberculosis, we can expect broad geographic dissemination of resistant virus.

The cost of antiretroviral therapy is also likely to impair the ability to use treatment as a means of controlling the epidemic. It has been estimated that the cost of treating only 50% of the world's population of existing and new HIV infections over the next decade would be in the range of $1.4 trillion US. Not only is it unlikely that these sums of money will be available, but even smaller amounts dedicated to the HIV epidemic could severely deplete funding for other serious and life-threatening diseases.

These observations are not presented to suggest that treatment should be relegated to the 10% of HIV-infected persons who reside in developed countries, while those in developing countries forgo the benefits of combination drug treatment. Rather, they argue that the very nature of HIV, the high mutation rate, the rapid emergence of multiple-drug-resistant HIV, and the inability to eradicate HIV, are complementary factors that are likely to increase the severity of the epidemic over the next decades. Indeed, the very success of antiretroviral treatment has potentially lengthened the lifetime potential for transmission of HIV, including multiple-drug-resistant strains.

Unlike other epidemics that produced disease and death directly related to the causative organism, HIV plays a direct and indirect role in the resurgence of other multiple-drug-resistant infections such as tuberculosis.[21] Although detailed cause and effect studies have not been performed, epidemiological data from India and China demonstrated dramatic increases in tuberculosis several years before documented increases in HIV infection.[22] In both countries, ongoing surveillance for tuberculosis, and the absence of surveillance for HIV, made it difficult to determine their relationship. However, in the United States, epidemiological data has forged a strong link to these infections and suggest that the immunodeficiency induced by HIV increases the susceptibility to tuberculosis, making treatment more difficult. Multiple-drug-resistant tuberculosis is more prevalent in HIV-infected persons, and it certainly is transmissible as evidenced by the spread to healthcare workers, airline passengers, and airline personnel.[23]

There are also unknown consequences of the association of the high mutation rate of HIV and the failure to develop a controlling immune response. Unlike bacteria, which appear to retain genetic integrity over long periods of time, some viruses, especially HIV, have genetic similarity to recent common ancestors.[24] In the past bacterial, viral, and fungal mutations have occurred against the background of a stable immune system and have evolved mechanisms to avoid attacks by immune mechanisms by invading microenvironments. Some protozoans such as malaria use major antigenic change as a mechanism for avoiding immunologic destruction while others, such as hepatitis C virus, use molecular mimicry. All of these evasive mechanisms result in a more favorable environment for the survival of the specific organism and in general do not result in enhanced survival of unrelated organisms. The induction of a prolonged and severe immunodeficiency by HIV is unique, and the biologic consequences of this widespread immunodeficiency will almost certainly not be recognized for several additional decades. HIV infection complicates the ability to predict future pathogen proliferation dynamics within the host as described by Levin *et al.* in relation to the immunologic pressures that determine the "abundance, diversity, and distribution of a pathogen" within an infected host or in the global ecology. Indeed, since it is likely that the immunodeficiency produced by HIV will alter both the pathogen dynamics of past and current microorganisms and also provide an opportunity for new and unknown microorganisms to adapt to human hosts, we have yet to experience the full impact of HIV infection.

The lack of a controlling immune response to HIV permits ongoing viral replication and transmission. This is fundamental to understanding the continued escalation of the HIV epidemic. Previous viral disease epidemics, though responsible for waves of deaths associated with susceptibility to infection, came under control spontaneously as populations became immune to new infection. Even for infections such as smallpox, decades passed without any new epidemics occurring until a new population of susceptibles emerged. Not so for HIV, to which individuals remain either susceptible or infectious.

It is intriguing, but worrisome, to speculate about the consequences of prolonged replication of a virus such as HIV in the absence of adequate immune control. Several scenarios could be postulated. A mutation to a more virulent (more infectious) strain might occur, or there might be a mutation to a less virulent strain. Either mutation could result in expansion of the HIV epidemic. A more virulent strain, while producing death more rapidly, might also be associated with more rapid spread to larger numbers of individuals. Such mutations are not without precedent. The 1918 epidemic of influenza virus was associated with a mutation of that virus to one which rapidly spread worldwide and resulted in the deaths of 20 million persons in just one year.[25] A mutation to a less virulent strain would prolong the lifetime exposure potential and could also result in significantly greater spread of the virus, although over a longer time span. Either mutation could be devastating.

There are other reasons why it is difficult to extrapolate from past epidemics to predict the impact of HIV on the future on the world's population. Technology has played an important role in the dissemination of infection, and the impact of travel has been well documented for measles, syphilis, the black plague, and smallpox. But the spread of these epidemics was "contained" by limitations in travel, the smaller global population (500 million in the 1600s to 7 billion in this decade), and ultimate self containment of the epidemics by the development of an immune population. Most of the new regions of the HIV epidemic can be linked to travel and to the identified means of transmission—unprotected sex, intravenous drug use, unscreened blood products, and multiple sexual partners. Once established in an area, heterosexual and perinatal HIV transmission follow. But along with HIV, other opportunistic infections may spread as well. With airplane travel reaching over 1.5 billion people per year and outbreaks of tuberculosis that have occurred among airline passengers, including drug-resistant tuberculosis, HIV and associated opportunistic infections are likely to gain access to even the most remote regions of the world.[23]

The biology of the known routes of HIV transmission will also make the control of the epidemic difficult. This is particularly true for the pediatric population in developing countries where mother-to-infant HIV transmission and transmission through breast feeding are widespread.[26,27] In countries with a high seroprevalence of HIV, such as sub-Saharan Africa, over 30% of pregnant women are infected, giving rise to extremely large numbers of HIV-infected infants at birth. Breast feeding adds additional large numbers to those who initially escape HIV infection. Even though cessation of breast feeding could reduce the transmission rate of HIV, the high mortality rate and expense of formula feeding in most developing countries does not make this a viable option.

We are encouraged by the clinical studies that demonstrate significant reductions in HIV transmission by means of antiretroviral treatment of HIV-infected mothers and their infants.[28–30] In the United States it is believed that transmission rates are less that 3% with combination antiretroviral therapy. Reduction of perinatal HIV transmission to less than 10% in developing countries by increased use of counseling, testing, and inexpensive treatment could save the lives of 350,000 infants each year.

Behavior modification programs that are directed at transmission primarily by the sexual route are extremely difficult to implement.[31] Cultural, religious, and individual beliefs frustrate known methods of prevention such as abstinence, monogamy, delayed sexual experience, and use of condoms. Although some prevention programs have been successful in some countries such as Uganda, it is clear that there has been little progress in most of the sub-Saharan countries. HIV is transmitted by sexual intercourse, a process that is fundamental to the survival of the human race.

The long asymptomatic period during which transmission can occur is another biologic feature unique to HIV. Epidemics such as smallpox, the black plague, and typhus were associated with outward manifestations of infection that alerted noninfected persons to the presence of disease. HIV-infected persons may be asymptomatic for over 10 years during which time they may infect multiple individuals. In countries where HIV testing of blood products is not performed, hundreds of thousands of persons my be infected each year from unscreened HIV-infected blood donated by asymptomatic individuals.

The unique biology of HIV, the immaturity of the epidemic, the high mutation rate of the virus, the rapid emergence and transmission of multidrug-resistant virus, the difficulty in effecting behavior changes to reduce transmission, and the lack of an effective vaccine for prevention strongly suggest that we are only at the earliest stages of this epidemic. It is for this reason that every method of prevention must be employed to effectively reduce the "pool" of HIV-infected persons. Interruption of transmission of HIV from mothers to infants is necessary to both reduce the pool of HIV-infected infants and to ensure a future generation of children for countries and regions whose human resources are rapidly vanishing. Extraordinary progress has been made in preventing perinatal HIV transmission. Preventive treatment is now within the reach of all countries and many persons as economic barriers have been broken by cost-effective treatment.[32] There should be little tolerance for political leaders who rapidly deploy economic resources for human destruction while withholding life-saving health care from the powerless.[33]

REFERENCES

1. UNAIDS/WORLD HEALTH ORGANIZATION REPORT. 1999. The status and trends of the HIV/AIDS epidemic in the world. UNAIDS/WHO. New York.
2. KORBER, B., J. THEILER & S. WOLINSKY. 1998. Limitations of a molecular clock applied to considerations of the origin of HIV-1. Science **280:** 1868–1871.
3. AMMANN, A.J., G. SCHIFFMAN, D. ABRAMS, *et al.* 1984. B-cell immunodeficiency in acquired immune deficiency syndrome. JAMA **251:** 1447–1449.
4. PANTALEO, G., C. GRAZIOSI & A.S. FAUCI. 1993. New concepts in the immunopathogenesis of human immunodeficiency virus infection. N. Engl. J. Med. **328:** 327–335.
5. CAVERT, W. 1997. Preventing and treating major opportunistic infections in AIDS. What's new and what's still true. Postgrad. Med. **102:** 125–126.
6. MISRA, S.N., D. SENGUPTA & S.K. SATPATHY. 1998. AIDS in India: recent trends in opportunistic infections. Southeast Asian J. Trop. Med. Public Health **29:** 373–376.
7. DORNADULA, G., H. ZHANG, B. VANUITERT. *et al.* 1999. Residual HIV-1 RNA in blood plasma of patients taking suppressive highly active antiretroviral therapy. JAMA **282:** 1627–1632.
8. HANSON, C.V. 1994. Measuring vaccine-induced HIV neutralization: report of a workshop. AIDS Res. Hum. Retroviruses **10:** 645–648.
9. GRAHAM, B.S. & P.F. WRIGHT. 1995. Candidate AIDS vaccines. N. Engl. J. Med. **333:** 1331–1339.
10. STEIMER, K.S., C.K. SCANDELLA, P.V. SKILES, *et al.* 1991. Neutralization of divergent HIV-1 isolates by conformation-dependent human antibodies to Gp120. Science **254:** 105–108.
11. WILSON, C.C., R.C. BROWN, B.T. KORBER, *et al.* 1999. Frequent detection of escape from cytotoxic T-lymphocyte recognition in perinatal human immunodeficiency virus (HIV) type 1 transmission: the ariel project for the prevention of transmission of HIV from mother to infant. J. Virol. **73:** 3975–3985.
12. GIRARD, M., A. HABEL & C. CHANEL. 1999. New prospects for the development of a vaccine against human immunodeficiency virus type 1. An overview. C. R. Acad. Sci. III **322:** 959–966.

13. LEARMONT, J.C., A.F. GECZY, J. MILLS, *et al.* 1999. Immunologic and virologic status after 14 to 18 years of infection with an attenuated strain of HIV-1. A report from the Sydney Blood Bank Cohort. N. Engl. J. Med. **340:** 1715–1722.
14. RUPRECHT, R.M. 1999. Live attenuated AIDS viruses as vaccines: promise or peril? Immunol. Rev. **170:** 135–149.
15. PALMER, S., R.W. SHAFER & T.C. MERIGAN. 1999. Highly drug-resistant HIV-1 clinical isolates are cross-resistant to many antiretroviral compounds in current clinical development. AIDS **13:** 661–667.
16. FURTADO, M.R., D.S. CALLAWAY, J.P. PHAIR, *et al.* 1999. Persistence of HIV-1 transcription in peripheral blood monuclear cells in patients receiving potent antiretroviral therapy. N. Engl. J. Med. **340:** 1614–1621.
17. STEPHENSON, J. 1999. Hopes for HIV eradication dim as stopping HAART allows resurgence. JAMA **282:** 17–18.
18. SWARTZ, M.N. 1997. Use of antimicrobial agents and drug resistance. N. Engl. J. Med. **337:** 491–492.
19. RICHMAN, D.D. 1993. Resistance of clinical isolates of human immunodeficiency virus to antiretroviral agents. Antimicrob. Agents Chemother. **37:** 1207–1213.
20. YERLY, S., L. KAISER, E. RACE, *et al.* 1999. Transmission of antiretroviral-drug-resistant HIV-1 variants. Lancet **354:** 729–733.
21. GLEISSBERG, V. 1999. The threat of multidrug resistance: is tuberculosis ever untreatable or uncontrollable? Lancet **353:** 998–999.
22. YU, E.S., Q. XIE, K. ZHANG, *et al.* 1996. HIV infection and AIDS in China, 1985 through 1994. Am. J. Public Health **86:** 1116–1122.
23. World's Next Epidemic: Resistant Tuberculosis. Gazette World. 17 March 1999. Montreal, Canada.
24. LEVIN, B.R., M. LIPSITCH & S. BONHOEFFER. 1999. Population biology, evolution, and infectious disease: convergence and synthesis. Science **283:** 806–809.
25. SHORTRIDGE, K.F. 1999 Influenza—a continuing detective story. Lancet **354:** SIV29.
26. NDUATI, R., G. JOHN, D. MBORI-NGACHA, *et al.* 2000. Effect of breastfeeding and formula feeding on transmission of HIV-1: a randomized clinical trial. JAMA **283:** 1167–1174.
27. BULTERYS, M. & M.G. FOWLER. 2000. Prevention of HIV infection in children. Pediatr. Clin. N. Am. **47(1):** 241–260.
28. CONNOR, E.M., R.S. SPERLING, R. GELBER, *et al.* 1994. Reduction of maternal–infant transmission of human immunodeficiency virus type 1 with zidovudine treatment. Pediatric AIDS Clinical Trials Group Protocol 076 Study Group. N. Engl. J. Med. **331(18):** 1173–1180.
29. 1998. Administration of zidovudine during late pregnancy and delivery to prevent perinatal HIV transmission—Thailand, 1996–1998. Morbid. Mortal. Wkly. Rep. **47:** 151–154.
30. GUAY, L.A., P. MUSOKE, T. FLEMING, *et al.* 1999. Intrapartum and neonatal single-dose nevirapine compared with zidovudine for prevention of mother-to-child transmission of HIV-1 in Kampala, Uganda: HIVNET 012 randomised trial. Lancet **354:** 795–802.
31. CATES, W., JR. & G. DALLABETTA. 1999. The staying power of sexually transmitted diseases. Lancet **354:** SIV62.
32. MARSEILLE, E., J.G. KAHN, F. MMIRO, *et al.* 1999. Cost effectiveness of single-dose nevirapine regimen for mothers and babies to decrease vertical HIV-1 transmission in sub-Saharan Africa. Lancet **354:** 803–809.
33. DE COCK, K.M., M.G. FOWLER, E. MERCIER, *et al.* 2000. Prevention of mother-to-child HIV transmission in resource-poor countries: translating research into policy and practice. JAMA **283:** 1175–1182.

The Role of Antiretrovirals and Drug Resistance in Vertical Transmission of HIV-1 Infection

BLUMA G. BRENNER AND MARK A. WAINBERG[a]

McGill University AIDS Centre, Lady Davis Institute, Jewish General Hospital, Montreal, Quebec, Canada

ABSTRACT: Large-cohort studies in North America, Europe, and Thailand have shown that zidovudine/azidothymidine (AZT) monotherapy, given at the late stages of pregnancy, is of proven benefit in reducing mother-to-infant HIV transmission by 51% to 68%. AZT monotherapy will not be of long-term benefit for mothers because no single drug can counteract viral infection; benefits to babies will be short-lived if HIV-1 is acquired through breastfeeding after birth. Unfortunately, ongoing mutation of HIV under conditions of drug pressure allows for the evolution and selection of AZT-resistant viruses. Emergence of AZT-resistant variants in pregnant mothers (7–29%) and their infected offspring (5–21%) has been described in several studies. Drug resistance arises more frequently in those mothers who received AZT therapy before pregnancy. Recent advances in combination chemotherapy may provide alternative strategies in prevention of vertical transmission and drug resistance. Genotypic screening of the HIV-1 isolated from pregnant mothers may provide rational modifications in antiretroviral (ARV) strategies to circumvent vertical HIV transmission. This may be of advantage for resource-rich nations but not for underdeveloped nations with limited access to ARVs. Public health programs are vital to have an impact on the tragic pandemic of pediatric AIDS.

INTRODUCTION

Vertical transmission is the main mode of acquisition of HIV infection for children. Before 1993, the estimated rate of mother-to-child transmission ranged from 15 to 20% in Europe, 15 to 25% in the United States, and 25 to 35% in Africa.[1] Contributing factors attributed to vertical HIV transmission include clinical, immunological, and virological progression of disease in the mother; breastfeeding; and vaginal delivery.[2,3]

The groundbreaking American/French Pediatric AIDS Clinical Trial Group (PACTG) trial 076 showed that zidovudine/azidothymidine (AZT) could substantially reduce the risk of vertical HIV transmission.[4] In this study conducted between

[a]Address for correspondence: Dr. Mark Wainberg, McGill AIDS Centre, Lady Davis Institute/ Jewish General Hospital, 3755 Cote Ste-Catherine Road, Montreal, Quebec, Canada H3T 1E2. mdwa@musica.mcgill.ca

1991 and 1993, women with mildly symptomatic HIV disease and no prior treatment with antiretroviral drugs were given AZT on a continuous basis during the second and third trimesters and intravenously during labor, followed by daily treatment of infants for 6 weeks after delivery. Maternal-to-infant HIV transmission decreased by two-thirds with AZT treatment, with transmission rates of 7.6% of infants in the AZT group as compared to 22.6% in the placebo group. No significant adverse effects were seen in mothers or neonates. Recent results from PACTG Protocol 185 expanded these findings to include women with lower CD4 cell counts and prior AZT experience.[5]

These dramatic results led the USPHS to issue guidelines for voluntary HIV counseling and testing of all pregnant women and routine use of AZT for HIV-infected pregnant women. This directive has led to the increased use of pre- or post-natal antiretroviral therapy from existing levels of 21% in 1993 to 95% in 1997.[6] As a result, reductions in vertical HIV transmission have occurred to the point where most pediatric cases of HIV infection in the United States are from mothers who did not receive antiretroviral prophylaxis. It is now the practice in all Western countries to treat mothers with recommended antiretroviral drug (ARV) regimens regardless of their pregnancy status, thus possibly preventing transmission risk even further.[7–11]

A more pressing issue, perhaps, is that of treatment of mothers in underdeveloped and resource-poor nations with AZT monotherapy to prevent soaring rates of vertical HIV transmission. Results from an important Thailand study showed that a short-course treatment of administering AZT near the end of gestation and during delivery, but not to the newborn, resulted in a 51% reduction in rates of mother-to-infant transmission.[12]

It should be noted that short-term AZT monotherapy is of no clinical benefit for the women even if monotherapy were continued after delivery. In this context, AZT would not preserve its benefit during subsequent pregnancies if selection of AZT-resistant isolates were to occur. Despite the dramatic declines in mother-to-child HIV transmissions due to AZT monotherapy in pregnancy, many clinical, ethical, and cost-benefit issues questions must still be answered.[1,11–14] These include optimal timing of administration of AZT intervention, pharmakinetics and dosage, and determination of its effectiveness in different patient populations.[1] Concerns have been expressed about the possibility of long-term effects of exposure to ARVs during pregnancy, both for the mother and the infant (of whom four out of five are uninfected anyway) and the implications for antenatal screening.[1] In many resource-poor international settings, the current interventions are neither feasible nor affordable.[12,13]

Particularly problematic is the issue of breastfeeding. The United Nations Programme on AIDS recently announced that HIV-infected mothers in developing countries should consider alternatives to breastfeeding.[11] The proven benefit of AZT in preventing vertical transmission will be short-lived if babies who were born free of HIV acquire virus soon afterward by breastfeeding.

Clearly, it is essential to advocate the use of AZT and other ARVs to minimize vertical HIV transmission. Indeed, cumulative findings indicate that maternal viral levels are highly predictive of perinatal transmission risk.[15–17] ARVs exert major protective effects by reducing maternal HIV-1 levels before delivery. Further antiretroviral strategies are needed to prevent perinatal transmission in women with high or increasing virus levels and/or ARV-resistant virus.

AZT/ARV DRUG RESISTANCE

There is growing concern that the efficacy of AZT may decrease with time if the drug is given as monotherapy. The HIV-1 viral reverse transcriptase (RT) enzyme is responsible for copying viral RNA.[18] This enzyme has a high error rate and can generate between 0.2 and 1 point mutations during every viral replication event. The ability of HIV to mutate allows for the evolution and selection of viruses resistant to antiviral compounds, including AZT, under conditions of selective drug pressure. Many reports of transmission of AZT-resistant isolates have been published since the initial report of such an occurrence in 1989 in persons treated with AZT monotherapy for prolonged periods of time.[18,19] Resistance to AZT has been attributed to mutations at codons 41, 67, 70, 210, 215, and 219. In particular, mutations in codon 215 have been linked to high-level resistance to AZT in treated individuals.

To address the serious and growing concern as to whether AZT monotherapy will continue to reduce perinatal HIV transmission, a number of recent studies have assayed maternal samples from entry and delivery to determine (1) the prevalence of genotypic HIV variants resistant to AZT at entry, (2) if AZT resistance develops on study, and (3) the impact of AZT resistance on transmission of infection to infants.

The first case of pediatric infection with AZT-resistant viruses was reported in 1993.[20] Mother-to-child transmission of AZT-resistant viruses was first described in 1994, where the mother had received AZT for 15 months before pregnancy.[21] This case of transmission of the highly resistant virus, mutated at codon 215, was not attributable to AZT given at the end of pregnancy or during labor; rather, AZT drug resistance was present before gestation. In one case study, HIV infection with AZT-resistant genotypic variants arose after postnatal prophylaxis in a perinatally infected infant.[22] A recent case study has documented mother-to-infant transmission of primary HIV-1 infection during pregnancy.[23] A two-month-old child, seronegative at birth, presented with primary infection. Her mother had syphilis in the third month of pregnancy with negative HIV test results. Postpartum results indicated that the mother had undergone primary HIV-1 infection during pregnancy.

The prevalence and transmission of AZT-resistant viruses in mothers receiving AZT therapy during pregnancy are summarized in TABLE 1. It should be noted that transmission of genotypic markers associated with AZT resistance in mothers receiving AZT and in their infected offspring does not necessarily indicate that these viruses are completely phenotypically resistant to AZT. This is because advent of highly resistant T215Y/F mutations requires prolonged AZT therapy. The majority of observed AZT resistance in mothers and in their infected newborns were with K70R viruses conferring relatively low-level AZT resistance.

Retrospective genotypic analysis was performed on 96 of the women enrolled in the initial PACTG protocol 076 to determine levels of AZT-resistant variants with short-term AZT monotherapy during pregnancy.[24,25] None of the woman had high-level resistance to AZT at study entry or delivery; only two (3.2%) of 61 women carried the K70R mutation, associated with low-level AZT resistance. No women had T215Y/F mutations associated with high-level AZT resistance, although two women taking AZT before pregnancy carried the T215D or T215C substitutions. During the course of the PACTG 076 clinical study, only one of the 39 cases in the AZT arm of the study developed the K70R mutation and none harbored viruses with mutations

TABLE 1. Prevalence of genotypic markers associated with AZT resistance in mothers and HIV-infected newborns

Virus source	Sample size (n)	No. of cases of resistant viruses	AZT-resistant genotypic profile	Reference
Maternal	61	4 (6.5%)	K70R ($n = 2$); T215D/C ($n = 2$)	24,25
Infant	7	1 (14%)	K70R	
Maternal	14	3 (21%)	K70R ($n = 2$); M41L, T215Y ($n = 1$)	26
Infant	6	1 (17%)	T215T/S →T215Y in gestation	
Maternal	24	7 (29%)	70, 210,215,219	27,28
Infant	24	5 (21%)	70,210,215,219	
Infant	54	5 (9%)	K70R ($n = 3$), T215Y ($n = 1$), 41,210,215 ($n = 1$)	6
Maternal	16	4 (25%)	K70R ($n = 2$); 41,215 ($n = 2$)	8
Infant	1[a]	1 (5%)	41,215	

[a]This was the only case of maternal–infant transmission in 20 AZT-treated cases.

at codon 215. Only one of the seven infants infected with HIV carried K70R mutated virus from her K70R-infected mother.

In an important study of 24 pairs of AZT-exposed women and their HIV-infected infants,[27,28] a significant proportion ($n = 7$, 29%) of the cohort harbored viruses with AZT-associated genotypic mutations (TABLE 1). Transmission of AZT-resistant viruses to newborns occurred in only those cases ($n = 5$, 20%) where mutated AZT-resistant viruses were the predominant quasispecies in the virus mixture.

AZT is rarely used today in monotherapy, and AZT combination regimens are not always the treatment of choice for HIV-infected women. ARV cocktails, including nucleoside (NRTI) and nonnucleoside (NNRTI) inhibitors of viral reverse transcriptase, as well as protease inhibitors (PIs), have dramatically reduced viral load and disease progression in infected persons. The long-term effects of these highly potent regimens in pregnancy and infant well-being will require scrutiny.[29] Moreover, as triple drug combinations become commonplace, so too has the prevalence of viruses carrying genotypic markers suggestive of resistance to one or more classes of ARVs. HIV viruses with two- and three-class multidrug resistance (MDR) have been recently observed in newly infected individuals. Studies at four major centers, including our own, have begun to monitor the prevalence of resistant viruses by studying adults undergoing primary infection (TABLE 2).[30–33] These studies emphasize the growing public health problem of HIV drug resistance. The ramifications of ARV-resistant variants in vertical HIV transmission remain to be seen.

FUTURE DIRECTIONS IN ARV INTERVENTIONS

An estimated three million children have been infected with HIV-1 since the onset of the AIDS pandemic, with 90% of the reported cases occurring in Africa.[34] The incidence of childhood HIV-1 infection in Africa now projected at greater than 500,000 cases annually.[35] In the last two years, important progress has been made in

TABLE 2. Prevalence of HIV-1 variants carrying genotypic resistance mutations to nucleoside (NRTI) and nonnucleoside (NNRTI) reverse transcriptase inhibitors, protease (PI) inhibitors, and multidrug resistance (MDR) in cohorts with primary infection

Drug mutations at select codon sites	Montreal[30] (*n* = 80) 97–99	Geneva[31] (*n* = 82) 96–98	NY[32] (*n* = 80) 95–99	Five USA cities[33] (*n* = 141) 89–98
NRTIs	16.5%	10%	12.5%	
AZT-all	8.8%	9%	7.5%	
AZT- 41	3.8%	4.9%	5%	
67	2.5%	3%	8.8%	
70	1.2%	—	3.8%	
210	2.5%	1.3%	1.3%	
215	5%	8.5%	2.5%	2.1%
219	2.5%	—	1.3%	2.1%
3TC-184	5%	2.4%	5%	2.1%
ddI-74	1.3%	—	—	
ddC-69	2.9%	—	—	
d4T-50	1.3%	—	—	
NNRTI	11.3%	>1%	8.8%	0.7%
Primary PI	3.8%		2.5%	
30	1.3%	—	—	
48	1.3%	—	—	
82	1.3%	11.4%	1.3%	
90	3.8%	1.4%	2.5%	
Three-class MDR	3.8%	1.3%	3.8%	2.1%

the prevention of vertical HIV transmission with inexpensive anti-viral interventions. In a recent Côte D'Ivoire study, a short-course AZT regimen has shown a 37% efficacy at 6 months postpartum, in a breastfeeding cohort where treatment was provided from 36 weeks' gestation until delivery.[36] The UNAIDS-sponsored PETRA trials in sub-Saharan Africa report a preliminary 51% efficacy rate of an AZT-3TC combination regimen, given from 38 weeks' gestation until delivery.[37] The HIVNET 012 trial has been initiated in Kampala, Uganda in July 1999 to determine the efficacy of a single-dose nevirapine regimen.[38] If proven effective, this regimen may have an enormous impact in less-developed countries with high seroprevalence.

Taken together, most studies indicate that ARVs can play pivotal roles in preventing vertical HIV transmission. Unfortunately, vertical transmission of viruses carrying mutations that confer low-level resistance to AZT has been observed (TABLE 1). The prevalence of AZT- and ARV-resistant viruses in HIV-infected women can be expected to increase in frequency in the future. Whether HIV drug resistance influences the rate of mother-to-infant transmission, only time will tell. Genotypic screening of pregnant HIV-infected mothers may be warranted to adjust treatment strategies to avoid or reduce the risk of vertical transmission. Selective and rational modifications of drugs combinations may be effective in minimizing the development of resistance. There are growing concerns about the consequences of resistant viruses for infants. Clearly, HIV drug resistance is likely to emerge as a major public health problem that must be addressed in strategies for prevention of pediatric AIDS.

ACKNOWLEDGMENTS

This work was sponsored by FRSQ, CANFAR, MRC Canada.

REFERENCES

1. NEWELL, M.L. & D.M. GIBB. 1995. A risk–benefit assessment of zidovudine in the prevention of perinatal HIV transmission. Drug Safety 12(4): 274–282.
2. NEWELL, M.L. & C. PECKHAM. 1993. Risk factors for vertical transmission of HIV-1 and early markers of HIV-1 infection in children. AIDS 7: S91–S97.
3. MOFENSON, L. 1994. Epidemiology and determinants of vertical HIV transmission. Semin. Pediatr. Infect. Dis. 5: 252–265.
4. CONNOR, E.M., R.S. SPERLING, R. GELBER, et al. 1994. Reduction of maternal–infant transmission of human immunodeficiency virus type 1 with zidovudine treatment: Pediatric AIDS Clinical Trials Group Protocol 076 Study Group. N. Engl. J. Med. 331: 1173–1180.
5. STIEM, E.R., R.S. LAMBERT, L.M. MOFENSON, et al. 1999. Efficacy of zidovudine and human immunodeficiency virus (HIV) hyperimmune globulin for reducing perinatal HIV transmission from HIV-infected women with advanced disease. Results of pediatric AIDS clinical trial protocol 185. J. Infect. Dis. 179: 567–575.
6. FISCUS, S.A., A.A. ADIMORA, V.J. SCHOENBACH, et al. 1999. Trends in human immunodeficiency virus (HIV) counseling, testing, and antiretroviral treatment of HIV-infected women and perinatal transmission in North Carolina. J. Infect. Dis. 180: 99–105.
7. RACHLIS, A.R. & D.P. ZAROWNY. 1998. Guidelines for antiretroviral therapy for HIV infection. Canadian HIV Trials Network Antiretroviral Working Group. Can. Med. Assoc. J. 158: 496–505.
8. FRENKEL, L.M., L.E. WAGNER, L.M. DEMETER, et al. 1995. Effects of zidovudine use during pregnancy on resistance and vertical transmission of human immunodeficiency virus type 1. Clin. Infect. Dis. 20(5): 1321–1326.
9. MATHESON, P.B., E.J. ABRAMS, P.A. THOMAS, et al. 1995. Efficacy of antenatal zidovudine in reducing perinatal transmission of human immunodeficiency virus type 1. The New York City Perinatal HIV Transmission Collaborative Study Group. J. Infect. Dis. 172: 353–358.
10. SPOONER, K.M. 1998. Antiretroviral therapy in human immunodeficiency virus-infected individuals. Adv. Intern. Med. 43: 373–402.
11. WAINBERG, M.A. 1999. The endless tragedy of pediatric AIDS. J. Hum. Vir. 2: 1–2.
12. VUTHIPONGSE, P., C. BHADRAKOM, P. CHAISILWATTANA, et al. 1998. Administration of zidovudine during last pregnancy and delivery to prevent perinatal HIV transmission—Thailand 1996–1998. Morbid. Mortal. Wkly. Rep. 47: 151–154.
13. ROGERS, M.F. 1997. The challenges of implementing recommendations for prevention of HIV perinatal transmission: how have we done so far. Natl. Conf. Women HIV, Pasadena, California, May 4–7, p. 128.
14. COTTON, D. & H. WATTS. 1995. Management of HIV infection during pregnancy: new options, new questions. AIDS Clin. Care 7: 45–47.
15. FANG, G., H. BURGER, R. GRIMSON, et al. 1995. Maternal plasma human immunodeficiency virus type 1 RNA level: a determinant and projected threshold for mother-to-child transmission. Proc. Natl. Acad. Sci. USA 92: 12100–121004.
16. DICKOVER, R.E., E.M. GARRATTY, S.A. HERMAN, et al. 1996. Identification of levels of maternal HIV-1 RNA associated with risk of perinatal transmission. Effect of maternal zidovudine treatment on viral load. JAMA 275: 599–605.

17. PAEDIATRIC EUROPEAN NETWORK FOR TREATMENT OF AIDS (PENTA). 1998. HIV-1 viral load and CD4 cell count in untreated children with vertically acquired asymptomatic or mild disease. AIDS **12:** F1–F8.
18. WAINBERG, M.A. & G. FRIEDLAND. 1999. Public health implications of antiretroviral therapy and HIV drug resistance. JAMA **279:** 1977–1983.
19. LARDER, B.A., G. DARBY & D.D. RICHMAN. 1989. HIV with reduced sensitivity to zidovudine (AZT) isolated during prolonged therapy. Science **243:** 1731–1734.
20. FITZGIBBON, J.E., S. GAUR & L.D. FRENKEL. 1993. Transmission from one child to another of a human immunodeficiency virus type 1 with a zidovudine-resistance mutation. N. Engl. J. Med. **329:** 1835–1841.
21. SIEGRIST, C.A., S. YERLY, L. KAISER, *et al.* 1994. Mother to child transmission of zidovudine-resistant HIV-1. Lancet **344:** 1771–1731.
22. SRINIVAS, R.V., W.T. HOLDEN, T. SU & P.M. FLYNN. 1996. Development of zidovudine-resistant HIV genotypes following postnatal prophylaxis in a perinatally infected infant. AIDS **10:** 795–797.
23. VAN TINE, B.A., G.M. SHAW & G. ALDROVANDI. 1999. Mother-to-infant transmission of the human immunodeficency virus during primary infection. N. Engl. J. Med. **340:** 1548.
24. EASTMAN, P.S., D.E. SHAPIRO, R.W. COOMBS, *et al.* 1998. Maternal viral genotypic zidovudine resistance and infrequent failure of zidovudine therapy to prevent perinatal transmission of human immunodeficiency virus type 1 in pediatric AIDS Clinical Trials Group Protocol 076. J. Infect. Dis. **177:** 557–564.
25. EASTMAN, P.S., D.E. SHAPIRO, R.W. COOMBS, *et al.* 1997. Maternal genotypic zidovudine (ZDV) resistance and failure of ZDV therapy to prevent mother–child HIV-1 transmission. *In* Program of the 4th International Conference on Retroviruses and Opportunistic Infections. Washington, DC, January 22–26, p. 160.
26. JAPOUR, A.J., S. WELLES, K. MCINTOSH, *et al.* 1996. ZDV resistance (ZDVR) mutations in ZDV exposed mother infant pairs: preliminary findings from the women and infants transmission study. (WITS). Int. Conf. AIDS **11:** 370.
27. COLGROVE, R.C., J. PITT, P.H. CHUNG, *et al.* 1998. Selective vertical transmission of HIV-1 zidovudine resistance mutations. *In* Program of the 5th International Conference on Retroviruses and Opportunistic Infections. Chicago, IL, February 1–5, p 129.
28. COLGROVE, R.C., J. PITT, P.H. CHUNG, *et al.* 1998. Selective vertical transmission of HIV-1 antiretroviral resistance mutations. AIDS **12:** 2281–2288.
29. FISCUS, S., A.A. ADIMORA, V.J. SCHOENBACH, *et al.* 1998. Can zidovudine monotherapy continue to reduce perinatal HIV transmission? The North Carolina experience 1993–1997. Int. Conf. AIDS **12:** 624.
30. SALOMON, H., M.A. WAINBERG, B. BRENNER, *et al.* 1999. Prevalence of HIV-1 viruses resistant to antiretroviral drugs in 81 individuals newly infected by sexual contact or intravenous drug. AIDS **14(2):** F17–23.
31. YERLY, S., L. KAISER, E. RACE, *et al.* 1999. Transmission of antiretroviral-drug-resistant HIV-1 variants. Lancet **354:** 729–733.
32. BODEN, D., A. HURLEY, L. ZHANG, *et al.* 1999. HIV-1 drug resistance in newly infected individuals. JAMA **282:** 1135–1141.
33. LITTLE, S.J., E.S. DAAR, R.T. D'AQUILA, *et al.* 1999. Reduced antiretroviral drug susceptibility among patients with primary infection. JAMA **282:** 1142–1149.
34. UNAIDS. 1998. Mother-to-child transmission of HIV: UNAIDS technical update. UNAIDS. Geneva.
35. WHO. 1996. Childhood diseases in Africa. WHO. Geneva.
36. WITKOR, S., E. EKPINI & J.M. KARON. 1999. Short-course oral zidovudine for prevention of mother-to-child HIV transmission in Abidjan, Côte d'Ivoire: a randomized trial. Lancet **353:** 781–785.
37. SABA, J. 1999. *In* Program of the 6th Conference on Retroviruses and Opportunistic Infections. Chicago, IL, Jan 31–Feb 4.
38. MARSEILLE, E., J.G. KAHN, F. MMIRO, *et al.* 1999. Cost effectiveness of single-dose nevirapine regimen for mothers and babies to decrease vertical HIV-1 transmission in sub-Saharan Africa. Lancet **354:** 803–809.

The Best of Times and the Worst of Times: Implications of Scientific Advances in HIV Prevention for Women in the Developing World

GEETA RAO GUPTA[a]

International Center for Research on Women (ICRW), Washington, D.C. 20036, USA

If Charles Dickens were alive today and if he were asked to provide a social commentary on the situation of HIV/AIDS today as compared to the past, he would most certainly have described these times as the "best of times and the worst of times." We have therapies and treatments today to substantially improve the quality of lives of those living with HIV and AIDS in the countries that can afford them. We have more than a few countries we can cite as examples where concerted action supported by political will has shown results in combating the epidemic. We have prevention strategies that work. There are larger sums of private and public sector monies and interesting private and public partnerships being devoted to research to develop vaccines, including strains of the virus that are found only in the developing world. We have a more visible and growing advocacy movement for the development of microbicides. And, finally, we have not just one but two available, low-cost proven ways to prevent the transmission of HIV from mothers to their infants. Compared to years past, all this certainly qualifies for the first part of the Dickens' descriptor: "the best of times."

Simultaneously, in most of the developing world, which bears the burden of more than 95% of the world's HIV infection, the HIV/AIDS epidemic continues to rage on. The rates of infection in some cities in sub-Saharan Africa today, ranging from 20 to 30%, exceed our worst nightmares. And many countries today are face to face with the reality of a staggering erosion in child survival rates and declines in life expectancy. To make matters worse, the new biomedical options to prevent infection are accompanied by new complexities and conundrums. Some of these are ethical, some epidemiological, some economic, and many of them are related to those ubiquitous hurdles—inequality and poverty. Such is the magnitude of these complexities and challenges that sometimes it seems that, unless they are addressed, the benefits of new prevention technologies may not outweigh the costs. It is this sense of frustration in having solutions available at hand that are so difficult to implement—the frustration of being slowed down by hurdles that prevent the quick implementation of a new prevention technology in a context in which the epidemic mercilessly rages on—that makes these the worst of times.

Ironically, it is this dilemma, reconciling the best with the worst, that will perhaps, in the long run, provide us with some benefit. It will force us to take the time

[a]Address for correspondence: International Center for Research on Women (ICRW), 1717 Massachusetts Avenue, NW, Suite 302, Washington, DC 20036. Voice: 202-797-0007; fax: 202-797-0020.

geeta@icrw.org

to examine each aspect of a proposed biomedical intervention and the context within which we seek to implement it. At this meeting, we will discuss ways by which we can ensure widespread availability of the two low-cost regimens of antiretrovirals that were recently proved to be efficacious in preventing the transmission of HIV infection from an infected mother to her child. We will also be trying to sort through all the confusing data on the pros and cons of breastfeeding just when we've had some success convincing folks that "breast is best"! We will grapple with human rights issues and try to balance those with public health priorities. We will discuss how voluntary testing and counseling can be provided in prenatal settings that are poorly staffed and resourced. And we may at different points in time wonder whether any of this is worth it given the limited resources available. My plea that as you wade through the confusion, contradictions, and challenges and as we try to transform the available antiretrovirals into a feasible, acceptable, and accessible intervention, please take the time to reflect upon lessons that we have learned in the past.

For example, let us not forget the M in MTCT, like we once forgot the M in MCH. In those early days of maternal and child health programs, pregnant women and nursing mothers were provided nutritional and health interventions, but were forgotten by the health system once they delivered or weaned their babies. We soon learned how short-sighted that was even if child survival and health was the only outcome measured—children need healthy and productive mothers throughout childhood, not just in infancy. Moreover, it was a wasteful use of resources because the gains achieved in terms of the nutritional and health status of the mother with each pregnancy were lost between pregnancies, so that programs would start more or less from square one with each new pregnancy. And finally, the importance of ensuring the health of mothers for their own sake, in addition to ensuring positive health outcomes for their children, was the most significant missing element in those programs.

So, let us not forget that it is mothers who are a critical element of any successful prevention effort that seeks to reduce the transmission of infection from mothers to infants. For example, because voluntary testing and counseling (VCT) is a part of such an intervention, it must be motivated not by a desire to ensure compliance, but to provide full information in a way that protects the rights and choices of women. The success of VCT must not be measured by the number of women who agree to be tested or agree to take the particular antiretroviral, but by the unbiased quality of the counseling and support offered to women and their families. Three decades of family planning have taught us that being motivated by larger public health or demographic goals and imposing those on individual women's choices can result in outcomes that are quite the opposite of what is expected. Let us learn from those experiences. Let us borrow from the rich legacy of the International Conference on Population and Development held in Cairo in 1994 at which 179 nations recognized the value of women's right to information and choice in ensuring the success of reproductive health programs.

And let us acknowledge rather than be blind to the risks that our proposed intervention imposes on women. Asking pregnant women to determine their IIIV status exposes them to stigma and discrimination at a time when they are most vulnerable and require the most protection. Despite all our efforts to reduce the fear and ignorance that fuels discrimination and stigma, it is a cruel reality that individuals whose positive HIV status is exposed are often ostracized, marginalized, abandoned, and sometimes even killed. For pregnant women, who because of their gender are less likely to have the resources to cope with abandonment and are faced with the prospect of protecting and caring for another life yet to begin, such potential consequences are worse than death.

And let us also face with honesty, rather than deny or avoid, the overwhelming tragedy of using resources to save an infant's life, with none available to save that infants' primary nurturer and caretaker—the mother. Let us be aware of the sobering reality that an infant without the mother is likely to be at risk. But this epidemic—and those of you who have faced it head-on in communities and clinics, know this well—this epidemic has been anything but easy in the choices it poses. This is yet another example. The appropriate path to follow is to ensure that antiretrovirals are one of many prevention options available to women who seek to protect their children from infection. The most significant option must continue to be primary prevention because the best way to ensure that an infant is not infected is to protect the mother herself. In our excitement over biomedical options such as antiretrovirals let us not forget the value of primary prevention.

Most importantly, let us not get caught in trying to take sides between the well-being of mothers and that of children. Who could ever win such an ugly battle? Let our well-meaning advocacy for technologies and services to protect women not be interpreted as pitting mothers against their babies. At the Geneva conference when hecklers interfered with a presentation on the recent developments in antiretrovirals for perinatal transmission, a young African woman sitting next to me leaned over and said, "If you women want to fight for our rights as women, don't expect me as a pregnant woman to join you. Much as I would like to see resources directed toward ways to help me live and watch my child grow and be rid of my infection," she said, "as a pregnant woman I will fight first for the well-being of my unborn child, and I am grateful that such a medical option exists." Let us pay heed to her words and respect the complex realities of an infected mother's choices and her courage as she makes her decision. Let us advocate for better health services and medical options for women while we celebrate and support the effective implementation of programs to save infants' lives.

Next let us remember that mothers are women whose gender and the socioeconomic and cultural context in which they live defines their roles, as well as the amount of power they have in society. We know now through data gathered over the last three decades that gender norms limit women's access to information and restrict their mobility. We know that women are economically vulnerable because they do not have the same opportunities for education, training, or employment as men do. We know that of the 1.3 billion people who are trapped in absolute poverty worldwide, 70% are women. We have also learned the staggering extent to which domestic violence is a reality in the lives of many women worldwide. Overall, we now know that there is an imbalance in power between women and men that is apparent in heterosexual relations as well as in the economic and social spheres of life—with men having greater power than women. And, most importantly, we know that this imbalance in power has serious implications for women's ability to protect themselves from infection, to feel safe in determining their HIV status, to seek support and care when infected, and to make choices for their own welfare, independent of others. Each of these facts has implications for the success of a vertical transmission prevention intervention, and therefore to succeed, service providers and counselors must, at a minimum, be aware of these realities while we conduct the research necessary to find out how these facts affect women's ability to follow the regimens we propose.

As a long-term strategy, I recommend that we as AIDS researchers, community workers, and activists advocate for improvements in women's economic and social status. Gender inequity is fueling the epidemic. Empowering women is no longer an option, it is essential. I would like to propose four key strategies to accomplish this goal. Interestingly, and, I must admit, not coincidentally, the acronym for these is the same as the popular acronym for the strategies that came to define the child survival movement worldwide and resulted in significant reductions in infant and child mortality. The acronym I refer to is GOBI—which in the child survival lexicon stood for growth monitoring, oral rehydration, breastfeeding, and immunization. The GOBI for women represents G for gender-sensitive prevention technologies and services (such as microbicides and services that address women's gender-based constraints); O for opportunities for employment and income generation (that allow women the leverage to negotiate protection or take independent action); B for building social support for changes in gender norms; and I for information and education. Let us together commit ourselves to promoting each of these because without these changes in women's status the implementation of biomedical technologies will continue to be a challenge.

One social reality that persists in countries in the North and South alike and is less amenable to change, is that society favors women who are mothers. As my Nigerian friend Eka Williams, President of the Society for Women and AIDS in Africa recently explained to me, "While women in the West are now trying to make it in a man's world, in Africa," she said, "it is a reality that women have to make it in a woman's world—and motherhood is the membership card that allows you into that world." In South Asia, where I come from, the membership requirements are more stringent— you must have a son to prove that you are woman deserving of some status and respect! Why are we surprised then when some women, despite living in high-prevalence settings, refuse to have themselves tested before they get pregnant or when they are pregnant? And why are we astonished when infected women choose to have several children? The results of an HIV test, in many ways, have no bearing on a woman's decision to have a child. That decision is not a choice if the woman has to belong to the society in which she lives.

Breastfeeding, like motherhood, is a strong social norm and expectation for women in many developing countries. In a recent study in Dakar, Senegal, women were asked how people would react if a woman was unable to breastfeed her child. One woman said such a mother would be treated as a handicapped person, while another commented that an African woman who does not breastfeed is seen as a bad mother who rejects her child. Thus, if our advice to not breastfeed is to be followed, we must find a way to help mothers overcome these cultural barriers and expectations—and we cannot do this by working with mothers alone. It is critical that we involve the older women and the men in their communities, too, and find ways to help families and communities understand, accept, and support an infected mother's decision.

Despite all these social and cultural barriers, in countries in which antiretrovirals are already being offered to pregnant women, many women are stepping out to be tested and treated just to protect their unborn children. It speaks volumes for their courage. Let us not interpret their actions as representing the absence of any barriers in those settings, but rather as testimony of the mountains that women will climb to protect their families.

In order to support them, let us not forget the damage that can be caused by titles that stigmatize. We as a community have taught the world the need to avoid stigmatizing terminology—we have gone from prostitutes to sex workers; from risk groups and vectors of disease to risk behaviors, why is it then that we continue to feel comfortable with the use of the term mother-to-child transmission? What could be more blatantly accusatory? Why do we use this term when we know that the majority of women in prenatal clinics are at risk not because of their own sexual behavior but because of the sexual behavior of their male partners? Would it not be more fair then to at least share the blame by using the term parents-to-child transmission? I am not suggesting a change in nomenclature just for purposes of political correctness, but rather to promote a more fundamental change in the way we view the parties who are responsible for the health and well-being of a child—not just the mother, but rather the mother and the father. After three decades, family planning providers now recognize the need to include men, reach out to them, and ensure that they share the responsibility of planning a family. We cannot afford to make the same mistake. We must recommend counseling of both partners: only then can we hope for women to have the support they need to make the nontraditional and potentially stigmatizing choices that we are expecting them to make—to be tested, to consider the option of voluntary childlessness, to take drugs during pregnancy, and not to breastfeed.

It is clear, then, that the effective introduction of a biomedical technology requires much more than an efficient clinic-based intervention. It requires a broader, community-based effort that acknowledges and addresses women's needs and concerns, the needs and concerns of their male partners, and the perspectives of the communities in which they live. In reviewing much of what has been written since the first clinical trials of AZT began, I am struck by the absence of women's voices and community-based research. In order to design an effective community-based information, education, and counseling program to complement the availability of an antiretroviral prevention intervention, it is essential that we take the time to find out what women and their families living in affected communities know, feel and think about such an intervention. Just two weeks ago, with support from Glaxo-Wellcome and UNAIDS, ICRW in collaboration with in-country researchers initiated just such a study in Botswana and Zambia, using rapid assessment procedures to gather data on the perspectives of women and the communities in which they live. Many more such studies must be supported in other parts of the developing world. It is only by talking to women and communities and involving them that we will come up with practical solutions to the many conundrums that we face today.

Let me conclude on an optimistic note. First of all, let us take the time to rejoice in the new biomedical advances and commit ourselves to mobilize the political will and resources necessary to be able to make those available to all mothers and children in need. Then, let us view the many challenges we are faced with as opportunities to create the changes that we should have accomplished a long time ago. Let us use this opportunity to strengthen existing prenatal and maternal care services. Let us use the opportunity to engage men and other members of communities in a discussion about the well-being and health of the women and children in their communities. Let us use the opportunity to talk to communities about the high costs of stigma and discrimination. And most importantly, let us use the opportunity to strengthen women's socioeconomic status. Investing in women by providing them with education, training and skills, technologies and services that are women-friendly, employment, and social support guarantees healthy and productive women, as well as healthy and productive children, families, and communities. And that is the message we must communicate strongly, without any caveats.

Role of Nongovernmental Organizations in the Prevention and Care of HIV Disease in Women and Children

It Makes a Difference

SUNITI SOLOMON[a] AND AYLUR KAILASAM GANESH

Y.R.G. Centre for AIDS Research and Education, T. Nagar, Chennai 600 017, India

> *When the old man walked along the beach at dawn, he noticed a young woman ahead of him pick up a starfish and fling it into the sea. Catching up with the young lady, he asked her why she did this. The answer was that the stranded starfish would die if left to the morning sun.*
>
> *"But the beach goes on for miles and there are millions of starfish," countered the old man. "How can your efforts make any difference"?*
>
> *The young woman looked at the starfish in her hand and threw it to the safety of the seas. "It makes a difference to this one," she said.*
>
> LOREN EISELEY,
>
> ADAPTED FROM *UNEXPECTED UNIVERSE*

In India the first infections of HIV were detected in 1986.[1] Sentinel surveillance shows that currently 24.6/1000 are HIV positive.[2] Heterosexual transmission is responsible for 73.6% of infections,[2] and the virus has spread to both urban and rural populations.[3,4] It has spread from groups with high-risk behavior to the general population, including monogamous housewives.[5]

As the epidemic continues to expand to all corners of the country and all strata of the society, it is clear that every sector of society must respond. AIDS has ceased to be just a medical concern, but has challenged the economic, social, political, and religious spheres as well. Nongovernmental organizations (NGOs), the voluntary sector, are emerging as a powerful force in the effort to contain the epidemic.

An analysis of strengths, weaknesses, opportunities, and threats (TABLE 1)[6] clearly shows the strength of the NGOs lies in:

(a) the ability to make a quick, flexible response as well as to design and carry out programs faster than the government;

(b) strongly committed individuals with access to the "hard to reach" communities like injecting drug users (IDUs) and sex workers;

[a]Address for correspondence: Y.R.G. Care Centre for AIDS Research and Education, 1, Raman Street, T. Nagar, Chennai 600 017, India. Voice: 91 44 826 4242; fax: 91 44 825 6900. yrgcare@vsnl.com

TABLE 1. Comparative features of nongovernmental organizations (NGOs) and government

	NGO	Government
Strengths	Quick	Resources
	Rapport with the community	Legislation
	Motivation	
	Flexibility	
Weaknesses	Financial dependence	Outsider
	Lack of reach to a large geographic area	Slow
Opportunities	Underserved areas	Uniform public health program
	Marginalized communities	
Threats	Sustainability	Rejection
	Lack of management experience	Political commitment
	Expertise	

(c) community members on their staffs who attract community participation in HIV/AIDS prevention and care efforts. These communities often view the government as an outsider and NGOs are able to act in ways that are more difficult for the slower moving bureaucracies of the government agencies.

The major threats to an NGO are:

(a) the administrative systems are not designed for large-scale projects;

(b) "burn-out" among NGO volunteers leading to attrition is great because of their emotional involvement with persons with HIV/AIDS; and

(c) their tendency to work in isolation leads to unsustainable programs unless they network with each other and the government. They may be successful in small-scale programs, but will not be effective in "scale-up" projects.

For a success story to emerge, there should be a strong collaboration between the government agencies, nongovernmental organizations, and the private sector, all working towards one goal: to prevent the spread of HIV and to provide care and support for PLHA.

NGO, GOVERNMENT, PRIVATE SECTOR INTERLINK

NGOs, government, and the private sector interact in the areas of education, care, social mobilization, infant food, pharmaceuticals, and policy funding. And yet, each of the three sectors (NGO, government, and private) brings a unique strength in the role that it plays. For example, in India the government is the largest provider of health care. In Madras 65,000 out of 90,000 (66.6%) of the deliveries are conducted in public sector hospitals. Similarly, the government sets the policies and determines the priorities for spending.

The next largest player is the private sector, with roles in health care, pharmaceuticals, and production of infant food.

The NGOs, more specifically the AIDS service organizations (ASOs), however, facilitate education about HIV in the general community and mobilize support to make prevention feasible. NGOs have the freedom to handle subjects like sex education. They use facts and participatory techniques, which makes the educational programs more enjoyable and meaningful. This sector has always been a principal player in care and support because of its ability to reach the community and understand and respond to their needs.

An example of such a success story is the family welfare program in India. The target was to reduce the birth rate from 29/1000 to 21/1000 by the year 2000. By teamwork among government agencies, NGOs, and the private sector, they succeeded in lowering the birth rate in Tamil Nadu state to 17.5/1000 by 1998.[7]

PREVENTING THE SPREAD OF HIV INFECTION TO WOMEN AND CHILDREN: NGO ROLE

Primary Prevention of HIV Infection in Women

Because perinatal transmission begins with infected mothers and their partners, primary prevention of HIV can contribute markedly in preventing perinatal transmission by reducing the number of women infected with HIV. There are many approaches to primary prevention, including STD/HIV/AIDS education and sexuality programs for adolescents to eliminate myths and misconceptions. NGOs are most suited to conduct sex education programs for adolescents. In Asian countries where most marriages are arranged and men and women do not reveal their HIV status because of stigma, there should be a strong partner notification system to prevent women from acquiring HIV from infected spouses. Because the stigma is great for a "barren" woman, a wife might opt to become pregnant to save the marriage in spite of knowing her husband is HIV positive. NGOs have a vital role in demystifying the cultural issues and helping the women to understand options such as artificial insemination or adoption of children.

Voluntary Counseling and Testing

Before vertical transmission of HIV from mother to child can be prevented, the infected women need to be identified. There are 20 million live births in India, and a seroprevalence of HIV ranging from 1 to 3.5% in the various states.[8] Between 50 and 100 new antenatal care (ANC) women attend public hospitals. Promoting testing and counselling for HIV infection within the antenatal clinics, along with other health counseling, is a good strategy. Counselling and testing is more feasible if such procedures are developed in collaboration with NGOs and other community-based organizations. This will also increase the involvement and understanding of the larger community.[8] The NGO staff can visit the women in their homes and encourage couple and family counseling, so that women do not get blamed for not getting pregnant and their basic rights are protected. NGOs can also form a liaison between the family and hospital and increase institutional deliveries without discrimination.

Antiretroviral Therapy and Non-Antiretroviral Therapy Protocols

NGOs, especially AIDS service organizations (ASOs), can obtain antiretroviral drugs from national and international institutions and provide them to HIV-positive pregnant women who cannot afford to buy them. NGOs could also spend time counseling women on supportive methods like good nutrition, vitamins, and antioxidants, which act as immunomodulators to help reduce HIV transmission to the infant.

Many women feel that breastfeeding develops a bond between them and their infants and are reluctant to deny breast milk to the child. NGOs are in a good position, because of their rapport with the community, to counsel the woman and her family about the risks of breastfeeding for an HIV-positive mother. They could help in educating the family about formula food, should they choose to use it.

The NGO Role Starts with Primary Prevention of HIV Infection in Women

The NGOs play an important role in empowering women and helping them to understand their rights. Women are not able to insist on condom use, mostly because of their subordinate role and economic dependence on their husbands. They believe many myths and have misconceptions about sexuality. They need to be encouraged to use female-controlled barrier methods.

A large number of women who are pregnant are anemic. According to the National AIDS Control Organization (NACO), a small percentage of HIV infection in India is still through blood transfusion, even though in October of 1989 the government mandated that every unit of blood be tested for HIV. Effective implementation and advocacy for a safe blood supply could be an NGO role.[8]

Widows and Orphans

Many young women, because of HIV, have become widows within a year or two of marriage—left to fend for themselves and their infant.[9] NGOs have an important role to play in helping these widows with short-stay homes and skill building to achieve economic independence. NGOs could also help with the education and adoption of orphans.

CONCLUSION

Clearly, NGOs have enormous potential to be effective in the effort to prevent and manage HIV in women and children. For this reason, NGOs should be included as partners in government programs on HIV/AIDS. Networking among NGOs should be encouraged, in order that they share their experiences, both failures and successes. With their flexibility, diversity, and motivation, NGOs must be accepted as equal partners with governments and donors alike in the effort to prevent HIV infection in women and children. NGOs may be smaller than the government, but they can effectively take care of the "starfish" that come to their doors.

REFERENCES

1. SIMOES, E.A.F., G. BABU, T.J. JOHN, *et al.* 1987. Evidence of HTLV III infection in prostitutes in India. Indian J. Med. Res. **85:** 335–338.
2. NACO. 1999. Surveillance for HIV infection/AIDS cases in India. National AIDS Control Organization, 31 July.

3. AIDS Prevention and Control Project, Voluntary Health Services (APAC-VHS). 1997. Chennai HIV risk behaviour sentinel surveillance survey in Tamil Nadu, 1997. APAC-VHS.
4. SOLOMON, S., N. KUMARASAMY, R.E. AMALRAJ & A.K. GANESH. 1998. Prevalence and risk factors of HIV-1 and HIV-2 infection in urban and rural areas of Tamil Nadu, India. Int. J. STD AIDS **9(2):** 98–103.
5. GANGAKHEDKAR, R.R., M.E. BENTLEY, A.D. DIVEKAR, *et al.* 1997. Spread of HIV infection in married monogamous women in India. JAMA **278:** 2090–2092.
6. MERCER, M.A., L. LISKIN & S.J. SCOTT. 1991. The role of non-governmental organisations in the global response to AIDS. AIDS CARE **3:** 265–270.
7. GANESH, A.K. & Y.R.G. CARE. 1999. Description of the situation of mother-to-child transmission of HIV at Chennai (Madras), India, a report compiled for WHO/ UNAIDS, August 1999.
8. NACO. 1997–1998. Country scenario. NACO.
9. SABA, J. 1997. Identification of HIV infection in pregnancy: another era. Acta Paediatr. (Suppl.) **421:** 65–66.
10. NEWMAN, S., P. SARIN, N. KUMARASAMY, *et al.* 2000. Marriage, monogamy, and HIV: a profile of HIV-infected women in South India. Int. J. STD AIDS **11(4):** 250–253.

Advances in Antiretroviral, Immune-Based, and Gene Therapy for HIV Infection in Mothers and Infants

Implications for Future Use in Developing Countries

ARYE RUBINSTEIN[a]

Department of Pediatrics, Microbiology, and Immunology, Albert Einstein College of Medicine, Bronx, New York 10461, USA

The Second International Conference on Global Strategies for the Prevention of HIV-1 Transmission from Mothers to Infants focused on existing effective measures to prevent HIV-1 transmission and on how these can be implemented in resource-limited countries. Conference participants were unanimous in their call for action. It is inconceivable that the most affected populations will not have access to proven therapies that can slow down the continuous growth in numbers of HIV-1-infected women and children. Social, economic, and ethical issues that interfere with the implementation of adequate health care policies and potential remedial actions were highlighted.

The Satellite Conference on Advances in Pediatric AIDS was structured as a look into the future and as a venue for a worldwide dialogue between health care providers and scientists. It provided information on cutting-edge advances in the prevention of HIV-1 transmission from mother to infant and in the treatment of an established infection in a child. In each instance emphasis was given to tailoring advances to meet the needs, the available financial resources, and the existing medical and public health structure in developing countries. The highlights of these presentations will be briefly described:

The experience in the United Kingdom and in the United States in antenatal testing and surveillance of HIV-1 infection in pregnant women has shown that less sophisticated methods that do not require complex laboratory equipment are quite effective. The uses of rapid finger-stick blood tests and/or saliva instead of blood are most suitable for developing countries and address some of the cultural impediments for wide population screening.

Shorter and shorter treatments for pregnant women and newborns have been studied in clinical settings in developing countries. Knowledge of the antiretroviral pharmacokinetics during pregnancy and in the newborn, as presented by Mark Mirochnick, is essential for the design of improved, safe, and effective drug use. Although the physiologic changes of pregnancy are generally not an indication to warrant adjustment of dosing, normal growth and development in newborns and infants

[a]Address for correspondence: Arye Rubinstein, M.D., Albert Einstein College of Medicine, 1300 Morris Park Avenue, Mazer 200, Bronx, NY 10461. Voice: 718-430-2319; fax: 718-430-8982.

rubinste@aecom.yu.edu

have a profound impact on the pharmacokinetics of antiretrovirals. Washout of transplacentally acquired drug is slow. It is also important to take note that, whereas placental transfer of reverse-transcriptase inhibitors is good, preliminary data on protease inhibitors suggest that these highly protein-bound drugs do not cross the placenta well. In a small, ongoing study the median ratio of cord blood to maternal serum nelfinavir concentration was 4.5%. Lower fetal drug concentrations of nelfinavir may increase the risk of HIV-1 transmission but at the same time decrease the risk of toxic or teratogenic effects.

Another important issue is the understanding of the differences between the oral versus intravenous dosing of antiretrovirals during labor. ACTG protocol 076 included a continuous zidovudine infusion during labor to maintain a constant serum level.[1] Most practitioners in the developing world would prefer oral administration during labor. The trough of oral zidovudine at 300 mg every 3 hours during labor appears to be too low, and a loading dose of 600 mg is being now investigated. In contrast, women in labor demonstrate an increase in nevirapine half-life and a decrease in bioavailability. Overall, there is an increase in the variability of the pharmacokinetics of nevirapine.

Several recent reports suggest that there is no mother-to-infant HIV-1 transmission with combination antiretrovirals during pregnancy.[2] Moreover, combination therapy is becoming common during pregnancy. The toxicity of such a regimen is still not fully studied. Presently it is recommended that efavirenz be avoided because of associated fetal malformations in pregnant monkeys and that indinavir be avoided because of the induction of indirect bilirubinemia in the first weeks of life. A group of French investigators has suggested that mitochodrial disease may develop in HIV-1-exposed but uninfected children whose mothers used zidovudine during pregnancy. An analysis of a large number of a similar cohort enrolled in the ACTG 076 protocol has not confirmed this finding.

Drug choices in the treatment of HIV-1-infected infants and children have been presented and discussed by Spector, Oleske, Wilfert, and Rubinstein. Guidelines for the use of antiretroviral agents in pediatric HIV infection have been developed by the US National Working Group and were published in the *Morbidity and Mortality Weekly Report* by the Centers for Disease Control and Prevention in April 1998. These guidelines are reviewed monthly and updated regularly.

A recent revolution in HIV-1 treatment converted HIV-1 infection from a rapidly fatal disease to a chronic disease, but no permanent cure has been obtained even after three years of viral suppression by effective, highly active antiretroviral therapy (HAART).

Specific pediatric issues are the long-term metabolic and toxic consequences of HAART and the need to control HIV-1 infection of the brain. Therefore, special attention has to be given to the kinetics of crossing the blood–brain barrier for each medication used in children.

All experts agreed that treatment should be initiated with three drugs for any child under the age of 12 months with clinical symptoms and/or immunological impairment. It is controversial whether asymptomatic children with normal immunity and low viral loads should be treated. A case presentation was made of an initially asymptomatic child with a viral load <400 PCR copies/ml who was therefore on no antiretroviral therapy. This child, nevertheless, developed an HIV-1 encephalopathy, suggesting that withholding therapy in young children should be avoided in most instances.

Adherence issues are a major problem among pediatric patients. Adherence to treatment among children has been reported to range from as low as 11% to as high as 83%. To optimize adherence and to ensure commitment to a complex and possibly life-long regimen, a family approach with a large psycho-social component and education for caregivers is needed. Attention also has to be given to methods that improve the palatability of drugs.

Incomplete or delayed viral suppression and the emergence of drug-resistant mutations are more prevalent in children, probably because of poor compliance. In children, as in adults, noncompliance with antiretrovirals is not always associated with an acute and significant viral rebound. Nevertheless it was suggested to implement in children a more stringent phenotypic and genotypic viral testing as the standard of care.

Obviously, issues of optimal care and compliance are viewed differently in developing countries. Stephen Spector stressed that no matter where children live, they should not receive suboptimal antiretroviral therapy. He called upon industrialized countries, the World Bank, and pharmaceutical companies to help provide antiretroviral therapy to countries with limited resources. In the interim it was recommended that treatment in developing countries should be targeted to children that are most likely to progress, especially those under one year of age.

Another issue for developing countries is routine immunization for infections other than HIV-1. High rates of invasive pneumococcal disease in African countries are attributable to the increased morbidity and mortality in HIV-1-infected subjects. Previous studies in adults have shown a reduced but present immunogenicity of a pneumococcal polysacharide vaccine. It was therefore believed that pneumococcal immunization of HIV-1-infected adults has the potential to be an appropriate and cost-effective public health intervention to decrease morbidity and mortality in developing countries lacking access to antiretrovirals. Dr. Gilks from Liverpool reported that immunization of Ugandan adults with a 23-valent pneumococcal polysacharide was ineffective. There was actually an increased rate of pneumococcal disease in vaccine recipients.[3] In our studies in children dating back to 1985, we have found a severely impaired immunogenicity of a pneumococcal vaccine and of a neoantigen, bacteriophage $\phi X174$.[4] In a more recent study we have shown that primary immunization with bacteriophage $\phi X174$ followed by two boosters in HIV-1-infected asymptomatic adults resulted in a progressive specific immune attrition and an increased viremia.[5] These findings may explain the failure of the pneumococcal vaccine in adults in Uganda. Most importantly, the immune attrition observed during vaccine boosters could be blunted by short courses of antiretrovirals before and during immunizations.[5] These results put in question the use of the U.S. recommendations for childhood and adult immunizations in developing countries in which most HIV-1-infected patients are not on concurrent antiretroviral therapies.

The rest of the conference revolved around futuristic immune-based therapies and gene therapy. It is now well appreciated that total viral eradication by HAART is most unlikely. Virally infected cells were shown to persist even after optimal therapy.[6,7] Furthermore, HAART, even when achieving nondetectable viremia, does not fully restore immunity.[7] It was therefore suggested that immune potentiation in combination with HAART may eradicate latent virus reservoirs.

Several approaches were used to validate this hypothesis and to determine which immune functions need to be induced or enhanced. Among the approaches included were immune evaluations in long-term survivors as well as the effect of various immune manipulations on viral loads. Some HIV-1-infected persons are able to control viremia without HAART in a setting of strong HIV-1-specific cytotoxic T lymphocytes (CTLs).[8,9] In HIV-1-infected patients intravenous transfer of CTL clones was associated with transient decreases in viral loads.[10] Conversely, in SIV-infected macaques, *in vivo* depletion of CD8[+] cells with a specific monoclonal antibody resulted in a dramatic acute increase in viremia.[11] The picture in infants is not clear. Spontaneous drops in viremia were noted in infants before the detection of CTLs. Therefore, factors other than CTLs may be implicated in the control of viremia.

William Shearer reported that pediatric HIV-1-infected long-term survivors have significantly higher CD4[+] and CD8[+] T cells and CD19[+]/CD20[+] B cells and higher serum IgG levels. It has also been shown that CD4[+] T-cell help is essential for both cellular and humoral immunity to work together. Patients who have CD4[+] helper T cells that recognize HIV-1 proteins have the highest anti-HIV-1 CTL and the lowest viral load.[12] Finally, periodic IL-2 courses given to patients on HAART improved CD4 cells quantitatively and qualitatively[13] and reduced the number of latently infected T cells.[14]

Meyers *et al.* described T-helper cell responses among HIV-infected antiretroviral-untreated children in Soweto, South Africa. They used peripheral blood mononuclear cells stimulated with PHA, tetanus, or with synthetic HIV-1 envelope peptides measuring IL-2 production. Surprisingly, they have noted that strong HIV-1-specific T-helper cell responses are present in early mild disease as well as in the late severe clinical course. Their conclusion was that the T-helper cell responses, when initiated at the time of infection, may protect against disease progression, but later on these responses may not have a prognostic value. Yet, prolonged HAART may occasionally restore vigorous HIV-specific CD4[+] T-cell responses in newly infected infants.[15,16]

As mentioned previously, neither was the picture well defined with regard to the CTL responses. Luzuriaga has shown that CTLs are diminished in the first months of life[17] and may not play a role at all in early control of viremia. Dr. Goulder reported on studies of CTL and T-helper responses in the African population, which is the population most severely affected by the global epidemic. He used two methods to detect CTLs: the Elispot and a flow cytometric equivalent of intracellular interferon-γ staining. The latter assay, in which intracellular interferon staining of cells is stimulated with particular HIV peptides, is almost as sensitive as the Elispot. These new assays are simple, inexpensive, do not require sophisticated equipment, and can therefore be performed in laboratories in developing countries. In the Elispot a small number of cells is needed, which lends itself for use with pediatric patients. In his studies, Goulder has shown that the clade-C Gag-specific CTL responses dominating the infected Zulu and Xhosa populations of Durban, South Africa are different from those in Caucasoids and do reflect differences in frequencies of HLA. The definition of the epitopes targeted by CTLs in the African population opens up the opportunity for immune-based therapies specifically targeted for these populations. Dr. Goulder gave the example of using infusions of autologous dendritic cells pulsed with the appropriate population-specific peptides as a mode of immunotherapy.

The role of the various immune responses was studied in the context of mother-to-child HIV-1 transmission. Overall, without any intervention 25% of infants born to HIV-1-infected mothers acquire the infection, while the majority of babies escape infection by their HIV-1-infected mother. This is certainly not explained by a transplacental barrier, because during pregnancy maternal lymphocytes cross the placenta.[18,19] In an experiment dating back to 1964, labeled maternal cells that were retransfused into mothers before delivery were always identifiable in umbilical cord blood.[18] In the context of ubiquitous bidirectional exchange of maternofetal cells and fluids, potent immunological defenses could explain the lack of more frequent HIV-1 transmission.

There are indications that cellular immunity plays a role in prevention of HIV-1 transmission. Women with $CD4^+$ T-cell counts over 600/ml tend not to transmit the infection to their babies. In contrast, low $CD4^+$ T-cell counts are associated with increased maternal HIV-1 transmission,[21] lower antibody titers to HIV-1 antigens, and lower levels of neutralizing antibodies.[22] The role of neutralizing antibodies was discussed. Virus-specific antibodies can protect individuals against a wide variety of viral infections including polio, measles, and respiratory syncytial virus. There is therefore no reason why HIV-1-specific neutralizing antibodies should not play some protective role. Furthermore, humoral and cellular immunity are closely tied together in HIV-1 infection, with none being extremely potent without the other.[23] For example, neutralizing antibodies are preferentially found in HIV-1-infected subjects with preserved T-cell function and normal $CD4^+$ T-cell numbers. These antibodies may, by reducing the infectivity of the initial viral inoculum, provide time for the cellular immunity to mature and allow the maternal cellular protective immunity to kick in. Some studies indicated that the presence of high-affinity antibodies to the V3 loop of the envelope's gp120 and/or neutralization of primary isolates by maternal serum is crucial for the prevention of transmission.[23–25] However, a recent study in our New York City Perinatal HIV Transmission Collaborative Study Group failed to confirm this correlation.[26] In this study autologous primary isolated antibodies were obtained from transmitting and nontransmitting mothers. No association was found between the presence of neutralizing antibodies in maternal sera and perinatal transmission of HIV-1.[26] In contrast, *in vivo* studies in chimps, macaques,[27–29] and in SCID-hu mice[30] were mentioned in which neutralizing antibodies provided protection from HIV-1 and SHIV challenge and accelerated clearance of cell free virions.[30]

Immunological interventions to prevent mother-to-infant HIV-1 transmission were discussed by several speakers. In clinical trials with intravenous gammaglobulin and hyperimmunoglobulin (HIVIG) including specific antibodies for HIV-1, there was a modest effect on virus transmission with HIVIG (ACTG protocols 082 and 175). The use of zidovudine with HIVIG reduced the transmission rate to 4.9% in zidovudine-naïve and -experienced mothers.

It was recognized that, although transplacental transfer of maternal antibodies to the fetus may convey improved immunity, this transfer occurs late in gestation. Therefore, maternal passive immunization should be scheduled to achieve peak responses in the third trimester of pregnancy or near term in order to interfere with HIV-1 transmission. The use of monoclonal antibodies with broadly primary isolate-neutralizing activity or HIVIG spiked with monoclonal antibodies may offer an additional benefit. No monoclonal HIV-specific antibody has yet been tested in pregnant women.

William Shearer summarized studies using, in children, a recombinant molecule that binds to the CD4 binding site of the virus (CD4-IgG). He tested this treatment in pregnant women.[31] The CD4-IgG was found to be safe, to cross the placenta, and to neutralize cross clade HIV-1 viruses. A newer version of CD4-IgG with a longer half-life and four gp120 binding sites is being tested.

William Borkowsky discussed the role of active immunization of HIV-1 infected pregnant women. Combining antiretrovirals with therapeutic immunization may help achieve a reduction in viral loads to below 50 RNA copies/ml, a level in which no transmission of HIV-1 was noted in previous studies. A vaccine delivered to pregnant women might result also in active "vaccination" of the fetus. Immunization of baboon fetuses at 90–150 days of gestation with recombinant hepatitis B surface antigen was shown to induce a vigorous specific fetal IgG response[32] without any indication for induction of tolerance. Gerdt *et al.* reported good immune responses to a DNA vaccine against bovine herpes virus 1 introduced into the amniotic fluid in the oral cavity of sheep fetuses. This vaccine induced high levels of serum antibodies, a cell-mediated immune response, and a local immunity in the oral cavity of fetal lambs.[33] In humans fetal IgM responses have been demonstrated to maternal immunization with tetanus toxoid[34] and with congenital infections such as toxoplasmosis, cytomegalovirus, and HIV-1 infection. Live vector HIV-1 vaccines such as avian pox virus and peptide vaccines, when administered to pregnant women, may cross the placenta and induce protective responses in the fetus. In turn, there may be transplacental transfer of induced neutralizing antibodies in the mother. The only vaccine evaluated in pregnant women was the VaxGen gp120. This vaccine yielded no appropriate responses.

The timing of HIV-1 transmission to the fetus/baby lends itself to a "hepatitis B strategy" of active–passive therapy. However, not all vaccines are immunogenic when given at birth. In humans vaccines such as tetanus and diphtheria have to be delayed to 1 month of age to obtain an appropriate immune response. Berkowsky reported that vaccination of newborns with recombinant gp120 vaccines, canarypox vector expressing gp160 and p24, showed some antibody and CTL responses to HIV-1 antigens beginning at 2 months of age. So far no clinical benefit from these vaccines was observed. A newer avipox vaccine that incorporates nonstructural gene epitopes with structural genes as well as DNA vaccines will soon be evaluated in newborns.

Berkowsky also discussed the role of vaccines in older children as an adjunct to antiretroviral therapy. The results with AIDS vaccines in adults and in children are so far disappointing, although some immune responses have been detectable. Recombinant gp120 and gp160 vaccines induced humoral and cellular immune responses in HIV-1-infected adults that infection itself did not stimulate.[35–38] Valentine *et al.*[39,40] reported the induction of significant levels of virus-specific proliferative responses after immunization of HIV-1-infected subjects with Remune (gp120-depleted, whole inactivated virus). Nevertheless, all the above-mentioned vaccines had at best a modest effect on CD4 cell counts, and none led to reduction in viral loads or to a clinical benefit. Studies with recombinant gp120 and gp160 vaccines in infants have also not yielded any clinical benefit. Nevertheless, more potent vaccines may have an important place in the armamentarium against HIV-1 infection in children.

Stem cell and gene therapy bear great potential for the treatment of the HIV-1-infected neonate and infant. Previous studies with discordantly infected twins showed that a bone marrow transplant from the uninfected twin to the infected twin resulted in a temporary immune reconstitution with subsequent HIV-1 infection and demise of donor cells. Consequently, donor cells have to be rendered resistant to HIV-1 infection before transplantation. Donald Kohn and associates described a phase I clinical trial with genetically engineered cells in HIV-1-infected children and adolescents. Four subjects underwent bone marrow harvest under general anesthesia. The bone marrow was processed to isolate CD34$^+$ cells that were subsequently transduced with the RRE (rev responsive element) to serve as a decoy to sequester REV protein. The transduced cells were then reinfused intravenously. Unfortunately the presence of gene-containing lymphocytes in the blood declined rapidly — within days. To attain some level of efficacy, it will be necessary to achieve higher levels of gene transfer. A variety of new retroviral vectors carrying anti-HIV-1 genes are under investigation. If successful, then gene therapy with such engineered cells could rescue HIV-1-exposed neonates from the dire consequences of HIV-1 infection without the need for open-ended pharmacological treatment.

In summary, the Satellite Conference on Advances in Pediatric AIDS dealt with cutting edge research in the pathogenesis of HIV-1 infection in children. It highlighted novel therapeutic experimental modalities to include antiretroviral therapies, passive and active immunization, and gene therapy. Taken together, recent advances may allow, in the near future, improved outcome in HIV-1-infected children and completely aborted mother-to-infant HIV-1 transmission. Foremost, emphasis has been given to the rapid adaptation of novel diagnostic and therapeutic modalities to developing countries and practical plans for international collaborations have to be implemented.

REFERENCES

1. CONNOR, E.M., R.S. SPERLING, R. GELBER, *et al.* 1994. Reduction of maternal–infant transmission of HIV-1 with zidovudine treatment. N. Engl. J. Med. **331:** 1173–1180.
2. STEK, A., M. KHOURY, F. KRAMER, *et al.* 1999. Maternal and infant outcomes with highly active antiretroviral therapy during pregnancy. Abstract. 6th Conference on Retroviruses and Opportunistic Infections. Chicago, IL.
3. FRENCH, N., J. NAKIYINGI, L.M. CARPENTER, *et al.* 2000. 23-Valent pneumococcal polysacharide vaccine in HIV-1 infected Ugandan adults: double blind, randomized and placebo controlled trial. Lancet **355:** 2106–2111.
4. BERNSTEIN, L.J., H.D. OCHS, R.J. WEDGWOOD & A. RUBINSTEIN. 1985. Defective humoral immunity in pediatric acquired immune deficiency syndrome. J. Pediatr. **107:** 352–357.
5. RUBINSTEIN, A., Y. MIZRACHI, L. BERNSTEIN, *et al.* 2000. Progressive specific immune attrition after primary, secondary and tertiary immunizations with bacteriophage $\phi X174$ in asymptomatic HIV-1 infected adults. AIDS **14:** F55–62.
6. ROSENBERG, E.S., J.M. BILLINGSLEY, A.M. CALIENDO, *et al.* 1997. Vigorous HIV-1 specific CD4$^+$ T cell responses associated with control of viremia. Science **278:** 1447–1450.
7. FINZI, D. *et al.* 1999. Latent infection of CD4$^+$ cells provides a mechanism for lifelong persistence of HIV-1, even in patients of effective combination therapy. Nature Med. **5:** 512–517.
8. GREENOUGH, T., F. BRETTLER, L. KIRCHHOF, *et al.* 1999. Immunological and virological characterization of individuals with long term nonprogressive HIV infection in a hemophilia cohort. 6th Conference on Retroviruses and Opportunistic Infections, Abstract 562.
9. ROSENBERG, E.S., B. WILKES, S. POON, *et al.* 1999. Preserving HIV-1 specific T cell help: will it prevent progression? 6th Conference on Retroviruses and Opportunistic Infections, Chicago. Abstract S41.

10. BRODIE, S., D. LEWINSOHN, A. PATTERSON, *et al.* 1999. In vivo migration of and antiviral activity of transferred HIV specific CTLs. Idem. Abstract 26.

11. JIN, X., D. BAUER, S. TUTTLETON, *et al.* 1999. Dramatic rise in plasma viremia after CD8$^+$ cell depletion in SIV infected macaques. Idem. Abstract 252.

12. LORI, F., D. ZINN, *et al.* 1999. Intermittent drug therapy increases the time to HIV rebound in humans and induces the control of SIV after treatment interruption in monkeys. Idem. Abstract LB5.

13. KOVACS, J.A., S. VOGEL, J.M. ALBERT, *et al.* 1996. Controlled trial of IL-2 infusion in patients infected with HIV-1. N. Engl. J. Med. **335:** 1350–1356.

14. CHUN, T.W., D. ENGEL, S.B. MIZELL, *et al.* 1999. Effect of IL-2 on the pool of latently infected, resting CD4$^+$ T cells in HIV-1 infected patients receiving HAART. Nature Med. **5:** 651–55.

15. AUTRAN, B., G. CARCELAIN, V. TUBIANA, *et al.* 1999. Effects of antiretroviral therapy on immune reconstitution. 6th Conference on Retroviruses and Opportunistic Infections, Chicago. Abstract S44.

16. LUZURIAGA, K. 1999. Pediatric antiretroviral therapy, Idem Abstract L1.

17. LUZURIAGA, K., D. HOLMES, A. HEREEMA, *et al.* 1995. HIV-1 specific CTL responses in the first year of life. J. Immunol. **154:** 433–443.

18. ZAROU, D.M., H.C. LICHTMAN & A.M. HELLMAN. 1964. The transmission of Cr-51 tagged maternal erythrocytes from mother to fetus. Am. J. Obstetr. Gynecol. **88:** 56–71.

19. CATLIN, E.A., J.D. ROBERTS, R. ERANA, *et al.* 1999. Transplacental transmission of natural killer-cell lymphoma. N. Engl. J. Med. **341:** 85–91.

20. SPERLING, R.S., D.E. SHAPIRO, R.W. COOMBS, *et al.* 1996. Maternal viral load, zidovudine treatment, and the risk of HIV-1 transmission from mother to infant. N. Engl. J. Med. **335:** 1621–1629.

21. SCARLATTI, G., J. ALBERT, P. ROSSI, *et al.* 1993. Mother to child transmission of HIV-1: correlation with neutralizing antibodies against primary isolates. J. Infect. Dis. **168:** 207–210.

22. DEVASH, Y., T. CALVELLI, D.G. WOOD, K.J. REAGAN & A. RUBINSTEIN. 1990. Vertical transmission of HIV is correlated with low affinity/avidity maternal antibodies to the gp120 principal neutralizing domain. PNAS **87:** 3445–3449.

23. CAROTENUTO, P., D. LOOIJ, L. KELDERMANS, *et al.* 1998. Neutralizing antibodies are positively associated with CD4$^+$ T-cell counts and T-cell function in long-term AIDS free infection. AIDS **12:** 1591–1600.

24. RUBINSTEIN, A., H. GOLDSTEIN, T. CALVELLI, *et al.* 1993. Maternofetal transmission of HIV-1: the role of antibodies to the V3 primary neutralizing domain. Pediatr. Res. **33:** S76–78.

25. UGEN, K., J. GOEDERT, J. BOYER, *et al.* 1992. Vertical transmission of HIV-1. J. Clin. Invest. **89:** 1923–1930.

26. HENGEL, R.L., M.S. KENNEDY, R.W. STEKETEE, *et al.* 1999. Neutralizing antibody and perinatal transmission of HIV-1. AIDS Res. Hum. Retrovir. **14:** 475–481.

27. SHIBATA, R., T. IGARASHI, N. HAIGWOOD, *et al.* 1999. Neutralizing antibody directed against the HIV-1 envelope glycoprotein can completely block HIV-1/SIV chimeric virus infection of macaque monkeys. Nature Med. **5:** 204–210.

28. MOORE, J.P. & D.R. BURTON. 1999. HIV-1 neutralizing antibodies: how full is the bottle? Nature Med. **5:** 142–144.

29. IGARASHI, T., C. BROWN, A. AZADEGAN, *et al.* 1999. HIV-1 neutralizing antibodies accelerate clearance of cell-free virions from blood plasma. Nature Med. **5:** 211–215.

30. GAUDUIN, M.C. *et al.* 1997. Passive immunization with a human monoclonal antibody protects hu-PBL mice against challenge by primary isolates of HIV-1. Nature Med. **3:** 1389–1393.

31. SHEARER, W.T., A.M. DULIEGE, M.W. KLINE, *et al.* 1995. Transport of recombinant human CD4-immunoglobulin G across the human placenta: pharmacokinetics and safety in six mother–infant pairs in AIDS Clinical Trial Group protocol 146. Clin. Diag. Lab. Immunol. **2:** 281–285.

32. WATTS, A.M., J.R. STANLEY, M. SHEARER, *et al.* 1999. Fetal immunization of baboons induces a fetal-specific antibody responses. Nature Med. **5:** 427–430.

33. GERDTS, V., L.A. BABIUK, S. VAN DRUNEN & P.J. GRIEBEL. 2000. Fetal immunizations by a DNA vaccine delivered into the oral cavity. Nature Med. **6:** 929–932.
34. GILL, T.J. 1983. Transplacental immunization of the human fetus to tetanus by immunization of the mother. J. Clin. Invest. **72:** 987–996.
35. VALENTINE, F.T., S. KUNDU, P.A.J. HASLETT, *et al.* 1996. A randomized, placebo controlled study of the immunogenicity of the HIV rgp 160 vaccine in HIV infected subjects with ≥400/ml CD4 T lymphocytes. J. Infect. Dis. **173:** 1336–1346.
36. ERON, J.J., M.A. ASHBY, M.F. GIORDANO, *et al.* 1996. Randomized trial of MN rgp120 HIV-1 vaccine in symptomless HIV-1 infection. Lancet **348:** 1547–1551.
37. TSOUKAS, C.M., J. RABOUD, N.F. BERNARD, *et al.* 1998. Active immunization of patients with HIV infection: a study of the effect of VaxSyn, a recombinant HIV envelope subunit vaccine, on progression of immune deficiency. AIDS Res. Hum. Retrovir. **14:** 483–490.
38. SANDSTROM, E., B. WAHREN & NORDIC VAC-04 STUDY GROUP. 1999. Therapeutic immunization with recombinant gp160 in HIV-1 infection: a randomized double-blind placebo-controlled trial. Lancet **353:** 1735–1742.
39. VALENTINE, F. *et al.* AND THE REMUNE STUDY GROUP. 1999. Immunological and virological evaluations of HAART compared to HAART plus an inactivated HIV immunogen. 6th Conference on Retroviruses and Opportunistic Infections, Abstract 346.
40. VALENTINE, F. *et al.* AND THE REMUNE STUDY GROUP. 1999. Immunological and virological evaluations of HAART compared to HAART plus an inactivated HIV immunogen. 6th Conference on Retroviruses and Opportunistic Infections, Abstract 346.

Global Strategies for the Prevention of HIV Transmission from Mothers to Infants

QUARRAISHA ABDOOL KARIM[a]

South African Medical Research Council, Southern African Fogarty AITRP, International AIDS Vaccine Initiative, Durbin, South Africa

ABSTRACT: The first part of this paper provides a brief overview of the global situation, the second will describe several scenarios that capture the key features of the emerging epidemics, and the third will present the specific challenges that these scenarios pose to us in terms of preventing the further spread of HIV.

INTRODUCTION

This is a defining moment in the history of the HIV pandemic. Since the last (and first) Global Strategies Conference, the results from five mother-to-child transmission studies have become available, namely, the short-course AZT trials in Thailand and Africa, HIVNET 012, Vitamin A, PETRA, and the Kenyan Breastfeeding Trial, dramatically increasing the menu of options for reducing infant transmission of HIV. This august gathering is meeting at a time when the problem of HIV infection is growing and the world is looking to us to come up with solutions to an important consequence of the epidemic, namely, reducing transmission of infection to infants.

Although the focus of this presentation is on the HIV epidemic, it should constantly be borne in mind that we are dealing with three inextricably linked epidemics—the largely asymptomatic HIV epidemic, the visible epidemic of AIDS, and the impact of the premature loss of lives on society. Furthermore, where heterosexual transmission of HIV occurs, there is a concomitant epidemic of HIV in infants due to mother-to-child transmission. The epidemiology and issues relating to mother-to-child transmission will be covered in other chapters in this volume, so I will not focus on the epidemic in infants here.

GLOBAL OVERVIEW

By the end of 1998, UNAIDS estimated that about 34 million persons worldwide had been infected with HIV and about 14 million had died of AIDS. The data on the global distribution of HIV emphasizes that no place on earth has been left untouched by this global pandemic. The uneven regional distribution of HIV infection is influ-

[a]Address for correspondence: Quarraisha Abdool Karim, South African Medical Research Council, Southern African Fogarty AITRP, International AIDS Vaccine Initiative, P.O. Box 171 20, Congella 4013, Durbin, South Africa.

karimq@mrc-ac-za

enced by numerous and varied factors such as time of introduction of the virus; size of population at risk; and the presence and scale of particular biological, social, political, and economic factors. Developing countries account for about 90% of new infections, with sub-Saharan Africa bearing a disproportionate burden of the HIV pandemic: 70% of new HIV infections and 80% of AIDS deaths occur among a tenth of the world's popoulation.

Sexual transmission remains the predominant mode of transmission, accounting for about 80% of HIV transmission. Mother-to-child transmission accounts for about 5–10% of HIV transmission, and intravenous drug use for about 5%; transmission through blood and blood products has been virtually eliminated in most parts of the world through stringent screening programs.

Before describing the various scenarios that epitomize the emerging HIV epidemics, it is important that the terminology used about prevalence and incidence rates be clarified.

Prevalence and Incidence

Most simply, the prevalence describes the amount of infection in a population at a point in time. Prevalence encompasses all infections, old and new, in a given population. In contrast, an incidence rate describes the number of new infections over a specified time period. In most instances the prevalence is calculated from data from a few specific subgroups.

Large studies that follow uninfected individuals over time enable measurement of incidence rates. These studies remain relatively rare in most countries. Through the HIVNET system and other multicenter trials of new prevention interventions, some incidence rate data has started to emerge, and we look forward to more of this type of information emerging over the next two to three years. In the interim, statistical techniques can be used to estimate incidence rates from repeat cross-sectional studies.

Even with good prevalence and incidence rate data, there are major gaps in our knowledge at the population level, such as the lack of behavioral data on sexual mixing and networking, the proportion of the population in high-risk categories or groups, and the proportion who are more vulnerable to HIV infection for other reasons.

Despite the imperfections in data sources and bearing in mind the primary purpose for collection of HIV data, that is, to prevent new infections through targeted interventions and planning, important trends can be discerned.

EMERGING HIV EPIDEMICS

From the first reported cases of AIDS in San Francisco, New York, and central and eastern Africa in the early 1980s, in less than two decades HIV has taken root and spread throughout the world. The HIV pandemic comprises a diversity of epidemics within and between countries. In several countries around the world, both developing and developed, true stabilization of the HIV epidemic has been observed— these will not be covered in this paper. In most parts of the world, HIV continues to spread. In focusing on emerging epidemics here, what I will be highlighting are disturbing emerging trends of concern to us.

Several countries and regions of the world have until recently remained insulated from HIV infection but are currently experiencing phenomenally high rates of infection; in yet other countries, a marked reduction or stabilization of HIV through some modes of transmission or communities may obscure newer modes of transmission or new subgroups that are acquiring HIV infection. Finally, there are countries where the HIV prevalence is low, but the impact in absolute numbers is disproportionate relative to the global burden of infection or where the emerging social millieu could enhance HIV transmission.

HIV Infection among Women

One of the overarching trends of deep concern is the increasing number of HIV infections in women, particularly young women. Women feature strongly in the emerging epidemics much more than they did in the first decade of the epidemic. UNAIDS estimated that at the end of 1998 there were 13.8 million women living with HIV; this represents about 43% of the global burden of HIV infection. The majority of women have been infected through unprotected sex. To date about 4.7 million women have died of AIDS, about 1 million just in 1998. Of the estimated 5.2 million new infections contracted among adults during 1998, 2.1 million or about 40% were among women. Biological, social, economic, and political factors contribute to the increased vulnerability of women. For many women, being married is their only risk factor for acquiring infection. There is also a growing association between coerced sex/rape and HIV transmission.

HIV Infection in South Africa

Currently southern Africa is experiencing one of the most rapidly growing epidemics. HIV is spreading predominantly through heterosexual contact with a concomitant epidemic among children infected through perinatal transmission. Compared to eastern and central African countries, southern Africa experienced a relatively late introduction to HIV. Several studies demonstrate that until about 1987, HIV infection was rare in southern Africa.

HIV seroprevalence among antenatal clinic attenders in the majority of the countries in southern Africa is >20%. Because this subgroup is a proxy marker for the spread of HIV in the general population, this figure is truly alarming.

I will focus on the country of South Africa as a case study to demonstrate more closely the nature of this rapidly unfolding HIV epidemic in southern Africa. Annual, anonymous, national antenatal HIV seroprevalence surveys have been conducted in South Africa since 1990. These surveys demonstrate a more than 30-fold rise in HIV infection within 9 years, from 0.76% in 1990 to 10.44% in 1995 to 23% in 1998. The HIV prevalence data provides an unequivocal picture of the unprecedented, explosively rapid spread of HIV infection in southern Africa.

HIV Incidence Rates in South Africa

Incidence rate data for women between the ages of 15 and 30 derived from repeat antenatal seroprevalence surveys, conducted in a rural community in the east coast of South Africa from 1992 until 1997, highlight the rapidly rising incidence rates

TABLE 1. Progression of HIV infection by age: 1992–1997

| | Year | | |
Age group	1992	1995	1997
20–24	6.9	21.1	34.7
25–29	2.7	18.8	27.8
30–34	1.4	15.0	23.4
35–39	0.0	3.4	12.9

that epitomize the progression of the HIV epidemic in South Africa. Incidence rates rose from 3.8% in 1993 to 7.4% in 1995 and 11.9% in 1997.

Young women in the general population in South Africa are experiencing rates previously seen only among high-risk sex worker populations. In a cohort of sex workers from truck stops in South Africa, the incidence of HIV was 11% in 1997.

Number of HIV-Infected South Africans

At the end of 1998 it was estimated that approximately 3.6 million adults and about 220,000 babies had been infected with HIV in South Africa. The age-specific data from several antenatal surveys demonstrate higher rates of infection among younger women. The large increases (in excess of 300%) in HIV prevalence from 1992 to 1997 in the 20- to 24-year-old age group highlights the importance of youth in the HIV epidemic (TABLE 1).

Age and Gender Distribution

Repeat, cross-sectional, community-based, anonymous HIV seroprevalence surveys conducted in rural areas of the east coast of South Africa in 1990–1992 demonstrated that HIV infection was 3.2 times more prevalent among women compared to men. These surveys also demonstrate an early rise of infection in women compared to men. Note also the peak HIV prevalence for women in the 20- to 24-year age group, while that for men is in the 25- to 29-year age group. Women are not only experiencing high HIV prevalence, but also they are becoming infected at an earlier age than men (FIG. 1).

The relative difference in HIV prevalence between men and women decreases as the epidemic progresses. A community-based, cross-sectional survey conducted in the same area in 1994 demonstrated a 2.3-fold difference in HIV prevalence between men and women.

HIV and Tuberculosis

The impact of the second epidemic is starting to be felt with increases in HIV disease, AIDS, and death. The most common HIV/AIDS-presenting opportunistic infection in South Africa is tuberculosis. The progression from asymptomatic to early disease is best reflected in the rise in new tuberculosis cases and the number of co-infections with HIV.

In a rural community in South Africa, co-infection with HIV in adult tuberculosis rose from 36% in 1993 to 59% in 1995 to 65% in 1997. New tuberculosis cases have

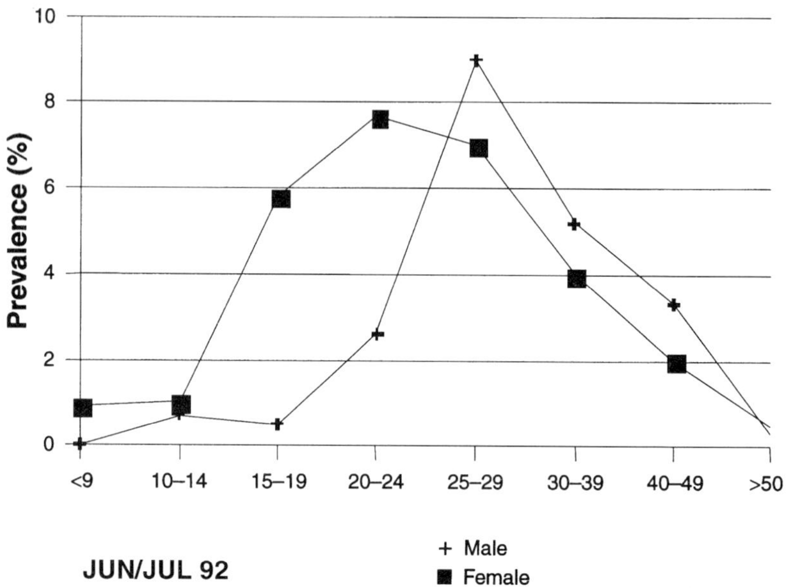

FIGURE 1. Age and gender differences in HIV infection in rural KwaZulu-Natal, 1992.

a similar age and gender profile to that seen in the HIV epidemic, with women presenting at a much younger age than men. The TB fatality rates are much higher where there is co-infection with HIV. The key features of this emerging epidemic are the late introduction of the virus, the rapid rise in infection, the high prevalence at plateau, and the high incidence rates in young people.

HIV Infection in Rwanda

Fanned by a decade of ethnic war and social upheaval including massacres, rape, and refugees of monumental proportions, HIV is spreading rapidly in rural areas of Rwanda. A survey conducted in this central African country in 1986 demonstrated a seroprevalence of 9.4%, whereas a survey 10 years later found that 15% of Rwandans were infected with HIV. About half the women in rural areas have been widowed and have lost children through the civil war.

While the prevalence among antenatal clinic attenders in urban areas has plateaued and remained at between 15 and 20% from 1990 to 1996, most of the new infections are occurring in rural areas. HIV seroprevalence has increased from 1.7% in 1986 in rural areas to 10.3% in 1997.

New infections in urban areas are increasing in the younger age group, while declining in the older age groups. In contrast, in rural areas the increases are mainly among older women. There has been an increase in HIV prevalence among rural Rwandan women in the 26- to 40-year age group from 2.8% in 1986 to 14.1% in 1997. The epidemic in Rwanda highlights the stabilization of the HIV epidemic in some subgroups, masking the introduction of new subgroups acquiring HIV infection.

HIV Infection in the United States

AIDS mortality data from the United States demonstrate the falling mortality rates due to AIDS as well as the impact of antiretriviral treatments on increasing survival among AIDS patients. Rosenberg and Biggar demonstrate the overall decline in HIV seroprevalence in the 18- to 27-year age group. Nevertheless, an examination of the gender analysis demonstrates a decline among men but an increase among women. Furthermore, an analysis of the mode of transmission illustrates how declines in HIV prevalence among men who have sex with men masks the increase among black men and women through heterosexual transmission.The HIV epidemic in the United States has evolved from an initial outbreak among men who have sex with men in a few cities to an important killer of young Americans. Currently, of all incident HIV infections in the United States:

- >2/3 are in ethnic and racial minorities;

- >1/2 are in heterosexuals;

- almost 1/3 are in women;

- although men who have sex with men still present a powerful risk factor for HIV infection, this behavior accounts for fewer infections and, in most instances, the infections are occurring among younger men.

The epidemic in the United States highlights the scenario in which reduction in HIV transmission through some modes of transmission is obscuring new modes of transmission and new subgroups that are acquiring HIV infection.

HIV Infection in Eastern Europe

In Russia and the Ukraine, the predominant mode of transmission is through intravenous drug use. Between 60,000 and 180,000 persons are currently estimated to be infected with HIV. Before 1994 HIV infection was rare in the Ukraine. Since 1994, the spread of HIV has been observed almost exclusively among intravenous drug users (IDUs). In the past 12 months the number of intravenous drug users infected with HIV in the Ukraine increased sixfold, from 1000 to 6000.

In the Ukraine and Russia, few data exist on the spread of HIV in the general population. Rapid bridging between the IDU population and non-drug-using general population of young adults is anticipated. Despite the lack of HIV data, there are indications that there may be rapid spread because of the recent major social, political, and economic changes, which have led to a sharp rise in the IDU population.

In addition, sharp rises in STD rates suggest imminent risk of HIV spread. In Russia, the declines in syphilis rates through the 1980s have been reversed, and they have increased rapidly since 1991 from < 10,000 cases in 1990 to close to half a million cases in 1997 alone.

Similar to the situation in Russia, in China the number of HIV-infected peersons grew 10-fold, from 10,000 people in 1993 to 100,000 in 1995.

HIV Infection in India

In terms of absolute numbers of HIV infection in South and Southeast Asia, India has the most infections. Relative to its total population of about 970 million people, the estimated 3 million HIV infections translates to a prevalence of < 0.5%! Sexual transmission is the main driving force. Of the estimated 1 million sex workers, 10% are in Mumbai alone. The HIV prevalence among sex workers in Mumbai is 30%.

Although almost all states report HIV infection, the epidemic is fairly localized. About 80% of the infections reported for Maharashtra are actually from the city of Mumbai. Of note is that 21 of the 32 states only contribute 4% of the total infections. The infections reported from Manipur are almost exclusively through intravenous drug use, which is an important risk factor. Of the estimated 2 million drug users, 50,000 are IDUs. HIV infection rose from 43.5/1000 to 333/1000 in the first 6 months of 1994 in this group.

STDs constitute a major health problem in India. STD surveys conducted in Tamil Nadu in 1992 demonstrate a high prevalence of STDs that could fuel the spread of HIV in this country. Already, this state contributes about 20% of reported HIV infections.

HIV Infection in Latin America and the Caribbean

The HIV epidemics in Latin America and the Caribbean reflect the heterogeneity observed worldwide. HIV/AIDS has taken its toll among men who have sex with men and intravenous drug users. There is evidence of increasing spread in the heterosexual population and in particular among the impoverished and illiterate segments of society. Data remain scant.

In Brazil, there are several routes of transmission, which accounts for the approximately half-million HIV infections in Brazil: Thus far, men who have sex with men and intravenous drug use have been the main routes of transmission. Rising rates among women demonstrate that heterosexual transmission is becoming more prominent. In urban areas the prevalence of HIV infection among pregnant women ranges from 1 to 5%, is about 5% among sex workers, and is from 33 to 60% among IDUs. The trend is increasing infection among women and among younger, more impoverished, and rural populations. Since 1992 in the Brazilian state of Sao Paulo, AIDS has been the leading cause of death among women aged 20–34.

THE CHALLENGES

Global Pandemic—a Complex Mosaic of Dynamic Epidemics That Need to Be Elucidated More Clearly

These range from epidemics confined to specific, defined high-risk subgroups to diffuse, widespread epidemics in the general population. The emerging epidemics highlight a strong association between HIV infection and youth, gender, mobility, and poverty. With each of these factors, the rapidity of the growth of the epidemic among women is increased.

Incidence Rate Data Indicate Both Prevention Opportunities Missed and Potential Benefits of Prevention

Australia and Thailand demonstrate low incidence rates as a result of strong intervention programs. On the other hand, southern Africa has missed most of this opportunity to have a decisive impact on the HIV epidemic. The opportunity exists in China, India, and Eastern Europe to avert the scenario being experienced in southern Africa.

Prevalence Rates Indicate the Need for Care, Destigmatization, and Compassion

Even with miraculous breakthroughs in terms of vaccines or treatment, there will be an enormous burden on already strained health care services. The need for preparation for the disease burden and impact is highlighted.

HIV serostatus remains unknown for the majority of persons and underscores the need for increased access to voluntary testing and counseling sites.

Despite ever-increasing numbers of HIV-infected people, there is prevalent social and legislative stigma and discrimination. The need for compassion cannot be sufficiently underscored.

The increasing numbers of infection in women has implications for infant transmission of HIV.

The Human Tragedy behind the Numbers: Young, Poor, Women, Marginalized, and Discriminated Against

While we look at the data presented here, we must not forget the faces behind these numbers—the young, the poor, women, the marginalized, and the discriminated against. The gender imbalance in society that fuels the continued vulnerability of women places an urgency for women-initiated methods such as vaginal microbicides and female condoms as well as social norms and legislation to protect and enhance women's status and rights.

Need for Universally Affordable and Available Vaccine and Antiretroviral Therapy

Bold international leadership is required to move forward on an AIDS vaccine. There is a dire need in most parts of the world for access to good-quality health care including affordable antiretrovirals.

In conclusion, the data presented here bear testimony to our technical capabilities as a human race and highlight a challenge for all of us to ensure implementation of what we know works at the magnitude and scale required to turn this pandemic around. While we bask in the euphoria of stabilized epidemics, reduction in AIDS mortality, and advances in reducing transmission of HIV infection to infants, I remind you of these words of the late Jonathan Mann, "The epidemic cannot be stopped in one country until it is stopped in all." We remain inextricably bound to each other in a global society where diseases know no boundaries and where we are all threatened if a single one of us is in danger.

BIBLIOGRAPHY

1. JOINT UNITED NATIONS PROGRAMME ON HIV/AIDS AND THE WORLD HEALTH ORGANISATION. 1998. Report on the status of the HIV/AIDS pandemic. UNAIDS and WHO. Geneva.
2. ABDOOL KARIM, Q. & S.S. ABDOOL KARIM. 1999. South Africa: host to a new and emerging HIV epidemic. Sex. Transm. Infect. **75:** 139–147.

3. ABDOOL KARIM, Q. & S.S. ABDOOL KARIM. 1999. Epidemiology of HIV infection in South Africa. Int. AIDS Soc. Newslet.: 4–8.
4. ROSENBERG, P.S. & R.J. BIGGAR. 1998. Trends in HIV incidence among young adults in the United States. JAMA **279:** 1894–1899.
5. ASTHANA, S. 1996. AIDS-related policies, legislation and programme implementation in India. Health Policy Plann. **11:** 184–197.

Prevention of Perinatal HIV Infection

What Do We Know? Where Should Future Research Go?

MARY GLENN FOWLER[a]

Epidemiology Branch, Division of HIV/AIDS—Surveillance and Epidemiology, Centers for Disease Control and Prevention, Atlanta, Georgia 30333, USA

ABSTRACT: Major progress has been made in reduction of perinatal HIV transmission in the United States and Europe following the PACTG 076 results using zidovudine (ZDV) for prevention of mother-to-infant HIV transmission. Internationally in the past two years, short-course antiretroviral trials have shown efficacy for both antenatal or intrapartum and postnatal interventions. Trials in Bankok, Thailand, and Cote d'Ivoire demonstrated that antenatal ZDV started at 36 weeks could reduce transmission by 50% among non-breastfeeding women and about 37% among breastfeeding women. Uganda trial results with one dose of nevirapine given to the mother at the onset of labor and to the newborn resulted in a 47% reduction in transmission when compared to a regimen of ZDV given intrapartum and for 1 week to the newborn. These recent international research findings provide evidence that both short-course antenatal/intrapartum and intrapartum/neonatal prophylaxis can effectively reduce perinatal HIV transmission in resource-poor settings. In order to avert the 1600 new infant HIV infections occurring daily, the world community must act to rapidly implement these international perinatal trial results.

INTRODUCTION

Research in the past five years has led to major advances in both prevention and treatment of HIV-1 in the United States and Europe. These trends are shown in major declines in both adult AIDS and mortality[1] and dramatic reductions in new pediatric AIDS cases in the United States since 1994 with the widespread implementation of zidovudine (ZDV) for prevention of perinatal HIV transmission (FIG. 1).[2] In the rest of the world, however, particularly in resource-poor settings, the pandemic continues unabated. At present, over 30 million men, women, and children are estimated to be HIV infected, of whom two-thirds reside in Africa.[3]

The toll of HIV disease internationally includes both illness and increased mortality, which are severely straining health care systems of resource-poor countries. Major upheaval of cultural and societal infrastructures are occurring as the infection spreads both in urban and rural areas, among the well educated and illiterate, and among political leaders and followers. The impact among young people and children

[a]Address for correspondence: Mary Glenn Fowler, M.D., M.P.H., Epidemiology Branch, Division of HIV/AIDS—Surveillance and Epidemiology, Centers for Disease Control and Prevention, 1600 Clifton Rd. NE, MS E-45, Atlanta, GA 30333. Voice: 404-639-5190; fax 404-639-6118.
mgf1@cdc.gov

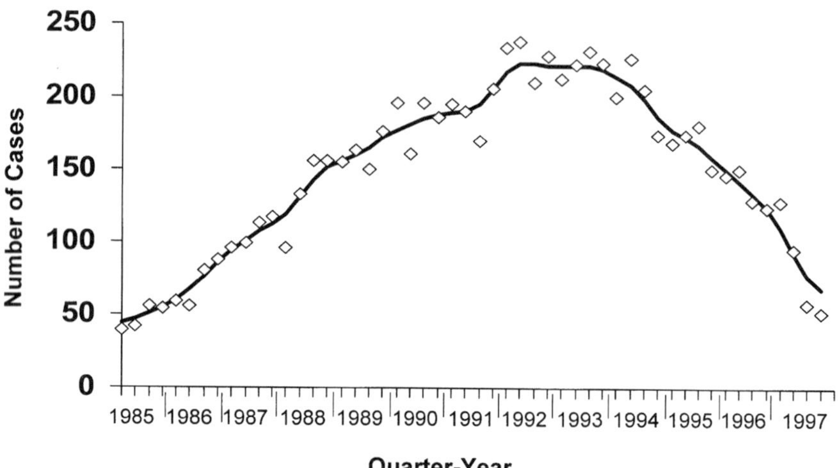

FIGURE 1. Number of perinatally acquired AIDS cases by quarter year of diagnosis, United States, 1985–1997. (Adjusted for reporting delays and redistribution of NIRs, data reported through September 1998. Source: M.L. Lindegren, CDC.)

has been particularly devastating. Worldwide, 1600 infants become HIV infected each day by mother-to-infant transmission; and over half a million children die each year from AIDS-related illnesses. Additionally, approximately 8.2 million children are estimated to have been orphaned because of the death of at least one parent from HIV.[3] Over the past decade, the gains in infant and child survival based on global immunization and oral rehydration programs have been severely eroded by the AIDS epidemic with child mortality rates rising sharply in most of sub-Saharan Africa. Driving these statistics are the high seroprevalence rates (10–45%) among women in major urban areas of southern and eastern Africa[4] and the current lack of implementation of perinatal HIV prevention trial findings. If international trends in heterosexual transmission of HIV are not reversed, a similar explosion of the perinatal HIV epidemic and its consequences are anticipated in Southeast Asia over the next 10 years.

This paper summarizes current understanding of risk factors for mother-to-infant transmission of HIV-1 including breastfeeding transmission, reviews results of recent international trials, and discusses future perinatal HIV research and implementation challenges.

RISK FACTORS FOR PERINATAL HIV TRANSMISSION

Studies from the early 1990s in the United States, Europe, and Africa reported a number of risk factors for transmission before the widespread use of zidovudine.[5,6] These included increased maternal illness severity, elevated viral load, immune factors such as low maternal CD4 counts and maternofetal HLA concordance, placental pathology including chorioamnionitis, increased duration of membrane rupture, maternal illicit drug use, preterm delivery, breastfeeding, and in developing countries anemia and low vitamin A levels.

Since the results of the PACTG 076 trial findings in 1994,[7] the widespread implementation of an intensive regimen of zidovudine prophylaxis given prenatally, intrapartum, and to the neonate for 6 weeks has resulted in substantial decreases in transmission in the United States.[8,9] Currently, rates in the 5–10% range are reported among infants born to HIV-infected women who received zidovudine. Likewise, the widespread use of highly active combination antiretroviral therapy in industrialized countries has resulted in even lower rates being reported with case series suggesting rates of 2% or lower.[10]

Evaluation of the relative importance of other risk factors in the presence of antiretroviral interventions are beginning to emerge. Not surprisingly, only a few other risk factors continue to be strong predictors of transmission. Both the Thai short-course ZDV trial[11] and the US PACTG 185 trial results[8] indicated that maternal viral load at delivery is still an important risk factor for transmission in the presence of ZDV. Other data among women with nondetectable viral load reported in three different studies suggests an extremely low risk for transmission (<1%) among a series of 171 women with undetectable viral loads (less than 400–1000 RNA copies/ml) around the time of delivery.[8,11,12] Recent studies also suggest that breastfeeding, duration of membrane rupture, and absence of elective cesarean section before labor continue to be independent risk factors for infant infection in the presence of zidovudine.[13,14]

The role of the placenta and obstetrical factors in perinatal transmission have also received continued scrutiny. In general, the placenta is an effective immunologic and physical barrier to perinatal HIV transmission: in the absence of antiretrovirals, only about 1 in 4 babies become infected. Nevertheless, inflammation related to chorioamnionitis and other insults to placental integrity can lead to breeches in this protection. Data from an observational placental study among HIV-infected women delivering in Zaire indicated that those with severe histologic choriomanionitis had an increased risk of transmission compared to women with mild or no chorioamnionitis,[15] and similar findings were noted in a smaller U.S. study, particularly among women with duration of membrane rupture greater than 4 hours.[16] These data indicate a potential role for prenatal treatment of chorioamnionitis as a further strategy to reducing perinatal transmission.

The role of cesarean section in reducing the risk of mother-to-infant HIV infection has been more clearly delineated in the past year. In a meta-analyses of approximately 8000 mother infant pairs, cesarean section before the onset of labor or rupture of membranes was associated with about a 50% reduction in risk of infant infection irrespective of maternal zidovudine receipt: rates reported were 19% for vaginal or nonelective cesarean section versus 10.4% for elective cesarean section in the absence of zidovudine; and 7.5% for vaginal or nonelective cesarean section versus 2% for elective cesarean section in the presence of zidovudine.[17] Similar findings were also reported in a European randomized trial of cesarean section versus other type of delivery.[18] These findings have led to a recent statement by the ACOG that HIV-infected women should be offered elective cesarean section at 38 weeks gestation as part of a multifaceted approach to prevention of perinatal HIV transmission.[19]

WHAT DO WE UNDERSTAND ABOUT BREASTFEEDING TRANSMISSION?

Rates of infant HIV infection are approximately doubled among breastfeeding women in various studies from around the world.[6,20,21] Although most risk factors for transmission are still not well understood, recent data from a Malawi study indicates that viral load in breast milk is associated with increased risk of transmission.[22] The timing and relative proportion of breastfeeding at various time periods has also been addressed in a number of recent published studies. A meta-analysis found that late acquisition by breast milk transmission after 2.5 months of age was about 3.2% per 100 person-years of breastfeeding;[23] and the research from Malawi[24] suggests a similar risk (about 3%) in the second year of life with a somewhat higher risk (about 7–8%) during months one to twelve. Recently, Nduati *et al.* reported that most infant infections related to breastfeeding occurred early and that transmission in the first 6 weeks of life accounted for about two-thirds of all breastfeeding transmission.[21] This data was based on findings from a randomized clinical trial of breast versus formula feeding in Nairobi, Kenya. Other data from a vitamin A trial in South Africa[25] suggest a possible protective effect of exclusive breastfeeding on risk of infant HIV infection when compared to mixed feeding.

WHAT DO THE INTERNATIONAL PERINATAL TRIAL RESULTS TELL US?

The overall aim of the international perinatal HIV prevention trials have been to test safe, deliverable, and sustainable interventions that can maximally reduce perinatal HIV transmission in resource-poor settings. General perinatal prevention strategies that have been assessed include prenatal vitamin A supplementation, chlorhexidene vaginal and neonatal wash, and use of formula. Antiretrovial trials have evaluated short-course antenatal and intrapartum zidovudine; zidovudine/lamivudine given prenatally, intrapartum, and postnatally; and nevirapine given intrapartum and postnatally. The results of the short-course antiretroviral and other perinatal prevention trials carried out in international settings can contribute greatly to our understanding of the relative impact of antieretroviral and other interventions targeted at the antenatal, intrapartum, and postpartum periods.

The short-course zidovudine trials were carried out among non-breastfeeding, HIV-infected women in Bangkok, Thailand[11] and breastfeeding, HIV-infected women in west Africa (Cote d'Ivoire and Burkina Faso).[13,26] In two of the trials, zidovudine was given for four weeks to the mother antenatally and intrapartum (Bangkok[11] and Abidjan, Cote d'Ivoire[13]) and in the trial in Burkina Faso/Ivory Coast[26] the women additionally received one week of zidovudine postpartum. Results at 3 months following delivery indicated a 50% reduction in perinatal HIV transmission risk for the zidovudine group compared to placebo group among non-breastfeeding women in Bangkok but only a 37% reduction in risk of transmission among breastfeeding women in west Africa. Also, there was no reduction in perinatal transmission risk between the two studies in the west Africa setting for those mothers who received postpartum zidovudine for 1 week compared to those who did not.

Most importantly, the reduction in risk from the peripartum interventions in west Africa showed little loss of efficacy by later breastfeeding transmission among infants through age 6 months.

The multisite PETRA trial[27] in Uganda, South Africa, and Tanzania utilized combination zidovudine/lamivudine (ZDV/3TC) in a factorial design. The most comprehensive arm (A) gave 4 weeks of ZDV/3TC antenatally, intrapartum, and then for 1 week to mother and infant. The other arms gave intrapartum and postpartum dosing (arm B) or intrapartum-only dosing (arm C), and each dosing regimen was compared to placebo. Findings at 6 weeks were a 50% reduction in transmission risk for those receiving ZDV/3TC in arm A; 38% reduction in arm B; and no difference in transmission risk for for those receiving intrapartum dosing only (arm C) when compared to placebo.

The most recent international perinatal trial results were from HIVNET 012 in Uganda.[28] This trial assessed the efficacy of a single dose of nevirapine (a potent long-acting nonnucleoside reverse transcriptase inhibitor) given to women at the onset of labor and to their neonates at hospital discharge. The nevirapine regimen was compared to intrapartum zidovudine given to women plus one week zidovudine given to their neonates. Findings at 3 months were a 47% reduction in risk of transmission for the group receiving nevirapine. This study and arm B of the PETRA ZDV/3TC trial strongly support the concept of neonatal prophylaxis as an effective perinatal HIV prevention strategy. Overall conclusions gleaned from the international trials are the following:

- Both antenatal/intrapartum and intrapartum/postnatal antiretroviral regimens can significantly reduce perinatal HIV transmission by one-third to one-half.

- Antenatal interventions appear to work primarily through viral load reduction but are less efficacious in breastfeeding settings than non-breastfeeding settings.

- Intrapartum strategies alone (except for elective cesarean section) do not appear efficacious based on results of PETRA ZDV/3TC and chlorhexidene studies.

- Intrapartum plus 1 week of zidovudine to the neonate cannot be recommended in breastfeeding settings based on the Uganda nevirapine study.

- Neonatal prophylaxis is an important prevention strategy based on the nevirapine and PETRA ZDV/3TC studies.

- There is little washout of the efficacy of peripartum antiretroviral regimens by six months among breastfed infants of HIV-infected women based on the short-course ZDV studies.

- Exclusive breastfeeding followed by weaning may prove useful in reducing the risk of transmission compared to mixed feeding but requires more research.

- Prolonged infant prophylaxis (including antiretroviral and active/passive immune agents) during the breastfeeding period needs to be assessed for infants of HIV-infected women who breastfeed.

FUTURE RESEARCH DIRECTIONS: OPERATIONAL RESEARCH AND CLINICAL TRIALS

One of the major challenges following the successful international perinatal HIV trial results is to translate these findings into public health practice in resource-poor settings. A number of efforts are currently under way.

In Thailand, the Ministry of Health has begun implementation of counseling and testing with the offering of short-course ZDV to HIV-infected women in two regions of northern Thailand serving approximately 160,000 pregnant women. Plans are to build on these experiences and move toward national implementation over the next year.

In Africa, the international organizations (UNICEF/UNAIDS/WHO) are helping to support counseling and testing for over 10,000 women in pilot projects in each of 9 countries with the offering of short-course antiretrovirals (ZDV or nevirapine) and formula to HIV-infected women. The pilot projects are at varied stages of implementation but most should be under way within the next 12 months. Based on the lessons learned from these pilot efforts, countries will attempt to implement these perinatal interventions widely in the framework of ongoing antenatal services.

In resource-poor settings, perinatal HIV clinical trial research efforts are now focused on prevention of transmission from breastfeeding. Future trials will evaluate the efficacy of giving short or longer course nevirapine given to breastfed infants of HIV-infected women. Other trials will assess whether hyperimmune globulin can protect the infant during the first several weeks of breastfeeding and whether a combination of peripartum antiretrovirals plus an HIV vaccine series could protect infants against breastfeeding transmission throughout the lactation period. Related research efforts include laboratory-based studies to yield better understanding of viral and immune factors in breast milk that influence risk of transmission.

For mid-developing countries, future studies should address whether combination short-course strategies (e.g., paring short course antenatal ZDV with nevirapine at delivery and to the neonate before hospital discharge) or other combination regimens in non-breastfeeding, HIV-infected women can reduce perinatal HIV transmission to less than 5%.

CONCLUSIONS

In the United States and Europe, the possibility of preventing almost all new cases of pediatric HIV infection is within reach. Worldwide, however, over a half a million infants will likely continue to become HIV infected each year despite efficacious perinatal prevention strategies. The call to action is clear. There is an urgency for international agencies, public health and political leaders, community leaders, nongovernment organizations, women, and families to work collectively and rapidly to translate the successful international perinatal HIV prevention trial results into public health practice. The time is now, the means are available, the challenges are immense, and the next generation will judge carefully whether or not this opportunity was used wisely.

REFERENCES

1. FLEMING, P.L., J.W. WARD, J.M. KARON, *et al.* 1998. Declines in AIDS incidence and deaths in the USA: a signal change in the epidemic. AIDS **12(Suppl. A):** S55–S61.
2. LINDEGREN, M.L., R.H. BYERS, P. THOMAS, *et al.* 1999. Trends in perinatal transmission of HIV/AIDS in the United States. JAMA **282:** 531–538.
3. UNAIDS. 1998. Report on the global HIV/AIDS epidemic, June 1998. UNAIDS/ WHO. Geneva.
4. US Bureau of the Census. 1999. Recent HIV seroprevalence levels by country: February 1999. Research Note No. 26.
5. MOFENSON, L.M. 1997. Mother–child HIV-1 transmission. Obst. Gyn. Clin. N. Am. **24:** 759–784.
6. EUROPEAN COLLABORATIVE STUDY. 1992. Risk factors for mother-to-child transmission of HIV-1. Lancet **339:** 1007–1012.
7. CONNOR, E.M., R.S. SPERLING, R. GELBER, *et al.* 1994. Reduction of maternal–infant transmission of human immunodeficiency virus type 1 with zidovudine treatment. N. Engl. J. Med. **331:** 1173–1180.
8. STIEHM, E.R., J.S. LAMBERT, L.M. MOFENSON, *et al.* 1999. Efficacy of zidovudine and human immunodeficiency virus (HIV) hyperimmune immunoglobulin for reducing perinatal HIV transmission from HIV-infected women with advanced HIV disease. Results of Pediatric AIDS Clinics Trial Group Protocol 185. J. Infect. Dis. **179:** 567–575.
9. COOPER, E.R., R.P. NUGENT, C. DIAZ, *et al.* 1996. After AIDS clinical trial 076. The changing pattern of zidovudine use during pregnancy, and the subsequent reduction in the vertical transmission of human immunodeficiency virus in a cohort of infected women and their infants. J. Infect. Dis. **174:** 1207–1211.
10. BECKERMAN, K.P., A.B. MORRIS & A. STEK. 1999. Mode of delivery and the risk of vertical transmission of HIV-1 [letter]. N. Engl. J. Med. **341:** 205–206.
11. SHAFFER, N., R. CHUACHOOWONG, P.A. MOCK, *et al.* 1999. Short-course zidovudine for perinatal HIV-1 transmission in Bangkok, Thailand: a randomized controlled trial. Lancet **353:** 773–780.
12. GARCIA, P.M., L.A. KALISH, J. PITT, *et al.* 1999. Maternal levels of plasma human immunodeficiency virus type 1 RNA and the risk of perinatal transmission. N. Engl. J. Med. **341:** 394–402.
13. WIKTOR, S.Z., E. EKPINI, J.M. KARON, *et al.* 1999. Short-course oral zidovudine for prevention of mother-to-child transmission of HIV-1 in Abidjan, Cote d'Ivoire: a randomized trial. Lancet **353:** 781–785.
14. SIMONDS, R.J., R. STEKETEE, S. NESHEIM, *et al.* 1998. Impact of zidovudine use on risk and risk factors for perinatal transmission of human immunodeficiency virus. AIDS **12:** 301.
15. ST. LOUIS, M.E., M. KAMENGA, C. BROWN, *et al.* 1993. Risk for perinatal HIV-1 transmission according to maternal immunologic, virologic, and placental factors. JAMA **269:** 2853–2859.
16. VAN DYKE, R.B., B. KORBER, E. POPEK, *et al.* 1999. The Ariel project: a prospective cohort study of maternal–child transmission of human immunodeficiency virus type 1 in the era of maternal antiretroviral therapy. J. Infect. Dis. **179:** 319–328.
17. THE INTERNATIONAL PERINATAL HIV GROUP. 1999. The mode of delivery and the risk of vertical transmission of human immunodeficiency virus type 1 — a meta-analysis of 15 prospective cohort studies. N. Engl. J. Med. **340:** 977–987.
18. THE EUROPEAN MODE OF DELIVERY COLLABORATION. 1999. Elective caesarian-section versus vaginal delivery in prevention of vertical HIV-1 transmission: a randomized clinical trial. Lancet **353:** 1035–1039.
19. ACOG COMMITTEE OPINION. 1999. Scheduled cesarean delivery and the prevention of vertical transmission of HIV infection. Number 219, August 1999. Published in Obstet. Gynecol. **94:** S1–3.
20. TESS, B.H., L.C. RODRIGUES, M.-L. NEWELL, *et al.* 1998. Infant feeding and risk of mother-to-child transmission of HIV-1 in Sao Paulo State, Brazil. J. Acquir. Immune Defic. Syndr. **19:** 189–194.

21. NDUATI, R., G. JOHN, D.A. NGACHA, *et al.* 1999. Breastfeeding transmission of HIV-1: A randomized clinical trial. X1th International Conference on AIDS and STDs in Africa. Ab 13ET5-2 (Monday Sept. 13).

22. LEROY, V., M.-L. NEWELL, F. DABIS, *et al.* 1998. International multicentre pooled analysis of late postnatal mother-to-child transmission of HIV-1 infection. Lancet **352:** 597–600.

23. SEMBA, R.D., N. KUMWENDA, D.R. HOOVER, *et al.* 1999. Human immunodeficiency virus load in breast milk, mastitis, and mother-to-child transmission of human immunodeficiency virus type 1. J. Infect. Dis. **180:** 93–98.

24. MIOTTI, P.G., T.E.T. TAHA, N.I. KUMWENDA, *et al.* 1999. HIV transmission from breastfeeding: a study in Malawi. JAMA **282:** 744–749.

25. COUTSOUDIS, A., K. PILLAY, E. SPOONER, *et al.* 1999. Influence of infant-feeding patterns on early mother-to-child transmission of HIV-1 in Durban, South Africa: a prospective cohort study. Lancet **354:** 471–476.

26. DABIS, F., P. MSELLATI, N. MEDA, *et al.* 1999. Six-month efficacy, tolerance, and acceptability of a short regimen of oral zidovudine to reduce vertical transmission of HIV in breastfed children in Cote d'Ivoire and Burkina Faso: a double blind placebo-controlled multicentre trial. Lancet **353:** 786–792.

27. SABA, J. 1999. Interim analysis of early efficacy of three short ZDV/ETC combination regimens to prevent mother-to-child transmission of HIV-1: the PETRA trial [abstract]. 6th Conference on Retroviruses and Opportunistic Infections. Chicago. Abstract booklet. S7: 212.

28. GUAY, L.A., P. MUSOKE, T. FLEMING, *et al.* 1999. Intrapartum and neonatal nevirapine compared with zidovudine for prevention of mother-to-infant transmission of HIV-1 in Kampala, Uganda: HIVNET 012 randomised trial. Lancet **354:** 795–802.

The Cost Effectiveness of a Single-Dose Nevirapine Regimen to Mother and Infant to Reduce Vertical HIV-1 Transmission in Sub-Saharan Africa

ELLIOT MARSEILLE,[a,g] JAMES G. KAHN,[b] FRANCIS MMIRO,[c] LAURA GUAY,[d] PHILIPPA MUSOKE,[e] MARY GLENN FOWLER,[f] AND J. BROOKS JACKSON[d]

[a]*Health Strategies International, Orinda, California 94563, USA*

[b]*Institute for Health Policy Studies, Department of Epidemiology and Biostatistics, Center for AIDS Prevention Studies, and AIDS Research Institute, University of California, San Francisco, California, USA*

[c]*Department of Obstetrics and Gynaecology, Makerere University, Kampala, Uganda*

[d]*Department of Pathology, Johns Hopkins University School of Medicine, Baltimore, Maryland, USA*

[e]*Department of Paediatrics, Makerere University, Kampala, Uganda*

[f]*HIV/AIDS Branch, Centers for Disease Control and Prevention, Atlanta, Georgia, USA*

INTRODUCTION

Mother-to-child transmission (MTCT) of the human immunodeficiency virus type 1 (HIV-1) infects about 1,600 children daily, the majority in sub-Saharan Africa.[1] Identifying economical interventions to reduce this ongoing devastation is an urgent public health priority.

Results of the HIVNET 012 trial using an "ultra short-course" regimen of nevirapine (NVP) in Kampala, Uganda were announced in July 1999. The regimen consists of a single 200-mg oral dose of NVP to the mother at the onset of labor and a 2-mg/kg dose to the infant within 72 hours of birth. This was compared with a previously untested zidovudine (AZT) regimen consisting of 600 mg AZT orally to the woman at the onset of labor and 300 mg every 3 hours until delivery followed by 4 mg/kg orally twice daily to the infant for 7 days after birth. Compared with the AZT control arm, the HIVNET 012 regimen demonstrated a 47.0% reduction of HIV-1 transmission in infants at 14–16 weeks of age. If the AZT regimen is itself efficacious, the efficacy of NVP would be even greater compared with that of a placebo. Therefore, 47.0% may underestimate the true efficacy of NVP. The regimen was well tolerated, and adverse effects in both mothers and infants were balanced between the NVP treatment group and the AZT control arms.[2] Because the HIVNET 012 regimen consists of only one dose to mother and one to infant, it is less expensive than other proven regimens and potentially more cost effective. This extended

[g]Corresponding author. Voice: 925-254-5379; fax: 415-820-6131.
emarseille@home.com

abstract summarizes the methods and key finding of a recent appraisal of the economics of the HIVNET 012 regimen in sub-Saharan Africa.[3]

METHODS

Overview of Model

Using a computer-based model, we assessed the cost effectiveness of a hypothetical program to provide the HIVNET 012 regimen to a cohort of 20,000 pregnant women in sub-Saharan Africa where breastfeeding is the norm. Outcome measures included program cost; pediatric HIV-1 cases averted; cost per case averted; and cost per disability-adjusted life-year (DALY). Efficacy and program cost data were derived from the HIVNET 012 trial. Other epidemiologic and economic data were obtained from published sources. The analysis compared the cost effectiveness of HIVNET 012 versus no drug therapy with that of other short-course antiretroviral (ARV) regimens, from the public sector payer's perspective. We also assessed two strategies for implementation of the HIVNET 012 regimen: (1) counseling and testing women for HIV prior to treatment ("targeted treatment"); and (2) offering NVP to all pregnant women ("universal treatment" with no HIV counseling and testing). Results were subjected to sensitivity analyses.

Value of Key Inputs

HIV-1 Prevalence. Model results were calculated for HIV-1 prevalence rates ranging from 3 to 40%.

HIV-1 Transmission Rates. The HIVNET 012 trial reported a perinatal and early postnatal transmission rate of 25.1% in the AZT arm. Late postnatal risk, from 2.5 to 24 months, was calculated via meta-analysis at 7.4% of those uninfected at 2.5 months, and this figure was adopted for this analysis.[4]

Cost of NVP. The combined cost of a 200-mg tablet of NVP for the mother and a 2-mg/kg suspension dose for the infant is $4.00 based on the wholesale list price of NVP at the Johns Hopkins Hospital Pharmacy in Baltimore, Maryland.

Cost of Voluntary Counseling and Testing (VCT) per Woman. A recent study of the cost of antiviral regimens for HIV-1 vertical transmission prevention in South Africa estimated the cost of VCT to be $7.30 per mother.[5] This figure is in the mid-range of published estimates and was adopted for the present study.[6–8]

Discounted Incremental Lifetime Cost of Treating HIV-Positive Child. For the base case analysis we adopted the conservative approach of setting incremental treatment costs of HIV-positive versus HIV-negative children at zero.

RESULTS

Under the universal treatment option with a 30% HIV-1 seroprevalence and base case estimates for model inputs, the HIVNET 012 regimen averts 603 cases of infant HIV-1; costs $83,300; and generates 15,862 DALYs. The associated cost-effectiveness ratios are $138 per case averted or $5.25 per DALY. At 15% seroprevalence the

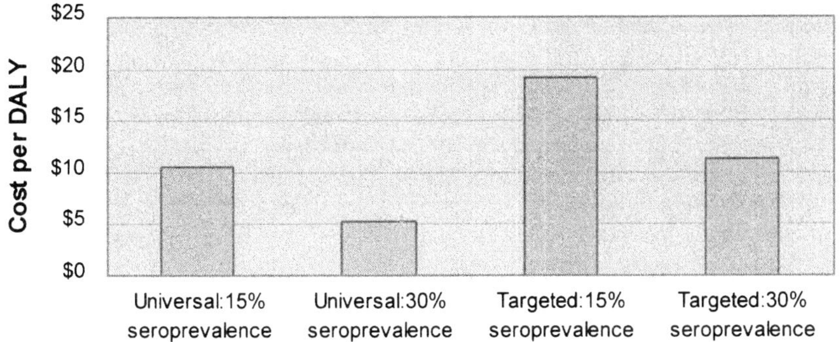

FIGURE 1. Cost effectiveness of the HIVNET 012 regimen by HIV-1 seroprevalence and by targeted versus universal treatment.

universal treatment option also costs \$83,300 and averts 302 cases at \$276 per case averted or \$10.51 per DALY. At 30% seroprevalence, the targeted treatment option costs \$141,900 and averts 476 cases at \$298 per case or \$11.29 per DALY. At 15% seroprevalence, the targeted treatment option costs \$124,500 and averts 246 cases at \$506 per case or \$19.18 per DALY (FIG. 1).

When HIV-1 seroprevalence exceeds 3.0%, the universal HIVNET 012 regimen is likely to be as cost effective as other well-accepted public health interventions (\$50 per DALY). For the targeted treatment option this threshold seroprevalence is 4.5%. Sensitivity analyses indicated that the high cost-effectiveness of HIVNET 012 is robust under a wide range of input values. It is also more cost-effective than the CDC/ Thai, PETRA-A, and PETRA-B regimens which have cost-effectiveness ratios of \$49.37, \$106.37, and \$42.76 per DALY, respectively, when HIV-1 prevalence is 30%.

DISCUSSION

The finding of higher cost-effectiveness associated with the universal treatment option is sensitive to the cost of NVP, to the cost of VCT, and to the assumption that there are no "external" benefits of VCT in reducing adult-to-adult (horizontal) HIV transmission. The potential horizontal transmission prevention benefits of VCT in sub-Saharan Africa have not been well documented,[9] but some research on the effects of VCT on behavior change suggests that it could be substantial.[10,11] Such reduction in HIV transmission, if it occurred, would affect the relative cost effectiveness of universal and targeted treatment. To illustrate, if 50% of the cost of VCT is attributed to horizontal transmission prevention, targeted treatment becomes more cost-effective across the relevant range of prevalence levels. However, if drug costs are also reduced by 50%, universal treatment again becomes more cost-effective above 16% HIV prevalence.

The single dose to mother and infant NVP regimen administered in the intrapartum and immediate neonatal periods represents a deliverable and cost-effective regimen for preventing mother-to-child transmission (MTCT) of HIV-1 in sub-Saharan

Africa, especially under the universal treatment option. Our findings also suggest that in this region the HIVNET 012 NVP regimen is more cost-effective than are the multi-dose regimens found effective in the CDC-Thai and the PETRA trials. In high seroprevalence areas, more lives could be saved for a given investment in MTCT prevention. These results also imply that in lower seroprevalence areas where multi-dose regimens are not routinely used, or cannot be used, NVP therapy could have a significant public health impact at a reasonable cost. If HIVNET 012 efficacy and safety are confirmed in future trials or improved upon with multi-drug single-dose regimens, the basis for wide implementation of antiviral drug-based MTCT control programs will have been greatly strengthened.

ACKNOWLEDGMENTS

This study was supported in part by the HIV Network for Prevention Trials, Division of AIDS, NIAID/NIH contract N01-AI-35173; in part by a National Institute of Mental Health Clinical Services Research Training Grant, Program T32 MH18261; and in part by the Societal Institute for the Mathematical Sciences through grant DA 09531 from the National Institute on Drug Abuse.

REFERENCES

1. UNAIDS, 1998. Mother-to-Child Transmission of HIV: UNAIDS Technical Update. UNAIDS. Geneva.
2. GUAY, L.A., P. MUSOKE, T. FLEMING *et al.* 1999. Intrapartum and neonatal single-dose nevirapine compared with zidovudine for prevention of mother-to-child transmission of HIV-1 in Kampala, Uganda. Lancet **354:** 795–802.
3. MARSEILLE, E., J.G. KAHN, F. MMIRO *et al.* 1999. Cost effectiveness of single-dose nevirapine regimen for mothers and babies to decrease vertical HIV-1 transmission in sub-Saharan Africa. Lancet **354:** 919.
4. LEROY, V., M.L. NEWELL, F. DABIS *et al.* 1998. International multicentre pooled analysis of late postnatal mother-to-child transmission of HIV-1 infection. Lancet **352:** 597–600.
5. KINGHORN, A. 1998. Projections of the costs of anti-retroviral interventions to reduce mother-to-child transmission of HIV in the South African Public Sector. HIV Management Services. Johannesburg.
6. LUTTER, C. 1998. Mother-to-Child Transmission of HIV in the Dominican Republic: Estimated Population Attributable Risk and Cost of the Integrated Preventive Package. PAHO. Washington, DC.
7. ALWANO-EDYEGU, M. & E. MARUM. 1999. Knowledge is Power: Voluntary HIV Counselling and Testing in Uganda. UNAIDS. Geneva.
8. AISU, T., M.C. RAVIGLIONE, E. VAN PRAAG *et al.* 1995. Preventive chemotherapy for HIV-associated tuberculosis in Uganda: an operational assessment at a voluntary counselling and testing centre. AIDS **9:** 267–273.
9. DE ZOYSA, I., K.A. PHILLIPS, M.C. KAMENGA *et al.* 1995. Role of HIV counseling and testing in changing risk behavior in developing countries. AIDS **9**(Suppl A): S95–101.
10. ALLEN, S., J. TICE, P. VAN DE PERRE, A. SERUFILIRA *et al.* 1992. Effect of serotesting with counselling on condom use and seroconversion among HIV discordant couples in Africa. BMJ **304:** 1605–1609.
11. SWEAT, M., S. GREGORICH, G. SANGIWA *et al.* 2000. Cost-effectiveness of voluntary counseling and testing in reducing sexual transmission of HIV-1 in Kenya and Tanzania. Lancet **356:** 113–121.

Access to Voluntary Counseling and Testing for HIV in Developing Countries

HOOSEN M. COOVADIA

Department of Paediatrics and Child Health, Faculty of Medicine, University of Natal, Private Bag X7, Congella, South Africa 4013

ABSTRACT: The counseling that precedes and follows testing of subjects for HIV has become, quite unexpectedly, a focal point for assessment of the ethical propriety, availability, and appropriateness of health services during the AIDS epidemic. It can be anticipated that in the worst affected regions, Voluntary Confidential Counseling and Testing (VCCT) will be an integral component of "...access to comprehensive, essential, quality health care" which is WHO's goal of "Health for All" in the next century. The role, purpose, location, and methods of VCCT, which were reviewed at the previous Global Strategies Conference in 1997, are summarized. Currently understood objectives of VCCT include acceptance of the test, provision of care for HIV-infected individuals (particularly pregnant women), prevention of HIV transmission, and psychosocial support. Many countries in Africa are gradually instituting VCCT as part of their Primary Health Care package. For example "...access to care, counselling and support" for HIV/AIDS and STDs is one of the top 10 national priorities in South Africa. However, closer examination in the country reveals personnel and skill shortages, inability of half the primary health care (PHC) clinics to provide antenatal services, and HIV testing being offered in only 56%. Condom availability is generally good, but termination of pregnancy is undertaken in a bare 27% of hospitals. In other regions of Africa, VCCT is also deficient in many respects: medical services are often unavailable, support is absent, availability is restricted and there are few trained counselors. Consequently, workloads are heavy. Requirements for effective counseling will be listed. The global determinants of inequities in accessing VCCT, such as the GNP and the crushing debt burden borne by poor countries, are discussed. A third of women worldwide receive no antenatal care, and just 60% of the roughly 133 million annual births throughout the world are attended by trained health personnel. Even when VCCT services are available, they are often not acceptable. The overwhelming majority of African women appear to accept HIV testing, but only a proportion (59–61% in recent intervention trials) return for the results. Obstacles to be overcome for provision of VCCT services are identified. Evidence for a positive impact of VCCT services includes facilitated decision-making, acceptance and coping with HIV, improved family and community acceptance, increased condom use, and reduced gonorrhea rates and HIV transmission.

GLOBAL TARGET

At a worldwide level, one of the targets of the World Health Organisation in its goal of "Health for All" in the next century is to "improve access to comprehensive, essential, quality health care."[1] This should include voluntary counseling and testing (VCT) for HIV at appropriate sites. It is anticipated that "by 2010, all people will have access throughout their lives to comprehensive, essential quality health care, supported by essential public health functions."

SOUTH AFRICA: VCT AS A PRIORITY

Within South Africa, one of the top 10 priorities for the National Department of Health is "access to care, counselling and support" for HIV/AIDS and STDs.[2] The problems encountered in achieving this objective are limited capacity, costs of treatment which can be high, lack of information on these diseases, and delays in appointment of appropriate staff.

A serious attempt has been made to make quantitative and qualitative assessments of access to health services in some developing countries. This effort has been strenuous in South Africa in an attempt to take stock of existing health resources so as to plan more effectively for the future. This audit[2] reveals the following information.

Most hospitals in the country had existing policies for HIV Informed Consent, Pre-Test Counselling, and Confidentiality; the average was 73% of all hospitals with urban (91%) and rural (63%) differences. The quality of VCT provided is not known, although when evaluated in research settings, it can be inadequate. Clinics (which should be the prime sites for VCT) had personnel shortages; the percentage of clinics with at least one person with skills update in HIV/AIDS was between 33% (Northern Cape) and 72% (Eastern Cape). A similar range prevailed for skilled personnel in STDs. More worrying was the fact that only 46% (urban) to 55% (rural) of clinics had Antenatal Services available. Family Planning Services were more widely available (± 80%). An average of 56% of these clinics offered HIV testing (range 20–100%); more than 80% offered testing for syphilis. Condom availability was generally good throughout the country (± 80% of Primary Health Care Clinics). VCT includes an option for termination of pregnancy; this service was available in only 27% of hospitals (urban 48% and rural 15%).

VCT: 1997

In order to place the subject of access to VCT in context, it is worthwhile to review the positions reached at the previous Global Strategies Conference in Washington in 1997.[3] VCT was seen as a tool for communication and education on the disease, as a means for access to other interventions such as anti-retroviral drugs, and as a process that prevents involuntary disclosure of HIV status. In a workshop on the topic of implementation of VCT, the following conclusions were reached:

1. VCT should develop within centers integrating HIV information, STD services, and family planning. This is a view supported by UNAIDS.[4]

2. (a) Group counseling and partner involvement should be encouraged.

   (b) Methods should be culturally sensitive (accounting for breastfeeding practices and partner notification) and confidential to prevent stigmatization.

   (c) Rapid tests for diagnosis (HIV, STD) would increase efficiency.

TABLE 1. Access to voluntary counseling and testing (VCT)

	GNP per capita ($) (1996)	% Population with access to safe H_2O^a adequate sanitation[b] (1990–1997)	Total fertility rate (1995)	Annual births (,000) (1997)	% Pregnant women immunized against tetanus (1995–1997)	% Births attended by trained health personnel (1995–1997)
World	5,051	72[a]; 44[b]	2.8	132,827	52	60
Industrialized countries	27,086	...	1.7	9,950	...	99
Developing countries	1,222	71; 44	3.1	119,457	52	55
Least developed countries	232	56; 36	5.3	24,219	48	28
Sub-Saharan Africa	528	50; 44	5.9	25,218	39	37

3. Best practices should be expanded from local to national, and an international network could facilitate exchange of experience, research, training, and types of care.

ACCESS TO VCT

Access to VCT is directly determined by availability of health services, antenatal clinics (ANC) in particular, and it is an expression at country level of the global inequities in wealth, skills, and resources, as measured by broad indicators such as Gross National Product per capita, growth rate per annum, debt service as a proportion of exports, provision of services, health indicators, etc.[5] (TABLE 1). Tallis,[6] in an appraisal of the psychosocial impact of a diagnosis of HIV among pregnant women in Kwazulu Natal, suggested that access to VCT was reduced by unemployment, poverty, illiteracy, migration, and erosion of basic human freedoms. HIV increases the powerlessness of women and worsens the lack of control over their sexuality and fertility, compromising their capacity to access health services and benefit from them.

It is known that about a third of women globally receive no antenatal care whatsoever.[7] Furthermore, only 60% of the roughly 133 million births throughout the world are attended by trained health personnel; this proportion ranges between virtually total coverage in the industrialized world to 28% in the least developed countries and 37% in sub-Saharan Africa.[5] As a surrogate marker of access to ANC, the percentage of pregnant women immunized against tetanus is 52% globally; this figure is as low as 39% in sub-Saharan Africa.[5] These inadequacies in the provision of health services essential for the introduction of VCT reveal the distance developing countries have to cover in order to implement any intervention for reduction of mother-to-child-transmission of HIV_1. The barriers to access to anti-retrovirals are worth comparing in this context.[8] Aside from the major problem of inadequate funds, the barriers include insufficient health services, lack of distribution channels, lack of

TABLE 2. VCT Centers available by country and HIV seroprevalence rates

Country	City	VCT Centers (million inhabitants)	HIV seroprevalence %
Burkina Faso	Bobo Dioulasso	2.5	9.2
Cote d'Ivoire[a]	Abidjan	0.4	14.0[b]
Kenya	Nairobi	3.0	15.0
	Mombasa	4.00	12.5[b]
Tanzania	Dar Es Salaam	1.3	12.0
Malawi[a]	Blantyre	5.0	30.0[b]
Zambia	Lusaka	6.7	27.5[b]
Zimbabwe	Harare	0	28.0
South Africa	Soweto	0.33	18.3[b]
	Durban	4.00	27.0[b]
Thailand	Bangkok	2.5	2.3

[a]Two studies.
[b]Unlinked anonymous testing. VCT, voluntary counseling and testing.
Adapted from Cartoux *et al.*

laboratories and technology, administrative delays, lack of medical training, and complexity of care and management.

A recent international postal survey of VCT in 11 cities in developing countries found that of the 8 cities with more than 2 million inhabitants each, four had only one VCT center available for the entire population.[9] The HIV seroprevalence rates were high in all these cities: 9–18% in 7 sites and > 28% in 5 sites (TABLE 2).

ACCEPTABILITY OF VCT

Even if ANC services and VCT were accessible and available, how acceptable would they be to women in developing countries. Recent evidence from trials in the third world to reduce mother-to-child transmission (MTCT) show some disturbing trends.[10–12] Overall, between 74 and 84% of pregnant women will accept HIV testing following pre-test counseling. In the international postal survey carried out during late 1997, the acceptance rates were also high: median 92%; range 53–99.7%.[9] Acceptability rates increased with the number of VCT centers available, a record of previous experience with such testing, VCT provided with ANC services, and non-government organization (NGO) support. Even outside a research setting within routine services African women generally accept HIV testing; in Kenya, East Africa, 99% agreed,[13] whereas in Burkina Faso, West Africa, this figure was 90%.[14] However, substantial numbers do not return for the result; return rates were between 59 and 61% in the MTCT trials,[10–12] 70 and 73% in those attending routine clinics,[13,14] and 82% (range 33–100%) in the international survey.[9] The reasons for the failure to return include the self-perception of being at high risk for HIV, fear of violence in the event of disclosure, financial difficulties, and a change of mind.[15,16] In a literature review of the subject, Chazal-Bertoletti[17] identified a number of factors influencing acceptability of HIV testing by pregnant women in developing countries. Predictors of uptake were perceived benefits, knowledge of MTCT and available treatment, midwives' attitudes, counseling services, and universal testing.

IMPROVING ACCESS TO VCT

In addition to the broader issues just discussed, improving access and return rates to counseling and testing include longer term measures such as a change in community attitudes and behaviors, couple counseling and testing, universal testing and shorter term support which reduces the financial costs of attendance, and shorter delays in obtaining HIV results. In Uganda, evaluation of a Rapid Test for HIV showed that the return rate increased by 20% when the delay was reduced from 21 days to 1 day.[15] In the UK, the quality of care (i.e., midwife) determined the uptake of HIV testing.[18] In industrialized countries, availability of VCT centers, acceptance rates, and return rates are generally high, although in some places the acceptability of HIV testing varies widely.[9]

In summary, the obstacles to be overcome in providing VCT services include lack of policy, lack of resources, unreasonable demands on counselors, difficult access to services, inappropriate atmosphere in the clinic, lack of privacy and confidentiality, and no follow-up support. HIV testing always requires informed consent; however, lack of access to pre-test counseling should not be a barrier to voluntary HIV testing.[4]

IMPACT OF VCT

Implementation of VCT services can produce a wider range of benefits. ANC services will improve, maternal and infant health can benefit, and education and training of appropriate health personnel become feasible.

The objectives of VCT include the following: (1) acceptance of the HIV test; (2) detection of HIV-infected individuals: to provide prophylactic and affordable care; (3) detection of HIV-infected pregnant women: to provide antiretroviral therapy where affordable, to offer termination of pregnancy or cesarean section where applicable, to increase choices for future pregnancies, to advise on breastfeeding, to make available prophylaxis against opportunistic infections, and to provide advice on nutrition and care for HIV-infected infants; (4) prevention of HIV transmission: by providing information, education, guidance, and continuing support; and (5) achievement of psychosocial benefits: to cope better and lead positive lives.

In general, in developing countries, particularly Africa, VCT services appear to fall short in many specific features. Medical services are often unavailable, continuing support (e.g., NGOs, counselors) is absent, availability is restricted outside research sites, there are few trained counselors, workloads are heavy, and training is limited. Pre-test group counseling is the norm and lasts about 15 minutes; post-test counseling is individualized and lasts about 26 minutes.[9]

The requirements for effective counseling services are careful selection of trainees, supervised placement, continued training and support, retention of trained staff, appropriateness of settings, and a network of referral services. Moreover, it is suggested that with the woman's consent counseling can be "… extended to spouses, sex partners and relatives … (concept of shared confidentiality)."[4]

A randomized controlled trial of VCT in three countries (Kenya, Tanzania, and Trinidad) involving 3,120 subjects has shown that VCT can induce behavioral change.[19] In the experimental group the prevalence of unprotected sex by women with nonprimary partners was reduced. A recent Zambian study demonstrated that VCT improved coping strategies, easing anxiety about the HIV infection.[20]

The impact of VCT services was recently summarized by UNAIDS[4,21–23] and includes the following: they help in decision-making about HIV tests;[23] encourage acceptance of and coping with HIV;[22] improve family and community acceptance;[22] increase condom use;[21] reduce the prevalence of gonorrhoea (in HIV-infected persons);[23] and reduce HIV transmission.[23]

REFERENCES

1. WHO. 1998. Health for All in the 21st Century. WHO. Geneva.
2. EDWARDS-MILLER, J. *et al.* 1998. Measuring quality of care in South African clinics and hospitals. *In* South African Health Review. A. Ntuli, Ed. :157–193. Health Systems Trust, 401 Maritime House, Salmon Grove, Durban 4001.
3. ROGERS, M. 1997. Implementation of HIV counselling and testing in the international setting. *In* Conference on Global Strategies for the Prevention of HIV Transmission from Mothers to Infants. N. Martin *et al.*, Eds. :169. Washington, DC.
4. UNAIDS. 1997. Counselling and HIV/AIDS. UNAIDS technical update. UNAIDS. Geneva. http://www.unaids.org; unaids@unaids.org
5. BELLAMY, C. 1999. Statistical Tables. *In* The State of the World's Children. UNICEF: 91–127. New York.
6. TALLIS, V. 1997. An exploratory investigation into the psychosocial impact of an HIV positive diagnosis in a small sample of pregnant women, with special reference to KwaZulu Natal. M. Soc. Sc. Dissertation, University of Natal, Durban, South Africa.
7. WHO. 1997. Coverage of Maternal Care: A Listing of Available Information. 4th Edition. WHO. Geneva.
8. HOGG, R.S. *et al.* 1998. One World, One Hope: The Cost of Providing Anteretroviral Therapy to All Nations. AIDS **12:** 2203–2209.
9. CARTOUX, M. *et al.* 1998. Acceptability of voluntary HIV testing by pregnant women in developing countries : an international survey. AIDS **12:** 2489–2493.
10. SHAFFER, N. *et al.* 1999. Short course oral zidovudine for perinatal HIV-1 transmission in Bangkok, Thailand : a randomised controlled trial. Lancet **353:** 773–780.
11. WIKTOR, S.Z. *et al.* 1999. Short course oral zidovudine for prevention of mother-to-child transmission of HIV-1 in Abidjan, Cote d'Ivoire: a randomised trial. Lancet **353:** 781–785.
12. DABIS, F. *et al* 1999. 6-month efficacy, tolerance, and acceptability of a short regimen of oral zidovudine to reduce vertical transmission of HIV in breastfed children in Cote d'Ivoire and Burkina Faso: a double-blind placebo-controlled multicentre trial. Lancet **353:** 786–792.
13. KIARIE, J. *et al.* 1996. Acceptability of Antenatal HIV-1 Screening. XI International Conference on AIDS. Vancouver, BC (Abstr. MoC 211).
14. CARTOUX, M. *et al.* 1996. HIV testing and counselling (HIV C&T) in African pregnant women in the context of interventions to reduce mother-to-child transmission (MTCT). XI International Conference on AIDS. Vancouver, BC (Abstr. ThC 411).
15. FRENCH, N. *et al.* 1997. HIV testing strategies at community clinic in Uganda. AIDS **11:** 1779.

16. TEMMERMAN, M. *et al.* 1995. The right not to know HIV-test results. Lancet **345:** 969–970.
17. CHAZAL-BERTOLETTI, E. 1998. Acceptability of HIV testing among pregnant women in Malawi. M.Sc. Dissertation, University of London, London.
18. SIMPSON, W.M. *et al.* 1998. Uptake and acceptability of antenatal HIV testing: randomised controlled trial of different methods of offering the test. BMJ **316:** 262–267.
19. COATES, T. *et al.* 1998. The Efficacy of Counselling and Testing in Reducing HIV Risk In Developing Countries. 5th Conference on Retroviruses and Opportunistic Infections. Chicago, IL.
20. KAYAWE, *et al.* 1998. Clients' Views on HIV Counselling and Testing. Is It Helpful? 12th World AIDS Conference, Geneva (Abstr.).
21. MUGULA, F. *et al.* 1995. A community-based counselling service as a potential outlet for condom distribution. International Conference on AIDS/STD in Africa. Kampala.
22. TASO UGANDA. 1995. The inside story: participatory evaluation of HIV/AIDS counselling medical and social services, 1993–1994. TASO. Kampala. Uganda.
23. ALLEN, S. *et al.* 1992. Confidential HIV testing and condom promotion in Africa: impact on HIV and gonorrhoea rates. JAMA **268:** 3338–3343.

Rapid Voluntary Testing and Counseling for HIV

Acceptability and Feasibility in Zambian Antenatal Care Clinics

J. P. BAKARI,[a] S. McKENNA,[b] A. MYRICK,[c] K. MWINGA,[d] G. J. BHAT,[e] AND S. ALLEN[a,f]

[a]*University of Alabama at Birmingham, Department of Epidemiology & International Health, Birmingham, Alabama 35294-2170, USA*

[b]*Stanford University School of Medicine, 300 Pasteur Drive, Stanford, California 94305, USA*

[c]*Harvard School of Public Health, Department of Immunology & Infectious Diseases, Boston, Massachusetts 02115, USA*

[d]*University Teaching Hospital, Department of Paediatrics and Child Health, Private Bag RW 1X, Lusaka, Zambia*

[e]*University of Zambia, Lusaka, School of Medicine, Lusaka, Zambia*

ABSTRACT: Voluntary testing and counseling (VTC) for HIV/AIDS is now widely accepted as an effective HIV prevention and control strategy among heterosexual couples in sub-Saharan Africa. The most appropriate format and venue for VTC remains a topic of debate among clinicians and public health professionals. Our research done in Lusaka, Zambia, took a tripartite approach to exploring the most acceptable format and venue for VTC: a community survey of attitudes towards VTC, a pre- and postcounseling knowledge survey, and a pilot study of same-day VTC in urban antenatal care clinics. A community survey of 181 individuals was conducted in July–August 1996 based on a structured questionnaire. A pre- and post-VTC intervention knowledge survey was conducted during the same period among 82 couples attending the Zambia-UAB HIV Research Project (ZUHRP) HIV VTC center in Lusaka. Finally, same-day HIV VTC was pilot tested in six antenatal clinic locations during February–May 1997 and June–August 1998. The community survey revealed that 98% of participants support promotion of HIV VTC in the community and 83.8% prefer the same-day testing format. The knowledge survey revealed misconceptions about discordance within a couple and perinatal transmission of HIV. Pilot testing in antenatal clinics was well received, with 84% of pregnant women requesting testing and 25% having positive HIV serologies. Women with primary school or less education, those seeking antenatal care in local clinics, and those seen before the third trimester of pregnancy were more likely to request HIV testing. Testing and counseling for HIV were shown to be feasible and effective in the antenatal clinic setting. Implementation of same-day HIV VTC in antenatal clinics is an effective strategy to prevent vertical trans-

[f]Address for correspondence: Susan Allen, University of Alabama at Birmingham, Department of Epidemiology & International Health, 845 19th St., Beville Bldg., Rm. 206, Birmingham, AL 35294-2170. Voice: 205-934-7193; fax: 205-934-1640.

sallen@uab.edu

mission and should be expanded to include couples to leverage a decrease in heterosexual transmission as well.

INTRODUCTION

Voluntary testing and counseling (VTC) for HIV/AIDS are now widely accepted as an effective HIV prevention and control strategy among heterosexual couples, particularly in sub-Saharan Africa where heterosexual transmission remains the primary source of new infections. In cities with a high prevalence of HIV, most infections occur in cohabiting couples; in order for these couples to adopt effective HIV risk reduction behavior, the HIV status of both partners must be known.[1] The most appropriate format and venue for VTC, however, remain a topic of debate among clinicians and public health professionals. Numerous formats are under discussion including: (1) same-day versus delayed result testing and counseling; (2) rapid HIV testing versus ELISA assays; (3) provision of incentives versus testing for free or with a nominal fee for cost recovery; (4) couples versus individual counseling; (5) long or repeated versus one-time counseling sessions; and (6) group versus individual education sessions, as well as a host of other considerations.

The selection of a testing and counseling format is inextricably linked to the testing and counseling venue. Private research or clinical facilities may offer increased confidentiality, whereas public facilities have increased accessibility. Antenatal care clinics have had priority consideration as an accessible point of entry for VTC since the ACTG 076 trial demonstrating the impact of Zidovudine on vertical transmission. The subsequent recommendation by the CDC in 1995 for providers to encourage HIV testing for all pregnant women further increased awareness of VTC. The recent announcement of the efficacy of Nevirapine, an easily administered and relatively inexpensive drug feasible for use in low-resource settings[2] lends urgency to implementing VTC at antenatal care clinics in sub-Saharan Africa.

Numerous published studies quantify the effectiveness of VTC by objective measures. Reduced HIV incidence, increased condom use among discordant couples, and decreased incidence of gonorrhea are well documented results of VTC interventions in African heterosexuals.[3–5] These studies justify the "why" of a testing and counseling intervention, but leave the details of "how" largely unanswered.

Studies have repeatedly shown that most adults want VTC when offered, but the reasons for refusal among the remaining minority are not well established. This is a critical gap, as reasons for declining HIV testing are important in determining the best format and venue for VTC. One large scale study in antenatal clinics in Burkina Faso and Cote d'Ivoire documented reasons for test refusal as "to seek agreement of the partner," "fear of AIDS," and "the need to make a decision later at home."[6] In light of sociogeographic differences between potential VTC sites, further study is needed to determine the generalizability to other African countries.

Client perceptions of HIV VTC need to be taken into account when developing appropriate interventions. In one study, clients reported hesitancy to refuse HIV testing, particularly in a hospital setting.[7] Typically, HIV VTC is conducted on two dates with pre-test counseling on the initial visit and post-test counseling up to 2 weeks later. Studies have inferred from HIV result-seeking rates below 50% that "readiness for VCT" is low and that clients may "not have fully understood the implications of being tested."[8,9] These studies did not examine the impact of offering same day testing, instead of delayed results, on willingness to seek test results.

Our research in Zambia has taken a tripartite approach to exploring the most acceptable format and venue for VTC: a community survey of attitudes towards VTC among those both seeking and declining HIV testing, a pre- and post-counseling survey of HIV knowledge, and a pilot study of same-day VTC in urban antenatal care clinics. By examining the issue from different angles within the same geographic location, it is anticipated that a more comprehensive model for VTC can be formed.

METHODS

The following studies were initiated by a National Institutes of Health-funded HIV research site established in Lusaka in collaboration with the University of California in San Francisco (from 1994–1996) and the University of Alabama at Birmingham (from 1996 to the present).

Community Survey

A private consulting firm was contracted in July 1996 to conduct a survey of community impressions of all commonly available HIV voluntary testing and counseling services in Lusaka, Zambia. The survey targeted participants in the same-day testing program offered at the HIV research site known as Zambia-UAB HIV Research Project (ZUHRP) as well as participants in the delayed results program offered at Kara Counselling Centre, a nongovernmental organization. Because VTC has long been a controversial topic, an experienced survey team without prior experience in HIV-related work was selected in an effort to collect data free from bias.

A total of 181 questionnaires were administered to random samples of participants stratified by decision to test or not to test and by testing site. Survey instruments were developed and administered in accordance with the following stratifications: one for community members who were invited to ZUHRP but did not attend ($n = 29$), one for couples who accepted the invitation to ZUHRP but were not tested ($n = 22$ individuals), one for couples tested at ZUHRP ($n = 99$ individuals), and one for couples tested at Kara Counselling Centre (another local testing center that only offers delayed results testing) ($n = 31$). All survey respondents were interviewed by an independent consultant from Afro-Development Services, Ltd. Interviews were conducted at ZUHRP and Kara with the exception of the 29 respondents who had not responded to the ZUHRP invitation; these individuals were interviewed in their home. Respondents were asked about personal demographics, impressions of HIV testing and counseling, and knowledge of HIV/AIDS. The survey administered to those participants tested at ZUHRP had additional questions regarding the quality of service experienced at ZUHRP, whereas those who chose not to be tested were asked the reason for their choice.

All respondents were randomly selected from among ZUHRP or Kara center attendees. Couples who attended ZUHRP but declined to be tested were oversampled in order to obtain more data on the reasons for declining the test. To assess attitudes among couples who did not respond to ZUHRP invitations, a random sample was drawn from recently invited couples for whom addresses were known in such a way to include all areas from which participants were recruited.

The surveys were analyzed using cross-tabulations stratified by the four categories (invited to ZUHRP but did not attend, attended ZUHRP but not tested, attended ZUHRP and tested, and tested at Kara) and separately by gender, HIV status ($\pm$) and couple status (concordant +, concordant − and discordant) for those who were tested at ZUHRP. Chi square statistics were also calculated.

Client Knowledge Survey

A pre- and post-intervention knowledge survey was administered to 82 couples attending the ZUHRP HIV testing and counseling center in the Emmasdale township of Lusaka during the months of July and August 1996. ZUHRP invites couples from all over Lusaka to come for HIV testing and counseling. Whereas some couples are brought to ZUHRP by radio announcements and the project's prominent street sign, the majority of couples respond to invitations from community workers. Community workers were selected from prior participants in the ZUHRP testing and counseling program and given a 1-day training program. These community workers entered Lusaka neighborhoods with written invitations for couples to come to ZUHRP. The invitations informed the couples that they were welcome to participate in a 1-day HIV testing and counseling program. The invitation specified that couples would receive a free lunch as well as transportation to the center and money for the return trip home. Explanatory letters addressed to employers were also provided for those individuals who needed to request time off from work. The project was open 6 days a week in order to maximize the number of couples who could come for counseling and testing. Couples who accepted the invitation were given an appointment for the following week and were informed of the meeting point from which transport to the center would be provided.

The procedures used in this 1-day VTC session were the product of 10 years of experience in Rwanda and Zambia. All ZUHRP counseling staff had received certificates of completion of 6 weeks of training courses offered by Kara Counseling and/ or the Ministry of Health Counseling Unit. Once couples reached the project, they were welcomed by the ZUHRP counseling staff. An itinerary of the day was given, and couples were reminded that they would have the opportunity to get HIV testing if they wished. The group was shown a video about the impact of HIV in a family. At key points during the video and afterward, a trained HIV/AIDS counselor led a group discussion about essential knowledge regarding HIV and its implications for concordant and discordant couples. In this interactive discussion, the whole group of volunteer couples were given a definition of HIV, how the virus is transmitted, how it is diagnosed, how transmission can be prevented, etc. This information was provided in Nyanja, which is one of the two most common languages spoken in the Lusaka area.

Following the group session, couples were offered the opportunity to discuss their HIV testing options in private rooms with a trained counselor. All counseling sessions were conducted with both members of the couple present. If the couple decided to participate in the same-day testing program, informed consent was obtained and numbered vials of blood were drawn for HIV and syphilis testing. If the couples chose not to get tested, they were free to leave at any time. All couples regardless of testing decision were provided lunch and transportation fare to return home.

While rapid HIV testing and rapid plasma reagin (RPR) testing was being performed, couples were given a simple lunch and a presentation on family planning. In the afternoon, couples met with a counselor to receive their HIV and syphilis results with post-test counseling. All RPR-positive individuals were treated for syphilis. In addition, all couples were invited to return at any time for followup counseling.

To assess baseline HIV knowledge and the impact of the VTC program on knowledge about HIV, pre- and post-intervention questionnaires were done. Up to four couples a day were asked to participate in the knowledge survey as they entered the project grounds. These couples were chosen randomly by the ZUHRP counseling staff. Those couples who agreed to be participants were administered the first part of the survey in private counseling rooms before any HIV education was given.

The second part of the survey was administered before the couples received their test results. For those couples who chose not to get tested, they completed the second half of the survey before they left the project grounds. Men and women were interviewed separately. Due to varying literacy levels of the Zambian population, ZUHRP staff read the survey question and answer choices aloud and asked for a verbal response from the participant.

The survey was divided into two parts: a knowledge assessment and a risk assessment. The knowledge assessment had nine questions that covered the basics of HIV transmission, and the risk assessment contained three questions regarding perceived risk and discordancy.

A total of 76 couple surveys were analyzed and four were excluded due to missing values. Survey responses were subsetted by gender and pre-/post-test answers, then analyzed using cross-tabulations, frequencies, and two-tailed Fisher's exact test for each of the questions.

Pilot Testing of VTC in Antenatal Care Clinics

In an effort to transfer knowledge from the free-standing ZUHRP clinic to antenatal clinics in the Lusaka area, a two-phase pilot program was conducted in February–May 1997 and June–August 1998. The pilot program was initiated by developing a supplemental training course for certified nurse-counselors who were based in antenatal clinics. To enroll in this ZUHRP training, participants were required to have completed one of two 6-week counseling training programs previously established by the Zambian Ministry of Health and Kara Counselling. The ZUHRP curriculum focused on same-day couples VTC strategy and included 3 days of didactic lectures, hands-on experience performing rapid HIV tests, and observed counseling sessions with real couples. In total, 150 antenatal care and delivery ward nurses and counselors were trained using the curriculum developed at ZUHRP. They then returned to their ANC clinic to implement same-day VTC with their pregnant clients.

The pilot VTC program was conducted in five antenatal care clinics in Lusaka as well as in the University Teaching Hospital. Approximately the first 30 women attending the antenatal clinic each day were invited to participate in a group discussion on essential knowledge regarding HIV and its implications for pregnant women (using an intervention similar to the one described in couples VTC above). After the group presentation, women were given the opportunity to talk with a counselor in a private room at the antenatal clinic. Nurse-counselors established a daily rotation of counseling and ANC duties. This ensured that staff dedicated to counseling did not have competing demands and also allowed all trained ANC staff to participate in counseling. After pre-test counseling, women deciding to participate in the same-day testing program gave informed consent, and anonymous linked numbered vials of blood were drawn for HIV and syphilis testing (as just described). The woman then proceeded with her regular antenatal visit. Post-test counseling was provided after the woman had completed the antenatal visit. All women were invited to ZUHRP for followup counseling regarding their personal result. In addition, all women were invited to bring their spouse for couples testing at ZUHRP.

Voluntary testing counseling for HIV was offered to 467 pregnant women in 1997 and 658 in 1998. As at ZUHRP, same-day HIV testing was conducted using a two-test algorithm. The first test was conducted using the HIV 1+ 2 Dipstick assay, a dot-immunoblot developed by the Program in Appropriate Technology and Health (PATH, Seattle, Washington). Positive and indeterminate results were then tested with the Capillus HIV-1/HIV-2 assay, a latex agglutination test developed by Cambridge Biotech Ltd (Galway, Ireland). This rapid HIV algorithm had proved to be more accurate than ELISA testing in a comparison conducted in a subset of 7,185 samples.[10] The difference in accuracy was largely attributable to human error, which is more of a problem with the multi-step ELISA done with >90 samples in a batch, compared with simpler rapid test technologies that can be done on one or a few samples at a time.

RESULTS

Community Survey

A total of 181 interviews were conducted in the Lusaka community by the private consulting firm described above; the sample was comprised of 29 people who declined the invitation or accepted but did not attend, 22 who attended the educational session but were not tested, 99 people who received HIV testing at ZUHRP, and 31 who were tested at the Kara Counselling Centre. Most of the survey participants were married (85%), with those tested at Kara showing a much larger proportion of single people ($n = 31$, 71% single or widowed versus 100% married at the ZUHRP center); this was an expected result, as ZUHRP does not conduct outreach to single people. The median age of the participants was 25 for those declining the invitation, 28 for those who attended but were not tested, 27 for those tested at ZUHRP, and 23 for those tested at Kara. The ages ranged from 16–56.

Overall, 98% of those interviewed thought HIV/AIDS counseling and testing was "good" and should be promoted in the community, including 90% of those who declined the invitation. Survey responses indicated that the most effective method of promotion for voluntary testing and counseling was through community workers. Overall, 69.8% of survey participants heard about testing from a community worker. Whereas 50% of discordant couples testing at ZUHRP heard about the service from a community worker, they were more likely than other couples to hear about testing in the popular media or from friends and colleagues ($p < 0.001$).

TABLE 1. Characteristics of community members surveyed ($n = 181$)

	Didn't come ($n = 29$)	Not tested ($n = 22$)	Tested at ZUHRP ($n = 99$)	Tested at Kara ($n = 31$)	p value
Knows someone with HIV	24 (89%)	13 (59%)	53 (54%)	22 (73%)	0.003
Reports "a lot" of knowledge about HIV	1 (4%)	4 (18%)	9 (9%)	5 (16%)	0.001
Previously tested for HIV			12 (12%)	3 (10%)	NS
Feels others would treat them differently if they were thought to be HIV positive	25 (86%)	9 (41%)	32 (32%)	18 (60%)	0.001
Heard of testing from community worker		16 (73%)	72 (73%)	18 (58%)	NS
Knows of other testing centers		5 (23%)	21 (21%)	4 (13%)	NS

Among couples interviewed at ZUHRP, men were more likely than women to know of other test sites ($p = 0.02$); however, there was no difference between how men and women heard of the testing center. Discussion between partners had a positive association with decision to test ($p <0.001$). In the community survey, 96% of couples who requested testing, 73% of those who came to the center but did not get tested, and 55% of those who declined the invitation to the center reported having discussed getting HIV tested with their partner. A strong association is therefore seen between discussion with partner and seeking testing.

A couple's decision to test was also associated with self-reported knowledge levels. Survey participants were more likely to seek testing if they had high perceived levels of knowledge about HIV ($p <0.001$). In fact, all of those participants who reported "no knowledge" or "don't know" their level of knowledge declined testing ($n = 13$).

There was a clear preference among survey participants for same-day testing over a delayed-results format (FIG. 1). Overall, 83.8% of those tested at either center preferred to receive their results on the same day. Clients tested at Kara were likely to prefer the same-day format (61% versus 94%, $p <0.001$), but were more likely to report feeling scared while waiting for their test result (35% versus 17% at ZUHRP, $p = 0.01$).

Overall, ZUHRP clients were pleased with the services provided. Greater than 80% reported that the community worker was pleasant and informative, counseling sessions and group discussions were understandable and of appropriate length, and the lunch and childcare services were of high quality.

Of the 22 ZUHRP attendees who elected not to be tested, half ($n = 11$) made the decision prior to pre-test counseling. The most common reason for declining testing was "needed more time to think about it" ($n = 10$, 46%). Other reasons included "spouse did not want to be tested" and "afraid of the results."

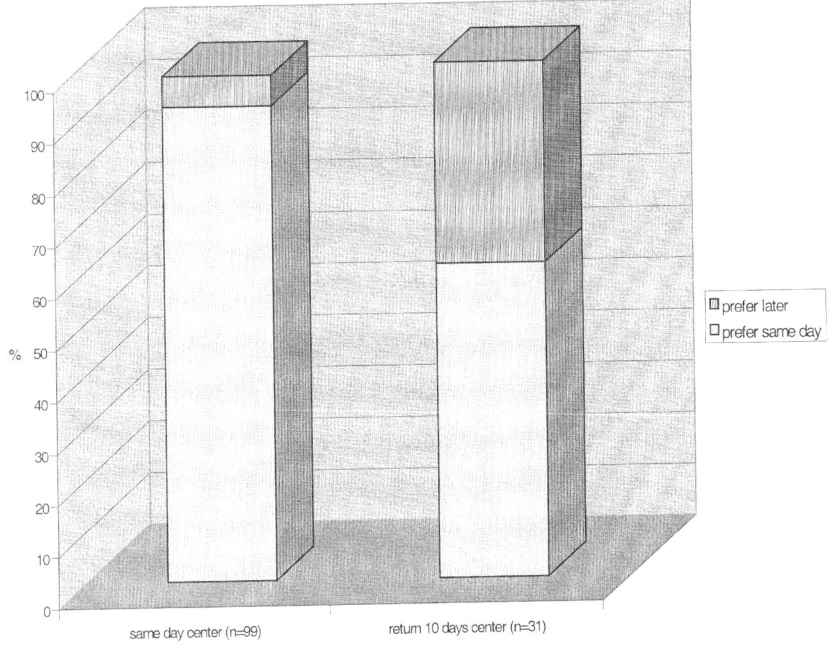

FIGURE 1. Preferred way to get HIV results.

Knowledge Survey

A total of 82 couples participated in the survey and 76 couples answered the survey completely, for a total of 152 study subjects. Of the 76 couples surveyed, 75% ($n = 57$) sought HIV testing and 24.5% of these were HIV positive. The gender balance among those testing positive was 53.6% ($n = 15$) female and 46.4% ($n = 13$) male.

Participants in this survey had a relatively high knowledge of HIV transmission and prevention before they received HIV counseling at ZUHRP. Overall improvement in knowledge after counseling was seen, however, in both men and women. Individuals were surveyed regarding the major modes of transmission: blood, semen, vaginal secretions, and perinatal transmission (FIG. 2). Although knowledge was high for transmission through unsafe sexual contact and dirty needles, there was a deficit in knowledge of perinatal transmission, evidenced by 13.2% of women and 14.5% of men who stated that HIV could not be transmitted from mother to child. An even larger percentage of respondents stated that only adults got HIV: 25.0% of women and 21.1% of men. These results did change after HIV counseling to only 4% of women and 5.3% of men who stated that HIV could not be transmitted from mother to child, and 12% of women and 10.5% of men who stated that only adults

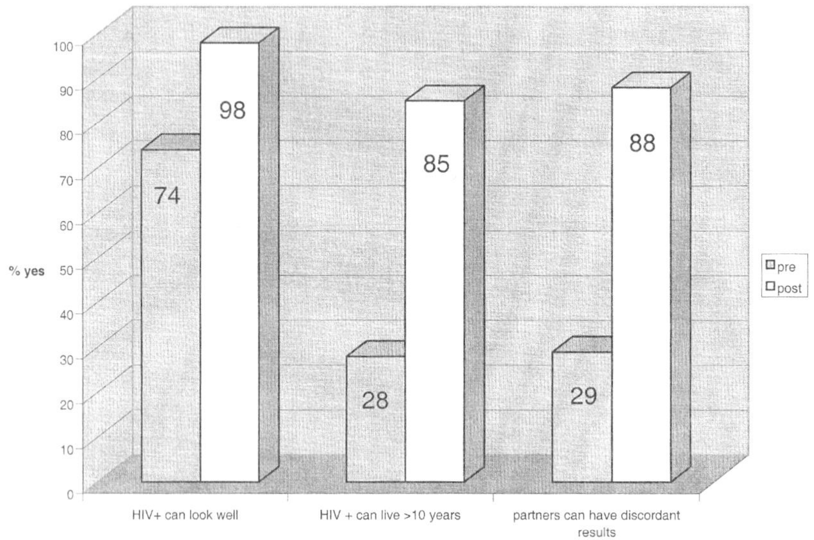

FIGURE 2. Knowledge about HIV/AIDS: impact of VTC program.

got HIV. In both cases, ZUHRP counseling reduced incorrect knowledge of transmission by at least one half.

An additional item regarding perinatal transmission was also problematic. Prior to counseling, 93.4% of women and 81.6% of men believed that if a mother had HIV, all her babies would have HIV. This number actually increased after counseling, indicating that couples were not receiving the message that with no drug intervention, 25–35% of babies born to HIV-positive mothers will be HIV positive.

Most couples surveyed felt that partners in a couple could not have different HIV test results (i.e., be "discordant"). Before ZUHRP counseling, only 25.0% of women and 32.9% of men recognized that discordance could exist. After counseling, this number increased to 88.2% for both men and women (p <0.001). Even for those respondents who felt that discordance could exist, most felt that it would only occur in a few couples or almost never (52.6% of women, 52.0% of men).

The misconception that HIV-positive individuals can easily be identified is another challenge in prevention efforts. In this study, 32.3% of female and 19.7% of male survey participants believed that an HIV-positive person could not look and feel healthy. Women respondents had a lower level of knowledge than men on this question (p = 0.065). Finally, 26.3% of women and 29.0% of men felt that an HIV-positive person could live for greater than 10 years. This number increased to 86.7% and 84.0%, respectively, after the postcounseling session.

The second component of the analysis compared knowledge level with serostatus. We specifically looked at the survey question asking the respondents to rate their risk level for HIV and at the serostatus of the individual. One of the most interesting results in this analysis was found among the Zambians who chose not to get tested for

TABLE 2. Pre- and postcounseling knowledge survey results ($n = 152$; male = 76 and female = 76)

	Pre	Post	
	Number (% yes)		p value
1. HIV is transmitted through sex without a condom			
Male	71 (93%)	75 (99%)	NS
Female	69 (91%)	75 (99%)	NS
2. HIV is transmitted through dirty needles			
Male	65 (86%)	74 (97%)	NS
Female	67 (88%)	75 (99%)	
3. HIV is transmitted from mother to child			
Male	64 (84%)	72 (95%)	0.06
Female	63 (83%)	72 (96%)	0.05
4. Condoms help protect against HIV infection			
Male	67 (88%)	73 (96%)	NS
Female	68 (90%)	75 (99%)	NS
5. Only adults get HIV			
Male	16 (21%)	8 (11%)	<.001
Female	19 (25%)	9 (12%)	0.04
6. If a mother has HIV, all her babies will have HIV			
Male	62 (82%)	69 (91%)	NS
Female	71 (93%)	69 (91%)	NS

HIV: 73.7% of those people who did not get tested felt that their chance of being HIV positive ranged from somewhat unlikely to impossible. This number dropped to 55.2% after counseling.

Women in this survey were more likely than men to misjudge their risk level. For example, 46.7% of HIV-positive women thought that their chance of being infected with HIV was impossible. After pre-test counseling, the number of HIV women thinking their risk was impossible dropped to 38.5% of respondents. HIV-negative women had a better perception of their risk: 21.4% of these women felt that their risk of being HIV positive was impossible, whereas most (31.0%) felt it was very unlikely.

While the women had the most dramatic mismatch between risk perception and serostatus, men had similar results. Of all men who classified their risk status as impossible or very unlikely, 20.5% were HIV positive. Indeed, these men who perceived themselves to be at low risk prior to counseling constituted 53.8% of HIV-positive men surveyed ($n = 13$). This number did not change significantly after counseling; however, there was an overall upward shift in perception of risk status, with the majority of men (54.4%) stating that their risk ranged from somewhat unlikely to somewhat likely.

Antenatal Clinic Pilot Testing

Voluntary HIV testing and counseling for HIV was offered to 1125 antenatal clinic attendees of whom 950 (84%) requested testing (TABLE 3). Most women (88%) were married, and the prevalence of HIV-positive antibody tests was 25% (236/950; 8 women had indeterminate results). High prevalence of HIV was associated with women's age 24–28 (37% versus 21% of women <24 or >28, $p = 0.001$), man's age 28–33 (39% versus 25% of men <28 or >33, $p = 0.03$), having a secondary or higher

TABLE 3. Demographic characteristics of antenatal clinic attendees

Characteristics	HIV tested ($n = 950$)		Not tested ($n = 175$)	
	Mean	C.I.	Mean	C.I.
Age	24.6	(24.1, 25.1)	25.2	(24.1, 26.5)
No. of pregnancies	2.5	(2.4, 2.6)	2.5	(2.3, 2.7)
No. of living children	1.5	(1.3, 1.8)	1.2	(0.8, 1.6)
No. of premature births	0.10	(0.06, 0.15)	0.07	(.00, .14)
Gestational weeks	22.7	(22.0, 23.3)	22.2	(20.1, 24.4)
Antenatal Clinic visit number	2.9	(2.7, 3.0)	3.9	(3.4, 4.4)
Spouse age	45.9	(42.7, 49.2)	39.3	(34.7, 44.6)

education (39% versus 25%, $p = 0.02$), presenting with the second or third pregnancy (32% versus 18% of first or fourth or higher, $p = 0.001$), being in the first or second trimester of pregnancy (25% versus 17% of third trimester, $p = 0.04$), and being tested at the University Teaching Hospital (30% versus 24% at the clinics, $p = 0.06$). One-quarter of women reported a previous miscarriage, which was associated with a moderately elevated HIV prevalence (35% versus 29%, $p = 0.3$). Positive syphilis serologies were found in 14% of pregnant women and were strongly associated with HIV (44% versus 22% HIV+, $p = 0.001$). Women seen at the UTH were older, more educated, and less likely to have syphilis than those seen in the clinics. Of interest was the finding that prevalence of HIV decreased significantly in pregnant women ≤19 years of age between 1997 and 1998 (11% versus 24%, respectively, $p = 0.02$).

Factors associated with willingness to test included type of healthcare facility offering testing, educational level of the woman, and stage of pregnancy. Local clinic attendees were more likely to request testing than attendees at the University Teaching Hospital (90% versus 72%, $p < 0.001$). Women with secondary school educations or higher (39% of the group) were less likely to request testing than those with primary or no education (71% versus 90%, $p = 0.001$). Thirty-four percent of pregnant women were in their third trimester, and were less likely to request testing than those at an earlier stage of gestation (82% versus 92%, $p = 0.001$).

There was no association between decision to test and age, number of living or dead children, premature births, pregnancies, or marital status or income.

DISCUSSION

Voluntary HIV testing and counseling is feasible, acceptable in the community,[10] and proven to save lives.[3,4] Same-day rapid testing specifically is preferred by clients and has demonstrated effectiveness in African settings.[11]

Testing of cohabiting couples accomplishes the dual purpose of reducing vertical and horizontal transmission. By providing this service in antenatal clinics, existing infrastructure can be utilized (although augmentation may be necessary) and a wide audience is accessible. To continue increasing the appeal of VTC, it must be noted that those survey participants with postsecondary education remain among the least frequent participants in VTC programs, as has been seen in other countries.[10] Targeted messages may be necessary to capture the attention and confidence of this group, which often includes those at highest risk for HIV.

Obstacles to couples testing indicated in the knowledge survey data include lack of knowledge about the possibility for discordant results, misinformation and fatalism about perinatal HIV transmission, and fear that having an HIV-positive result implies imminent death. The misconceptions regarding perinatal transmission could be due in part to the plot of the educational video shown which revolved around a young couple with discordant HIV results whose baby dies of AIDS. The visual image of the dying baby may counteract the factual information provided in counseling. Group and individual counselors as well as community outreach workers continue to seek new ways to convey this information in an effective manner. In addition, given the strong association between high self-reported knowledge of HIV and willingness to test, it is imperative that outreach workers maximize their opportunity to educate prospective clients at the time of issuing an invitation for HIV testing.

Practical obstacles may also be an important consideration in adapting antenatal clinic testing to accommodate couples. In particular, weekend hours, transport reimbursement, and childcare on site may be needed to decrease logistical constraints to testing. It is anticipated that the established, familiar practice of antenatal clinic attendance over time will facilitate participation in VTC programs by women, at least, and may decrease the need of incentives for men. In addition, offering couples testing in an established venue at predictable intervals may afford more opportunity for consultation between the partners prior to testing. With the primary reason for not testing in the antenatal clinic pilot studies being cited as "want to consult partner," offering couples testing may increase overall acceptability of VTC.

Incorporating rapid HIV testing into existing antenatal clinic infrastructure has been successfully tried in numerous African countries.[10] Several different interventions are now available for the prevention of mother-to-child HIV transmission. The low cost of Nevirapine has given rise to discussions regarding the cost-effectiveness of universal administration of Nevirapine to laboring women in high prevalence settings.[12] However, even given figures that could support universal administration, the authors concede that the cost-effectiveness balance of universal versus targeted implementation could shift when the cost of VTC is accrued to both prevention of vertical transmission and heterosexual transmission (an "added bonus" of testing and counseling in antenatal care clinics). Concerns regarding the long-term sustainability and potential for drug resistance in a universally administered Nevirapine regimen lend credence to the continued focus on implementation of testing and counseling in antenatal clinics. Regardless of the outcome of cost-effectiveness discussions, voluntary testing and counseling for couples remains a critical public health tool to reduce vertical and heterosexual transmission of HIV.

REFERENCES

1. ALLEN, S., E. KARITA, N. N'GANDU & A. TICHACEK. 1999. The Evolution of Voluntary Testing and Counseling as an HIV Prevention Strategy. L. Gibney *et al.*, Eds. Plenum Press. New York.

2. GUAY, L.A., P. MUSOKE, T. FLEMING *et al.* 1999. Intrapartum and neonatal single-dose nevirapine compared with zidovudine for prevention of mother-to-child transmission of HIV-1 in Kampala, Uganda: HIVNET 012 randomised trial. Lancet **354:** 795–802.
3. ALLEN, S., J. TICE, P. VAN DE PERRE *et al.* 1992. Effect of serotesting with counselling on condom use and seroconversion among HIV discordant couples in Africa. Br. Med. J. **304:** 1605–1609.
4. ALLEN, S.A., J. BOGAERTS, P. VAN DE PERRE *et al.* 1992. Confidential HIV testing and condom promotion in Africa: impact on HIV and gonorrhea rates. J. Am. Med. Assoc. **268:** 3338–3343.
5. KEOGH, P., S.A. ALLEN, C. ALMEDAL & B. TEMAHAGILI. 1994. The social impact of HIV infection on women in Kigali, Rwanda. Soc. Sci. & Med. **38:** 1047–1053.
6. CARTOUX, M., P. MSELLATI, N. MEDA *et al.* 1998. Attitude of pregnant women towards HIV testing in Abidjan, Cote d'Ivoire and Bobo-Dioulasso, Burkina Faso. DIT-RAME Study Group (ANRS 049 Clinical Trial). Diminution de la Transmission Mere Enfant du VIH. Agence Nationale de Recherches sur le SIDA. Aids **12:** 2337–2344.
7. ABDOOL KARIM, Q., S.S. ABDOOL KARIM, H.M. COOVADIA & M. SUSSER. 1998. Informed consent for HIV testing in a South African hospital: is it truly informed and truly voluntary? [published erratum appears in Am. J. Public Health **88:** 972]. Am. J. Public Health **88:** 637–640.
8. FYLKESNES, K.H.A., C. ROSENSVARD & P.M. KWAPA. 1999. HIV counselling and testing: overemphasizing high acceptance rates a threat to confidentiality and the right not to know. Aids **13:** 2469–2474.
9. TEMMERMAN, M., J. NDINYA-ACHOLA, J. AMBANI & P. PIOT. 1995. The right not to know HIV-test results [see comments]. Lancet **345:** 969–970.
10. CARTOUX, M., N. MEDA, P. VAN DE PERRE *et al.* 1998. Acceptability of voluntary HIV testing by pregnant women in developing countries: an international survey. Ghent International Working Group on Mother-to-Child Transmission of HIV. Aids **12:** 2489–2493.
11. MCKENNA, S.L., G.K. MUYINDA, D. ROTH *et al.* 18997. Rapid HIV testing and counseling for voluntary testing centers in Africa. Aids **11** (Suppl. 1): S103–110.
12. MARSEILLE, E., J.G. KAHN, F. MMIRO *et al.* 1999. Cost effectiveness of single-dose nevirapine regimen for mothers and babies to decrease vertical HIV-1 transmission in sub-Saharan Africa [see comments]. Lancet **354:** 803–809.

Subclinical Chorioamnionitis As a Targetable Risk Factor for Vertical Transmission of HIV-1

JEFFREY S.A. STRINGER[a] AND ROBERT L. GOLDENBERG

Center for Research on Women's Health, Department of Obstetrics and Gynecology, University of Alabama at Birmingham, Birmingham, Alabama 35233-2010, USA

INTRODUCTION

Significant strides have been made in recent years towards the reduction of perinatal HIV infection. Indeed, in the United States and other industrialized nations, coordinated efforts including early access to prenatal care, improved HIV counseling and testing services, and widespread availability of combination antiretroviral medications have brought the near eradication of vertically acquired HIV within the realm of possibility.[1] Remarkable progress has been made in the less developed world as well, where inexpensive and practical regimens of short-course zidovudine (ZDV)[2–4] and ultra-short-course nevirapine (NVP)[5] offer the possibility of measurable decreases in the global burden of pediatric HIV disease. These advances, although encouraging, are tempered by the sheer magnitude of the present epidemic; even if near perfect implementation of these new interventions were possible and a 50% decrease in perinatal transmission were realized globally, a staggering 300,000 children would still become infected each year worldwide.[6] Thus, there remains an urgent need within the field of perinatal HIV to continue the development of inexpensive and easily implemented interventions to decrease vertical transmission. Towards that end, this paper discusses chorioamnionitis as a risk factor for perinatal transmission of HIV, and how a simple and inexpensive antibiotic intervention in the mid-trimester and in labor might protect against vertical infection.

INFECTION AND SPONTANEOUS PRETERM BIRTH

Data evolving over the last 10 years have implicated chronic bacteriologic infections with organisms of relatively low virulence (e.g., *Ureaplasma urealyticum, Mycoplasma hominis, Gardnerella vaginalis, Bacteroides sp.,* and *Peptostreptococci sp.*) in the phenomenon of spontaneous preterm birth (SPB).[7–9] The likelihood of finding a chronic, upper genital tract infection by culture or histology in a given parturient varies inversely with gestational age at delivery; it is fairly uncommon at term and extremely common in cases of very early SPB. Indeed, the risk of very early SPB (i.e., birth weight <1,000 g) attributable to infection approaches 90%.[10] Women who deliver a preterm infant are at significantly increased risk of delivering another, and

[a]Address for correspondence: Jeffrey S.A. Stringer, MD, 1825 University Blvd, Mortimer Jordan Hall, Suite 120, Birmingham, AL 35233-2010. Voice: 205-934-7992; fax: 205-934-7999. stringer@uab.edu

there is some evidence that upper genital tract infection with the organisms just mentioned may even antedate a pregnancy.[11] We are currently studying this prospect longitudinally.

Acute chorioamnionitis differs from subacute or subclinical chorioamnionitis in its microbiology, histopathology, and clinical presentation, although the two are related in that the subclinical syndrome often precedes and can predispose to an acute episode.[7] Both involve ascending bacterial infection, with subsequent accumulation of neutrophils that are believed to be predominately maternal and derived from the decidual vessels.[12] The leukocytes migrate progressively through the chorion and amnion and sometimes into the amniotic fluid in response to cytokines and other chemotactic factors released by bacteria and host immune cells.[13]

The normal flora of the vagina is usually predominated by *Lactobacillus* species which maintain the mildly acidic vaginal pH and are believed to militate against colonization with more virulent organisms. Bacterial vaginosis (BV) represents a replacement of this flora with various anaerobic gram-negative species (e.g., *Gardnerella vaginalis* and *Mycoplasma hominis*). The presence of BV is consistently associated in the obstetric literature with an approximate twofold increase in SPB among low risk women[9] and a higher increase among women with other risk factors for SPB. Hauth and colleagues[14] achieved a measurable decrease in SPB among high risk women by treating with antibiotics in the mid-trimester. The effect of this intervention was exerted almost exclusively in BV-positive women and may be attributable to eradication of low-grade infection of the upper genital tract.

Although BV is commonly associated with SPB, a direct causal role has not been established. For example, a significant proportion of women who deliver preterm and whose placenta and membranes show evidence of chronic, low-grade inflammation do not have BV. Conversely, most women with BV do not deliver prematurely.[7] Thus, BV is believed to operate more as a marker for upper genital tract infection (the presumed real culprit in SPB) than as a causative agent per se. Other, more sensitive and specific markers of choriodecidual inflammation have been identified as well. For instance, the presence of various cytokines in amniotic fluid or cervicovaginal secretions is highly correlated with subclinical chorioamnionitis. The placental membrane protein, fetal fibronectin, when detected in the cervix or vagina during the mid-trimester, is highly predictive of choriodecidual inflammation and is perhaps the strongest known predictor of SPB.[15,16] Women with elevated levels of fetal fibronectin are significantly more likely to have either histologic or clinical chorioamnionitis and for their infants to develop neonatal sepsis.[17] Longitudinal study with the use of these newer markers has begun to reveal the chronicity of choriodecidual inflammation: the time between a positive fetal fibronectin assay and delivery with chorioamnionitis is typically at least 7 weeks.[17] Similarly, women with cytokine evidence of intraamniotic infection at 15–20 weeks' gestation may not deliver until as late as 32–34 weeks' gestation.[18]

TIMING AND MECHANISM OF PERINATAL HIV INFECTION

Although the timing of vertical transmission of HIV-1 has been described with increasing precision, the mechanism of infection remains elusive. Predominately for the sake of simplicity, investigators tend to consider antepartum and intrapartum viral transmission separately from postpartum (breastfeeding) transmission. The risks entailed by each component are generally conceived to be additive within individuals, although this has not been established with reasonable certainty. Based on characteristics of the neonatal immune response,[19] the timing of assay positivity,[20] and mathematical modeling,[21] the following relative proportions have been generated: Antenatal transmission, that is, transmission occurring prior to the day of delivery and documented by the presence of HIV DNA in the neonate within 48–72 hours of birth, is believed to account for as much as 25–35% of all non–breastfeeding-related transmissions. (In patients receiving antiretroviral therapy, this proportion may be lower.) The remaining 65–75% of non–breastfeeding transmission is attributed to intrapartum transmission and is diagnosed by HIV DNA negativity at delivery, followed by subsequent positivity.[22]

Two major mechanisms have been advanced to explain antepartum and intrapartum HIV infection. *Hematogenous infection* via maternal-fetal microtransfusion is compatible with the increased transmission risk observed with syphilitic villitis[23] or uterine contractions,[24] whereas *direct contact* of fetal mucosal surfaces with infected cervicovaginal secretions or maternal blood is compatible with the increased transmission risk observed with episiotomy, fetal scalp electrode use, and operative vaginal delivery.[25] We propose a third possibility, *transamniotic infection,* in which maternal leukocytes make their way into the amniotic fluid in response to bacterial infection and subsequently gain access to the fetus via the skin, mucous membranes, gut, or lung. This mechanism is compatible with the increased transmission risk observed with both overt and subclinical infection of the fetal membranes.[26] Infection by any of these three mechanisms could be potentiated by fetal immunologic immaturity.

Sharing of blood-borne elements between mother and fetus is known to occur. The phenomenon of maternal isoimmunization to fetal red cell and platelet antigens is a well-recognized consequence of transfusion from fetus to mother. Similarly, passage of formed elements from mother to fetus was documented as early as 1963 by Desai and Creger[27] who drew whole blood from a cohort of nine gravid women and reintroduced the white cells and platelets after fluorescent labeling. At the time of delivery, the presence of fluorescent forms was documented in the cord blood of six of their infants (four instances of platelet passage, four of granulocytes, and three of lymphocytes). These lines of evidence, coupled with the known ability of other viral species (e.g., rubella virus) to cross the placenta[28] lend considerable plausibility to the hematogenous mechanism of infection.

On the other hand, some viral species (e.g., herpes simplex virus types 1 and 2) are believed to be passed from mother to child primarily by direct contact of the fetus with infectious cervicovaginal secretions.[29] Presumably this line of thinking prompted Bhadrakom and others,[30] as part of the Thai-CDC short course zidovudine trial,[2] to measure viral load at birth in the nasal and oral fluids (obtained by lavage) of infants born to HIV-infected mothers. Based on the timing of DNA polymerase chain reaction positivity, they categorized infants as having sustained either intrauterine ($n - 21$) or intrapartum infection ($n - 31$) or having remained uninfected ($n = 306$). Virus was detected in the lavage specimens of 90% of intrauterine-infected infants (median titer 3292 copies/ml plasma), in 52% of intrapartum-infected infants (median titer 940 copies/ml plasma), and in 23% of uninfected infants (median titer undetectable.) No correlation was observed between the maternal plasma viral load and that of the infant oronasal lavage. Although it is conceivable that the detected virus may have originated from the infants themselves in those categorized as infected prior to labor, this seems an unlikely source in infants who were infected intrapartum. These data are provocative, because they point to a possible role of non-hematogenous antepartum infection.

A randomized trial of 0.25% chlorhexidine irrigation of the lower genital tract during labor did not produce a measurable decrease in HIV transmission except in a subgroup of women whose amniotic membranes had been ruptured for more than 4 hours.[31] Chlorhexidine clearly inhibits HIV replication at low concentrations *in vitro*.[32] Prolonged amniotic membrane rupture is a well known risk factor for ascending infection in labor, particularly with beta hemolytic *Streptococcus*. During labor, the fetus is exposed to the cervix and vagina for a relatively short period of time, and the majority of that exposure is to the occiput only. Thus, while chlorhexidine, a virucidal agent applied for the purpose of reducing infant exposure to HIV in the cervix and lower genital tract, did not reduce transmission, chlorhexidine, a bacteriocidal agent applied to the site where the causative agents of ascending chorioamnionitis reside, did reduce transmission in a subgroup of women at risk for ascending infection.

TRANSAMNIOTIC INFECTION AND ITS SIMILARITY TO BREASTFEEDING INFECTION

Postnatal seroconversion occurs in around 15% of infants breast-fed by HIV-infected mothers[33] and seems to be related to the duration of breastfeeding, although in a nonlinear fashion.[34] The mechanism by which postnatal infection occurs is incompletely characterized. Both cell-associated and cell-free virus can be isolated from breast milk,[35] although a relationship between breast milk viral titer and risk of postnatal infection remains to be definitively demonstrated. Likewise, it is unclear whether infection results from infant oropharyngeal, tonsillar, gut, or other exposure.

Recent data have suggested a possible role of bacterial infection and inflammation in the risk of breastfeeding transmission. Mastitis, both overt and subclinical, is characterized by the presence of leukocytes and increased sodium concentrations in expressed milk and has been linked to increases in both cell-free and cell-associated virus in colostrum and mature milk.[36,37] (Data on the precise attributable risk of this condition on postnatal infection have not been presented.) Similarly, the practice of mixed breast and bottle feeding, common in the less developed world, may bear a higher risk of infant seroconversion than exclusive breastfeeding,[38] an observation that has led some investigators to speculate a role of infant gastrointestinal inflammation. Taken together, these observations could indicate a critical role of bacterial coinfection in increased maternal viral delivery and perhaps in increased infant susceptibility to infection. It is interesting to note the similarities between postpartum transmission and our proposed mechanism of transamniotic infection. Perhaps even a common mechanism exists, whereby HIV gains access to the fetal gastrointestinal tract or lung by way of breast milk or amniotic fluid, a process that could be enhanced by concomitant bacterial infection in the form of mastitis or amnionitis.

HYPOTHESIS AND PROTOCOL DESCRIPTION

We hypothesize that in the presence of bacterial infection of the upper genital tract, maternal leukocytes are recruited by the local production of chemotactic factors and that these cells, many of which harbor HIV, may cross the amnion, gain entry into the amniotic fluid, and ultimately infect the fetus. These events may transpire in mid-pregnancy in response to the low-grade, progressive cascade that has been implicated in SPB. Alternatively, a similar mechanism may come into play proximate to and during labor, when more virulent organisms gain access to the exposed fetal membranes. We propose that appropriately timed antibiotic treatment that is specifically directed at the bacterial species described in the foregoing text will decrease choriodecidual inflammation, decrease the risk of spontaneous preterm birth, and decrease the risk of perinatal HIV transmission.

The *HIVNET protocol 024,* a phase III trial of antibiotics to reduce chorioamnionitis-related perinatal HIV transmission, is now underway in two sites in Malawi. Trial participants will be randomized to receive either two courses of antibiotics or two courses of placebo. All HIV-infected women will receive nevirapine per the *HIVNET protocol 012.*[5] Women randomized to antibiotics will receive an oral course of metronidazole 250 mg and erythromycin 250 mg, three times per day for a 7-day period sometime between 20 and 24 weeks' gestation. This regimen is aimed specifically at the organisms implicated in subacute chorioamnionitis. A second course of antibiotics will be administered to the same women at the onset of labor. This regimen is comprised of oral metronidazole 250 mg and ampicillin 500 mg and is taken every 4 hours until delivery. It is aimed at the organisms responsible for ascending infection and acute chorioamnionitis. The cost of both courses of antibiotics described is less than US $5 per woman.

CONCLUSIONS

The recent discovery of low cost, easily implemented interventions to protect children from HIV infection in the poor countries of the world is encouraging. However, important work remains to be done. Science's present understanding of the cellular and molecular mechanism of perinatal transmission remains poor. This trial is aimed at the treatment of a specific risk factor and promises to shed further light on understanding of the complex mechanism of perinatal infection. Secondary outcomes such as prematurity-related infant mortality and maternal febrile morbidity will be studied as well. If successful, this intervention may provide a low cost alternative or supplement to antiretroviral therapy to prevent perinatal HIV transmission.

REFERENCES

1. MOFENSON, L.M. 1999. Can perinatal HIV infection be eliminated in the United States? JAMA **282:** 577–579.
2. SHAFFER, N., R. CHUACHOOWONG, P. MOCK *et al.* 1999. Short-course zidovudine for perinatal HIV-1 transmission in Bangkok, Thailand: a randomised controlled trial. Lancet **353:** 773–780.

3. DABIS, F., P. MSELLATI, N. MEDA *et al.* 1999. Six-month efficacy, tolerance, and acceptability of a short regimen of oral zidovudine to reduce vertical transmission of HIV in breastfed children in Côte d'Ivoire and Burkina Faso: a double-blind placebo-controlled multicentre trial. Lancet 786–792.

4. WIKTOR, S., E. EKPINI, J. KARON *et al.* 1999. Short-course oral zidovudine for prevention of mother-to-child transmission of HIV-1 in Abidjan, Côte d'Ivoire: a randomised trial. Lancet **353**: 781–785.

5. GUAY, L.A., P. MUSOKE, T. FLEMING *et al.* 1999. Intrapartum and neonatal single-dose nevirapine compared with zidovudine for prevention of mother-to-child transmission of HIV-1 in Kampala, Uganda: HIVNET 012 randomised trial. Lancet **354**: 795–802.

6. UNAIDS/WHO. 1999. Report on the global HIV/AIDS epidemic: June 1998. [http://www.unaids.org/unaids/document/epidemio/june98/global_report/data/globrep_e.pdf]. Accessed September 20, 1999.

7. ANDREWS, W., R. GOLDENBERG & J. HAUTH. 1995. Preterm labor: emerging role of genital tract infections. Infect. Agents Dis. **1995**: 196–211.

8. HAUTH, J., W. ANDREWS & R. GOLDENBERG. 1998. Infection-related risk factors predictive of spontaneous labor and birth. Prenat. Neonat. Med. **3**: 86–90.

9. GIBBS, R., R. ROMERO, S. HILLIER *et al.* 1992. A review of premature birth and subclinical infection. Am. J. Obstet. Gynecol. **166**: 1515–1528.

10. CASSELL, G., J. HAUTH, W. ANDREWS *et al.* 1993. Chorioamnion colonization: correlation with gestational age in women delivered following spontaneous labor versus indicated delivery [Abstr.]. Am. J. Obstet. Gynecol. **168**: 425.

11. KORN, A., G. BOLAN, N. PADIAN *et al.* 1995. Plasma cell endometritis in women with symptomatic bacterial vaginosis. Obstet. Gynecol. **85**: 387–390.

12. KURMAN, R. 1994. Blaustein's Pathology of the Female Genital Tract. :992–1004. Springer-Verlag. New York.

13. ROMERO, R. & M. MAZOR. 1988. Infection and preterm labor. Clin. Obstet. Gynecol. **31**: 533–584.

14. HAUTH, J., R. GOLDENBERG, W. ANDREWS *et al.* 1995. Reduced incidence of preterm delivery with metronidazole and erythromycin in women with bacterial vaginosis. N. Engl. J. Med. **333**: 1732–1736.

15. GOLDENBERG, R., J. IAMS, B. MERCER *et al.* 1996. The Preterm Prediction Study: early fetal fibronectin testing predicts early spontaneous preterm birth. Obstet. Gynecol. **87**: 643–648.

16. LOCKWOOD, C., A. SENYEI, M. DISCHE *et al.* 1991. Fetal fibonectin in cervical and vaginal secretions as a predictor of preterm delivery. N. Engl. J. Med. **325**: 669–674.

17. GOLDENBERG, R., J. IAMS, B. MERCER *et al.* 1996. The Preterm Prediction Study: fetal fibronectin, bacterial vaginosis and peripartum infection. Obstet. Gynecol. **87**: 656–660.

18. WENSTROM, K., W. ANDREWS, J. HAUTH *et al.* 1998. Elevated second trimester interleukin-6 levels predict preterm delivery. Am. J. Obstet. Gynecol. **178**: 546–550.

19. KALISH, L., J. PITT, J. LEW *et al.* 1997. Defining the time of fetal or perinatal aquisition of Human Immunodeficiency Virus Type-1 infection on the basis of age at first positive culture. J. Infect. Dis. **175**: 712–715.

20. BRYSON, Y., K. LUZURIAGA, J. SULLIVAN & D. WARA. 1992. Proposed definitions for in utero versus intrapartum transmission of HIV-1 [letter]. N. Engl. J. Med. **327**: 1246–1247.

21. CHOUQUET, C., S. RICHARDSON, M. BURGARD *et al.* 1999. Timing of Human Immunodeficiency Virus Type 1 (HIV-1) transmission from mother to child: bayesian estimation using a mixture. Stat. Med. **18**: 815–833.

22. Newell, M.-L. 1998. Mechanism and timing of mother-to-child transmission of HIV-1. AIDS **12**: 831–837.

23. LEE, M.J., R.J. HALLMARK, L.M. FRENKEL & G. DEL PRIORE. 1998. Maternal syphilis and vertical perinatal transmission of human immunodeficiency virus type-1 infection. Int. J. Gynaecol. Obstet. **63**: 247–252.

24. PARAZZINI, F., for the EUROPEAN MODE OF DELIVERY COLLABORATION. 1999. Elective cesarean section versus vaginal delivery in preventing vertical HIV-1 transmission: a randomized clinical trial. Lancet **353**: 1035–1039.

25. ANONYMOUS. 1992. Risk factors for mother-to-child transmission of HIV-1. European Collaborative Study. Lancet **339:** 1007–1012.
26. ST. LOUIS, M.E., M. KAMENGA, C. BROWN *et al.* 1993. Risk for perinatal HIV-1 transmission according to maternal immunologic, virologic, and placental factors. JAMA **269:** 2853–2859.
27. DESAI, R. & W. CREGER. 1963. Maternofetal passage of leukocytes and platelets in man. Blood **21:** 665–673.
28. MILLER, E., J.E. CRADOCK-WATSON & T.M. POLLACK. 1981. Consequences of confirmed maternal Rubella at successive stages of pregnancy. Lancet **2:** 781–784.
29. WHITLEY, R., A. ARVIN, C. PROBER *et al.* 1991. A controlled trial comparing vidarabine with acyclovir in neonatal herpes simplex virus infection. Infectious Diseases Collaborative Antiviral Study Group. N. Engl. J. Med. **324:** 444–449.
30. BHADRAKOM, C., R. CHUACHOOWONG, N. SHAFFER *et al.* 1999. Detection of HIV in nasal/oral secretions of newborn infants of HIV-infected women, Thailand. Presented at the second conference on global strategies for the prevention of HIV transmission from mothers to infants, Montreal, Sept. 1–6, 1999.
31. BIGGAR, R.J., P.G. MIOTTI, T.E. TAHA *et al.* 1996. Perinatal intervention trial in Africa: effect of a birth canal cleansing intervention to prevent HIV transmission. Lancet **347:** 1647–1650.
32. HARBISON, M.A. & S.M. HAMMER. 1989. Inactivation of human immunodeficiency virus by Betadine products and chlorhexidine. J. Acquired Immune Defic. Syndr. **2:** 16–20.
33. DUNN, D.T., M.L. NEWELL, A.E. ADES & C.S. PECKHAM. 1992. Risk of human immunodeficiency virus type 1 transmission through breastfeeding. Lancet **340:** 585–588.
34. MIOTTI, P., T. TAHA, N. KUMWENDA *et al.* 1999. HIV transmission through breastfeeding: a study in Malawi. JAMA **282:** 744–749.
35. LEWIS, P., R. NDUATI, J.K. KREISS *et al.* 1998. Cell-free human immunodeficiency virus type 1 in breast milk. J. Infect. Dis. **177:** 34–39.
36. SEMBA, R.D., N. KUMWENDA, D.R. HOOVER *et al.* 1999. Human immunodeficiency virus load in breast milk, mastitis, and mother-to-child transmission of human immunodeficiency virus type 1. J. Infect. Dis. **180:** 93–98.
37. GUAY, L.A., D.L. HOM, F. MMIRO *et al.* 1996. Detection of human immunodeficiency virus type 1 (HIV-1) DNA and p24 antigen in breast milk of HIV-1-infected Ugandan women and vertical transmission. Pediatrics **98:** 438–444.
38. COUTSOUDIS, A., K. PILLAY, E. SPOONER *et al.* 1999. Influence of infant-feeding patterns on early mother-to-child transmission of HIV-1 in Durban, South Africa: a prospective cohort study. South African Vitamin A Study Group. Lancet **354:** 471–476.

Genital Tract Infections and Perinatal Transmission of HIV

TAHA E. TAHA[a] AND RONALD H. GRAY

School of Hygiene and Public Health, Johns Hopkins University, 615 N. Wolfe Street, Baltimore, Maryland 21205, USA

ABSTRACT: In areas of the world where genital tract infections (GTIs) are common, the prevalence of HIV and the rate of mother-to-child transmission (MTCT) of HIV are also high. Although observational studies suggested that GTIs are associated with MTCT of HIV, no controlled clinical trial has confirmed this finding. It is likely that GTIs that cause either discharges or ulcers during pregnancy increase perinatal transmission of HIV. Several potential biological mechanisms might facilitate perinatal transmission. For example, chorioamnionitis, increased viral shedding in cervicovaginal secretions, increased HIV acquisition during pregnancy, inflammatory cytokine production, preterm labor, prolonged rupture of membranes, ascending infection, and increased intrapartum infectious secretions are factors that can be associated with GTIs. Several studies have shown that treating clinical conditions associated with inflammation might alter HIV shedding. It is conceivable that preventing ascending infection or reducing exposure of the infant to infectious material during birth could reduce MTCT. This can possibly be achieved by antimicrobial therapy during pregnancy and intrapartum. Such an approach is practical, is less expensive, and has secondary benefits related to prevention of adverse pregnancy outcomes associated with GTIs. Antibiotics might also complement reductions in MTCT of HIV obtained by antiretrovirals given to the mother around the time of delivery. In addition, antibiotics could reduce infectious causes of morbidity and mortality in infant and mother.

INTRODUCTION

Background and Rationale

Practical and cost-effective interventions to reduce perinatal transmission of HIV and associated infant and child morbidity and mortality are urgently needed. To achieve this goal, putative risk factors that are amenable to modification or control need to be identified and interventions evaluated by randomized trials. Pediatric HIV/AIDS is threatening to reverse substantial gains in child survival achieved earlier as a result of successful immunization and other programs. Antiretroviral therapy is effective in reducing mother-to-child transmission (MTCT) of HIV. Whereas antiviral drugs are routinely recommended in industrialized countries, these drugs are not generally available or affordable in developing countries. In sub-Saharan Af-

[a]Corresponding author: Taha E. Taha, MD, PhD, Department of Epidemiology, School of Hygiene and Public Health, Rm E6011, 615 N. Wolfe St, Baltimore, MD 21205, USA. Voice: 410-614-5255; fax: 410-955-1836.

ttaha@jhsph.edu

rica, the MTCT of HIV is high and genital tract infections are common. Several conditions we refer to in our discussion are not conventionally sexually transmitted (e.g., bacterial vaginosis-associated organisms and Group B Streptococcus), but are more common in sexually active than among non-sexually active women. Therefore, in this article, we use the term genital tract infection (GTI) to include both sexually transmitted disease (STD) and non-sexually transmitted infections. The presence of GTIs could be a risk factor for MTCT. If an association can be established between GTIs and MTCT, an alternative preventive strategy would be to provide antimicrobial treatment to pregnant women. This approach is appealing, because GTIs are known to adversely affect reproductive outcomes and enhance heterosexual HIV transmission and acquisition.

The role of different factors in MTCT of HIV has not been fully defined. Multiple determinants and cofactors have been demonstrated or postulated, including viral load and viral characteristics, maternal immune response, obstetric events during labor and delivery, and maternal nutritional status. The interplay of these factors may explain the variation in reported MTCT rates and the generally higher MTCT rates in developing than in developed countries.

Numerous epidemiologic studies suggest that both ulcerative and nonulcerative STDs facilitate HIV transmission by increasing infectiousness of HIV-infected individuals or rendering HIV-uninfected individuals more susceptible to HIV infection. Potential biological mechanisms include increased shedding of the virus in genital fluids, recruitment of HIV target cells or HIV infected cells into the genital tract as part of the inflammatory process, stimulation of immune responses to an STD causing increased viral replication, and disruption of protective epithelial barriers.[1-5]

It is conceivable that GTIs may also be a factor in MTCT of HIV through chorioamnionitis, cervicitis, or birth canal ulcerations. In the United States, a history of maternal STDs has been associated with higher MTCT.[6] Studies in Zaire[7] and Uganda[8] have shown that placental membrane inflammation (chorioamnionitis and funisitis) was a major risk factor for MTCT, particularly among women who were not immunocompromised. In Uganda,[8] the investigators estimated that 34% of perinatal HIV transmission could be prevented by successful treatment of placental membrane inflammations due to cervicovaginal infections. In Zaire,[7] it was suggested that placental barrier defects could allow maternal-fetal transfer of cell-associated virus and that antimicrobial prophylaxis for chorioamnionitis may be a potential strategy to prevent vertical transmission. A large randomized community-based trial in Tanzania provided the first direct evidence that an improved STD treatment regimen can have a dramatic effect (a decrease of 38%) in lowering HIV incidence among adults.[9] However, no study has as yet provided direct evidence that treatment of GTIs results in reduced vertical HIV transmission. This could be attributed to difficulty in making GTI diagnoses (especially when asymptomatic), particularly in the developing world.

Current laboratory techniques allow for the detection of HIV DNA sequences after polymerase chain reaction (PCR) amplification in cervical and vaginal secretions. In Kenya, detection of endocervical HIV DNA in specimens from HIV-infected women was independently associated with *Neisseria gonorrhoeae*,[10] and HIV DNA detection in women correlated with microscopic evidence of cervical inflammation.[11] In Cote d'Ivoire, HIV detection in cervicovaginal lavage specimens of HIV-1 infected sex workers was more frequent in those with visible ulcers or with

N. gonorrhoeae and *Chlamydia trachomatis.* After treatment of STDs, detection of HIV-1 in cervicovaginal fluids was less frequent (but not significantly) among sex workers who were cured than among those not cured.[12] In Malawi, men with urethritis had a significantly higher median HIV-1 RNA concentration in seminal fluid than did men without urethritis. A significant decline in HIV shedding was noted after treatment in men with urethritis.[13]

In S. Africa, among men with genital ulcers (due to *Haemophilus ducreyi* or herpes simplex virus [HSV]), HIV shedding from the ulcers was associated with high plasma viral load, and successful bacterial or viral treatment was associated with reduction in viral shedding from these lesions.[14] In another study among HIV-infected women in S. Africa, the presence of a GTI (bacterial vaginosis, candidiasis, gonorrhea, chlamydia infection, trichomoniasis, or HSV infection) or high plasma viral load was associated with genital shedding, and successful syndromic treatment of the GTI was associated with significant reductions in vaginal shedding.[15]

These data suggest that treating the clinical condition associated with cervical/vaginal inflammation or ulcer might alter HIV shedding and thus possibly reduce MTCT by preventing ascending infection causing chorioamnionitis or by reducing exposure of the infant to infectious secretions during passage through the birth canal. Therefore, interventions aimed at GTI control may decrease MTCT and possibly the high rates of infant and child mortality attributed to perinatal HIV infection. Because MTCT rates are highest in geographic areas where GTIs and HIV are highly prevalent, control of GTIs could achieve a long-term goal of preventing heterosexual transmission of HIV and lead to fewer HIV-infected women of childbearing age. This paper discusses the association between GTIs and perinatal transmission of HIV and the potential use of treatment of GTIs as an intervention measure. To highlight the magnitude of HIV infection and GTIs, we include background data from two sub-Saharan African countries, Malawi and Uganda, where several cohorts of women were followed in urban hospital and rural community settings, respectively.

HIV, GTIs, and MTCT in Urban Malawi

HIV and STDs among pregnant and postpartum women in urban Malawi have been studied for the last 10 years. The HIV seroprevalence in pregnant women rose from 2% in 1985 to 31% in 1998.[16] The overall rate of seroconversion was 4.2 per 100 person years and was highest among young women (6.0 per 100 person years).[16] The rate of seroconversion was higher during pregnancy (7.9 per 100 person years; 95% CI 4.9–11.0) than postpartum (3.6 per 100 person years; 95% CI 2.9–4.3). The prevalence of GTIs among women attending the antenatal clinic of the Queen Elizabeth Central Hospital (QECH) in Blantyre, Malawi, was high. For example, in 1993 the prevalence of syphilis during pregnancy was 12.2%, gonorrhea 2.5%, trichomoniasis 28.6%, genital ulcers 6.7%, and genital warts 3.1%. The prevalence of these GTIs in 1990 was even higher.[16] In the same cohorts of women, the prevalence of bacterial vaginosis (BV) was 30% during pregnancy.[17] GTIs, especially BV, were significantly associated with the risk of maternal HIV seroconversion during both prenatal and postnatal periods.[18] Maternal STDs (active syphilis and cervicitis and vaginitis) were also significantly associated with increased child mortality.[19] The rate of MTCT of HIV was 28% by repeat PCR.[20]

TABLE 1. Disturbances of vaginal flora during pregnancy and incidence of mother-to-child transmission of HIV in Malawi (women enrolled in 1990)

Disturbance of vaginal flora	n	% children infected[a]	OR[b] 95% CI
None	14	14.3	1.0
Mild	102	23.5	1.9 (0.4–18.1)
Moderate	83	31.3	2.7 (0.5–26.7)
Severe[c]	144	27.8	2.3 (0.5–22.1)
Total	343	26.8	

[a]Baby tested for HIV at or after 12 months of age by serology.
[b]χ^2 trend test = 1.15; $p = 0.28$.
[c]Bacterial vaginosis.

A preliminary analysis of the rate of MTCT of HIV among women who had BV during pregnancy showed that the rate of perinatal HIV transmission was 14% among women who had normal vaginal flora and 28% among women with BV (a twofold increase) (TABLE 1). Although we did not detect a significant trend of association between HIV perinatal transmission of HIV and BV in this limited data (TABLE 1) and several children were lost to follow-up before testing for HIV infection by serology at or after 12 months, the findings suggest that BV may increase perinatal transmission. This is particularly important because BV and other GTIs were also associated with the risk of HIV acquisition during pregnancy.[18] Additionally, BV was significantly associated with preterm delivery especially among HIV-infected women in Malawi (FIG. 1). Overall, 33.8% of women with preterm birth had BV during pregnancy compared with 27.1% of term women (p <0.002). Among HIV-infected women who had pretem birth, 49% had BV compared with 41% who had term birth (p <0.03). Among HIV-uninfected women, there were no statistically significant differences in the frequency of BV during pregnancy among women who had term or preterm birth.

To reduce MTCT, the effect of cleansing the birth canal using a simple antiseptic (0.25% chlorhexidene solution) was studied in Malawi. This intervention did not lower MTCT of HIV [20] except in a subgroup of mothers with prolonged rupture of membranes in whom this intervention was associated with reduced MTCT of HIV. However, neonatal and maternal morbidity and mortality due to sepsis were significantly reduced.[21] A clinical trial to determine the effect of prenatal supplementation with vitamin A on MTCT of HIV was also conducted. This trial was based on earlier findings that women in Malawi with lower serum vitamin A were more likely to transmit HIV to their babies than were women with adequate serum levels of vitamin A.[22] Vitamin A supplementation had no significant effect on MTCT of HIV, at 6 weeks and 12 months; it also had no effect on breast milk HIV load level.[23] In this study, however, elevated breast milk sodium levels consistent with mastitis occurred in 16.4% of HIV-infected women and were associated with increased MTCT of HIV.

The Rakai STD Control for Maternal-Infant Health Study, Uganda

A community randomized trial of STD Control for HIV Prevention was conducted in rural Rakai district, Uganda, between 1994 and 1998.[24] Fifty-six communities

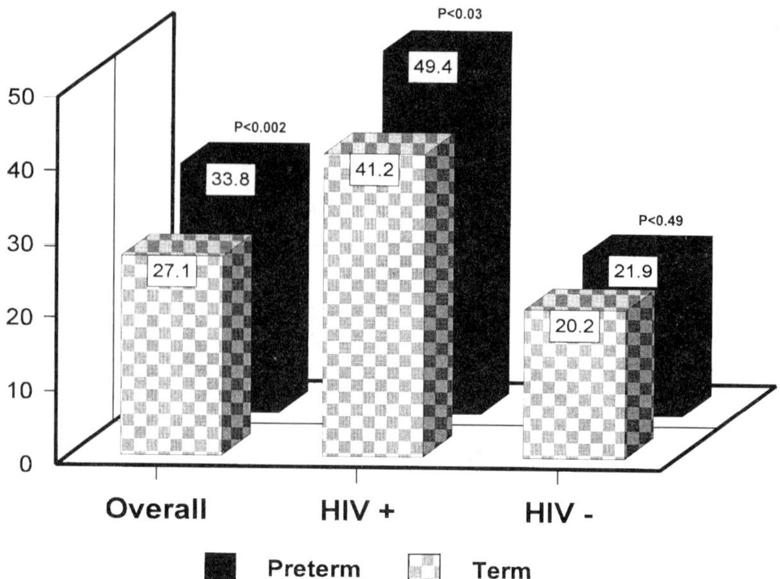

FIGURE 1. Percent of women with BV during pregnancy stratified by gestation and HIV status.

were aggregated into 10 clusters encompassing social and sexual networks, and clusters were randomly allocated to an STD control intervention arm and a control arm. All communities were visited at 10-month intervals over a period of 40 months. In the intervention arm, all consenting subjects received mass antibiotic treatment consisting of azithromycin 1 g, ciprofloxacin 250 mg, and metronidazole 2 g administered by directly observed therapy delivered in the home. Subjects with serologic syphilis were provided with intramuscular Benzathine penicillin in the home. These drugs are effective against syphilis, chancroid, gonorrhea, chlamydia, trichomonas, and bacterial vaginosis. In the control arm, consenting subjects received an anthelminth (mebendazole) and low dose iron/folate supplements. Treatments were repeated every 10 months for 5 visits. At the fifth and last visit, all control subjects were given the STD regimen.

Pregnant women were identified at each study visit and the treatment regimen was changed; ciprofloxacin (FDA category C drug) was replaced by cefixime in the intervention arm (FDA category B), and anthelminth (FDA category C) was withheld in the control arm. Because of these changes in treatment, women were carefully screened for pregnancy by interview and urine hCG testing. Pregnant women were then enrolled in a nested follow-up study to assess the effects of STD control on maternal and infant health. Enrollment took place at varying times during pregnancy, and the median length of gestation was 5 months.

In the maternal-infant study, information on sociodemographic, behaviors, obstetric history, and STD diagnoses was obtained at enrollment during pregnancy. After delivery, mothers and infants were followed up to determine outcomes of

TABLE 2. Maternal STDs postpartum, Rakai Study, Uganda

STDs	Intervention (%) (n = 1,813)	Control (%) (n = 1,714)	Cluster adjusted rate ratio (95% CI)	
HIV	15.7	14.6	1.11	(0.91-1.35)
Syphilis	3.4	3.3	1.02	(0.80-1.30)
Trichomonas	4.8	15.9	0.28	(0.16-0.47)
Bacterial vaginosis	36.5	49.3	0.73	(0.70-0.78)
Gonorrhea	0.7	2.2	0.43	(0.22-0.84)
Chlamydia	1.1	3.1	0.34	(0.14-0.84)
Upper genital tract infection	2.6	3.5	0.78	(0.52-1.17)

pregnancy, maternal STDs, infant anthropometry and gestational age, and infant ocular infections due to gonorrhea or chlamydia. Infants of HIV+ mothers were tested by PCR at birth and 4–6 weeks of age. Placentas were collected in 10% formol saline for histopathologic diagnosis of chorioamnionitis.

Of the maternal STDs at the time of enrollment during pregnancy, HIV prevalence was high in both arms (14.3% in the intervention and 11.8% in the control). The prevalence of syphilis (RPR/TPHA positive) was comparable in both study arms (4.5%), because syphilis was aggressively treated in all pregnant women. Trichomonas was lower in the intervention arm (12.3%) than in the control arm (18.8%) due to previous metronidazole therapy, and there were no differences in BV (44.5%), gonorrhea (1.3%), or chlamydia (3.3%) between study arms at enrollment during pregnancy. In the postpartum follow-up, however, the rates of trichomonas, BV, gonorrhea, and chlamydia were significantly reduced in the intervention than in the control arm (TABLE 2). HIV and syphilis rates were comparable between the study arms. In a subsample of placental histopathologic specimens assessed thus far, the prevalence of severe/moderate chorioamnionitis was 20.5% among HIV-positive mothers compared with 11.8% in HIV-negative mothers. HIV incidence was significantly higher during pregnancy (3.2 per 100 person years) than postpartum (1.6 per 100 person years) among the Rakai women, as has been observed in Blantyre, Malawi. However, despite substantial reduction of STDs associated with the mass antibiotic treatment during pregnancy, no reduction was observed in maternal HIV acquisition either in pregnancy or postpartum. Infant PCR data are not yet available to assess the impact of the intervention on MTCT.

FACTORS INFLUENCING MTCT OF HIV

In developing countries, the rate of MTCT of HIV ranges between 13% and 42%, with most studies reporting 25–30%. In developed countries, rates of 14–25% have been reported.[25] The rates are higher in Africa than in Europe or the United States, possibly due to variability in the distribution of associated risk factors related to transmission.

Perinatal transmission can occur prepartum (*in utero*), intrapartum, or postpartum. Although the exact timing and mechanism of transmission are not known, it ap-

TABLE 3. Factors influencing mother-to-child transmission of HIV

Antepartum	Intrapartum	Postpartum
Clinical HIV status	Mode of delivery	Breastfeeding
Viral load	Membranes ruptured >4 hr	Patterns of feeding
Viral characteristics	Obstetric procedures	Antiretrovirals
Immunological factors	Obstetric complications	
Nutritional factors	Multiple births	
Duration of pregnancy	Placental factors	
Other infections	Preterm/low birth weight	
Behavioral factors	Antiretrovirals	
Antiretrovirals		

pears that most of the transmission occurs late during pregnancy or at the time of delivery.[26] In breastfeeding populations, it is estimated that about 23% of the transmission is *in utero*, 65% is intrapartum, and about 12–14% is due to breastfeeding.[27,28] In a non-breastfeeding cohort in Thailand, about 75% (18% absolute rate) of the babies were assumed infected intrapartum and 25% (5.5% absolute rate) *in utero*.[29] TABLE 3 lists factors that are reported to influence MTCT of HIV.[26,30–34] Although these variables are presented separately as antepartum (*in utero*), intrapartum, or postpartum factors, it should be emphasized that a single factor could influence transmission at more than one period. Moreover, the role of these variables could be additive depending on the mechanism of action. Therefore, multiple interventions affecting transmission at different time points during pregnancy or delivery (antepartum and intrapartum) could, potentially, be beneficial. If the contribution of early intrauterine transmission is common in a specific community (based on the underlying risk factors), interventions that are taken at the time of delivery (e.g., antiviral drugs) might be less effective in reducing the MTCT of HIV.

ASSOCIATION OF GENITAL TRACT INFECTIONS AND MTCT OF HIV

Heterosexual transmission of HIV is dependent on infectiousness of the index case and susceptibility of the exposed host.[35,36] In addition, the efficiency of transmission is influenced by the mode of exposure. For perinatal transmission it appears that about a quarter of exposed babies are infected in the absence of any interventions. Infectiousness of a biological secretion depends on the concentration of the virus in the secretion and the virologic factors facilitating transmission such as advanced clinical or immunological HIV disease, which appear to increase HIV-1 in genital secretions.[37] Increased concentration of HIV in blood is associated with increased perinatal and sexual transmission.[31,38] Infectiousness is also higher with concurrent local inflammation in the genital tract.[35] Perinatal transmission is therefore probably influenced by most of the factors facilitating other modes of HIV transmission as well as by additional factors related to pregnancy (high levels of estrogen and progesterone, and local cervical factors such as increased vascularity, exudation, and ectopy[39]) and the processes of labor and delivery.

Role of Selected Factors Associated with MTCT of HIV and GTIs

Placental Factors. The role of the placenta appears to be important in perinatal transmission of HIV. However, several quantitative aspects related to maternal-fetal transmission through this organ are not known and need further evaluation.[33] Although HIV can be identified in the placenta, the placental-fetal barrier could protect against transmission of the virus, and a recently described placental human chorionic gonadotropin (hCG)-associated factor (HAF) with antiviral activity *in vitro*[40] may protect against transplacental HIV infection.

Chorioamnionitis, inflammation of the fetal placental membranes, is defined histologically by the presence of polymorphonuclear leukocytes in the membranes of the chorion and amnion and the amniotic fluid.[41] Either ascending infection (transcervical migration of vaginal microorganisms into the decidua, chorioamnion, or amniotic fluid) or hematogenous spread is a possible mechanism. Chorioamnionitis can also be due to spontaneous or mechanical rupture of the membranes, and several pathogens produce bacterial sialidase or collagenase enzymes that are known to decrease collagen synthesis or weaken collagenous tissues[42] and therefore could compromise the integrity of the membranes. Additional mechanisms include contact-dependent cytotoxicity (mediated by lysing of membranes)[43] or production of inflammatory cytokines that can stimulate prostaglandin synthesis and precipitate contractions leading to premature rupture of fetal membranes.[44] Organisms associated with chorioamnionitis include BV-associated bacteria, STDs such as *N. gonorrhoeae*, *C. trachomatis*, *Trichomonas vaginalis*, and *Group B Streptococcus*. Infection confined to the vagina (e.g., trichomoniasis) and the resulting metabolic products might also affect the integrity of the membranes. Chorioamnionitis is frequently asymptomatic, but can lead to intrapartum fever, prolonged rupture of membranes, and/or premature labor. Most cases of chorioamnionitis occur while the membranes are intact.

Inflammatory acute or chronic processes (e.g., due to GTIs) could lead to chorioamnionitis and increased perinatal transmission. Such associations between chorioamnionitis due to GTIs during pregnancy and MTCT of HIV have been consistently reported in several studies from both developing and developed countries[30,33,34,45–49] GTIs could attract placental macrophages (the Hofbauer cells), the initial line of antimicrobial defense,[41] and therefore increase susceptibility to HIV infection and possibly facilitate peripartum transmission of HIV. Hematogenous spread of syphilitic infection of the placenta is known to cause focal proliferative villitis and vasculitis and could involve the umbilical cord, causing funisitis; these inflammations are accompanied by lymphocyte and plasma cell infiltrations.[41] The association between GTIs and vertical transmission of HIV could also be due to increased viral shedding with cervicitis or ulceration, decreased mucosal barrier, increased viral load or virus activation, and impaired ability of these women to limit infective exposure *in utero*.[3,6]

Premature delivery among HIV-infected women might be mediated by the occurrence of chorioamnionitis,[50] a condition that has been reported more frequently among HIV-infected mothers.[51–53] Premature rupture of membranes (PROM), which may cause chorioamnionitis or result from preexisting chorioamnionitis, is associated with MTCT of HIV and is more common in HIV-positive women. PROM could enhance HIV transmission to the baby through mechanisms related to prematurity. Additionally, duration of rupture of fetal membranes for >4 hours could lead to HIV transmission to the baby through ascending infection. Infants born prematurely to HIV-seropositive mothers have been reported to be at higher risk of HIV infection.[53,54] On the other hand, preterm birth is strongly associated with GTIs such as BV, a condition reported to be more frequent among HIV-infected than HIV-uninfected women.[17,55] The mechanism of the association between preterm birth and HIV perinatal transmission is unclear. Possibly, premature labor can be precipitated by HIV infection of the mother. Alternatively, premature infants may be at increased risk of intrapartum transmission due to diminished immunocompetence and limited maternal transfer of protective antibodies that are mainly transported in late pregnancy[48,54] or due to disruption of the fragile dermis of premature infants. Fetal cell susceptibility to HIV infection could also vary by gestational age.[34]

Role of Confounding Factors. To determine the independent relationship between GTIs and MTCT of HIV, variables that could confound apparent associations need careful evaluation. This is particularly important, because no clinical trial has been reported. However, findings from randomized trials of STD mass treatment in pregnant women should help to demonstrate if control of STDs can lower HIV perinatal transmission rates. Of the potential confounders, we review the role of malaria, behavioral practices, and nutritional factors.

Malaria. The role of infectious diseases such as malaria, which preferentially infect the placenta and lead to similar adverse pregnancy outcomes including perinatal transmission of HIV,[56,57] need to be considered when studying the effect of GTIs on the placenta and possibly vertical transmission of HIV in developing countires. Although both malaria and HIV infection produce similar cellular immune responses,[58] several studies have failed to reveal an interaction between these two infections.[59–61] More recent data, however, suggest that systemic infections such as malaria increase the blood burden of HIV, and treatment of malaria reduces HIV concentration.[62] Since viral load has been implicated in MTCT of HIV,[29,31] infections that increase viral burden or factors that decrease viral level could be important.

Behavioral Factors. Strongly associated with GTIs are behavioral factors such as unprotected sexual intercourse and multiple sexual partners. These background factors should be taken into account, because unprotected sexual intercourse and multiple partners are reported to be associated with MTCT of HIV (strain diversity, cervical/vaginal inflammation, and association with chorioamnionitis). For example, in Butare, Rwanda, unprotected sexual intercourse with two or more partners, especially during pregnancy, increased the risk of transmission of the virus from mother to infant after adjusting for immunological status and GTIs, possibly through increasing the diversity of HIV variants in the mother.[63] In Brazzaville, Congo, women who had an unstable relationship with their primary partners (infant's father) had a higher risk of transmission of HIV to their babies than did women who had a longer term relationship, independent of the HIV clinical condition of the mother.[64] In a study from New York on HIV-seropositive women enrolled during pregnancy, the rate of perinatal HIV-1 transmission was 9.1% among women with no unprotected intercourse during pregnancy, 22.2% among those with moderate frequency, and 39.0% among those with high frequency. The rate of perinatal transmission remained significantly higher among women who had unprotected sexual intercourse after controlling for potential confounders.[65] In addition to strain diversity, two other mechanisms could explain the increased perinatal transmission associated with heterosexual behavior during pregnancy.[66] First, inflammation of the vagina and cervix could be increased with frequent intercourse either by microabrasions or through STDs when intercourse was not protected. Second, frequent intercourse might increase the risk of chorioamnionitis or affect the integrity of the placenta. Other investigators also reported that coitus during pregnancy (especially if the partner was harboring pathogenic organisms) could cause ascending infection and therefore chorioamnionitis.[67] The timing of these pathophysiological mechanisms is important, because most of the HIV transmission to the baby occurs during late pregnancy and intrapartum.

Nutritional Factors. The concentration of HIV in the genital tract is increased by vitamin A deficiency,[68,69] and maternal vitamin A deficiency has been shown to be associated with MTCT.[22] Lack of vitamin A could compromise T-cell and B-cell function and might contribute to increased viral load or decreased maternal antibodies crossing the placenta. Also, lack of vitamin A could increase vertical transmission by affecting the integrity of the placenta, increasing the susceptibility of the birth canal to trauma, or increasing the level of viremia in breast milk.[70] Vitamin A is also important for the integrity of mucous membranes and protection from infection. Nevertheless, a randomized trial of vitamin A supplementation failed to reduce the MTCT of HIV.[23] Although it has been suggested that vitamin A is a risk factor for HIV vertical transmission, little is known about the role of other micronutrients. However, a randomized trial suggested that multivitamin supplementation (excluding vitamin A) increased maternal T-cell counts in HIV-infected mothers.[71]

Summary of Mechanisms Related to GTIs Associated with HIV Transmission to the Newborn (FIG. 2)

Prepartum (in utero) factors:

- Chronic chorioamnionitis leading to preterm labor and/or ascending infection.
- Increased HIV viral shedding in cervicovaginal secretions (increased about fourfold during pregnancy.[72,73]
- Increased HIV acquisition during pregnancy; since HIV viremia is high after recent infection, this high viral load could increase the MTCT of HIV.

Intrapartum factors:

- Increased MTCT of HIV intrapartum through skin and mucous membrane contact with maternal cervicovaginal fluid during labor, ingestion or inhalation of infectious fluids, and ascending infection to the amniotic fluid.[34]
- Acute chorioamnionitis.

POTENTIAL INTERVENTIONS TO REDUCE MTCT OF HIV THROUGH TREATMENT OF GENITAL TRACT INFECTIONS

Persuasive evidence exists that GTIs are important in causing chorioamnionitis. As summarized in FIGURE 2, there are several potential mechanisms through which GTIs can enhance transmission of HIV from mother to child. As discussed by oth-

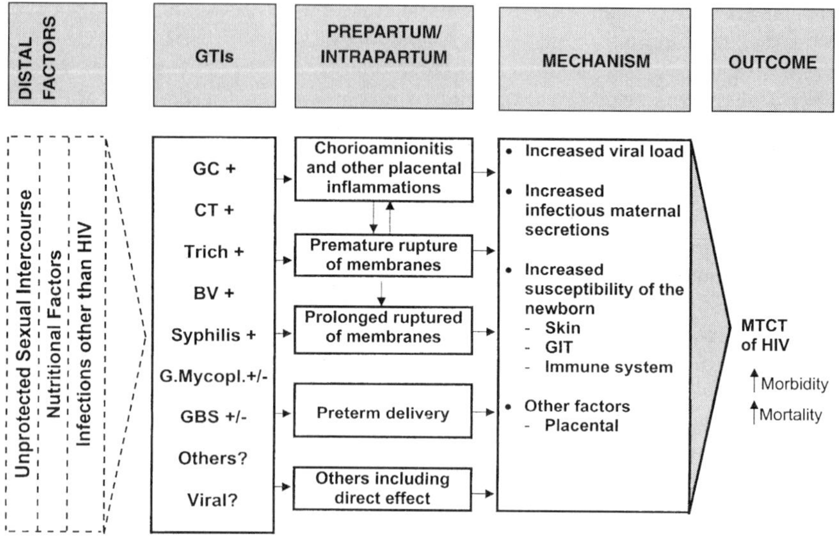

FIGURE 2. Genital tract infections and potential factors influencing MTCT ofHIV.

ers,[74] antimicrobial treatment of these conditions during pregnancy and at delivery could prevent chronic and acute chorioamnionitis and therefore reduce the chances of the virus being transmitted. Randomized trials to evaluate this type of intervention are underway in Malawi and Uganda. Based on results of these studies, treatment strategies during pregnancy, such as screening and selective therapy or mass therapy of common infections, need to be considered.

Other preventive interventions based on our data of higher HIV acquisition during pregnancy than postpartum include counseling of women to avoid unprotected sexual intercourse and multiple partners during pregnancy. As explained earlier, the high initial viremia following seroconversion may increase the MTCT of HIV.

The chlorhexidine trial in Malawi[20] has shown that use of a simple inexpensive microbicide (0.25% chlorhexidine) can significantly reduce neonatal and maternal sepsis and early neonatal mortality.[21] Although the main objective is to reduce the MTCT of HIV, secondary benefits pertaining to improvement of reproductive health in general could be anticipated by adopting less costly and sustainable measures such as the use of antibiotics. In addition, nutritional supplementation with vitamin A and multivitamins should be part of the routine care, because they have shown benefits to the mother and the child and are inexpensive.

The recent finding that a single dose of Nevirapine (a non-nucleoside HIV reverse transcriptase inhibitor antiviral drug given to the mother immediately before delivery and to the baby before discharge after delivery) has reduced perinatal HIV transmission by about 50% is encouraging. It might be asked if it is necessary to pursue alternative interventions such as treatment of GTIs inasmuch as effective, practical, and inexpensive antiretrovirals such as Nevirapine are available? As we alluded to in an earlier section of this paper, antimicrobial treatment could reduce the fraction of transmission that is antepartum. Moreover, current antiviral drugs are unlikely to reduce non-HIV infectious complications in the baby. It will be most beneficial to combine these regimens and to consider the additive effects of alternative interventions both antepartum and postpatum. A similar approach of combining antibiotic treatment antepartum and intrapartum and Nevirapine intrapartum and postpartum is now being developed to be implemented in several sites in sub-Saharan Africa. If successful, such "combination therapy" will cover the transmission continuum from antepartum to postpartum in addition to potential improvements in reproductive outcomes by safeguarding against potential infectious complications to the mother or the child.

ACKNOWLEDGMENT

The authors are grateful to the research teams in Uganda and Malawi for allowing the use of data from their respective projects.

REFERENCES

1. WASSERHEIT, J.N. 1992. Epidemiological synergy: interrelationship between human immunodeficiency virus infection and other sexually transmitted diseases. Sex. Transm. Dis. **19:** 61–77.
2. LAGA, M., A. MANOKA, M. KIVUVU et al. 1993. Non-ulcerative sexually transmitted diseases as risk factors for HIV-1 transmission in women: results from a cohort study. AIDS **7:** 95–102.
3. LAGA, M., M.O. DIALLO & A. BUVE. 1994. Inter-relationship of sexually transmitted diseases and HIV: where are we now? AIDS **8**(Suppl 1): S119–S124.
4. QUINN, T.C. 1996. Association of sexually transmitted diseases and infection with the human immunodeficiency virus: biological co-factors and markers of behavioral interventions. Int. J. STD & AIDS **7**(Suppl 2): 17–24.
5. HITCHCOCK, P.J. 1996. Screening and treatment of sexually transmitted diseases. AIDS Patient Care & STDs. Feb. :10–15.
6. NAIR, P., L. ALGER, S. HINES et al. 1994. Maternal and neonatal characteristics associated with HIV infection in infants of seropositive women. J. Acquired Immune Defic. Syndr. **6:** 298–302.
7. ST. LOUIS, M., M. KAMENGA, C. BROWN et al. 1993. Risk for perinatal HIV-1 transmission according to maternal immunologic, virologic, and placental factors. JAMA **269:** 2853–2859.
8. WABIRE-MANGEN, F., R.H. GRAY, F.A. MMIRO et al. 1999. Placental membrane inflammation and risks of maternal-to-infant transmission of HIV-1 in Uganda. J. Acquired Immune Defic. Syndr. **22:** 379–385.
9. GROSSKURTH, H., F. MOSHA, J. TODD et al. 1995. Impact of improved treatment of sexually transmitted diseases on HIV infection in rural Tanzania: randomized controlled trial. Lancet **346:** 530–536.
10. MOSTAD, S., M. WELCH, B. CHOHAN et al. 1996. Cervical and vaginal HIV-1 DNA shedding in female STD clinic attenders. Abstr. We.C.333. XI International Conference on AIDS, Vancouver, Canada.
11. KREISS, J., D. WILLERFORD, M. HENSEL et al. 1994. Association between cervical inflammation and cervical shedding of human immunodeficiency virus DNA. J. Infect. Dis. **170:** 1597–1601.
12. GHYS, P.D., K. FRANSEN, M.O. DIALLO et al. 1997. The associations between cervico-vaginal HIV shedding, sexually transmitted diseases, and immunosuppression in female sex workers in Abidjan, Cote d'Ivoire. AIDS **11:** F85–F93.

13. COHEN, M., I. HOFFMAN, R. ROYCE *et al.* 1997. Reduction of concentration of HIV-1 in semen after treatment of urethritis therapy: implications for prevention of sexual transmission of HIV-1. Lancet **349:** 1868–1873.
14. BALLARD, R.C., Y. HTUN, Y, DANGOR *et al.* 1999. HIV and genital ulcer disease - determinants of HIV shedding from lesions and consequences of therapy. Abstr. 055. Thirteenth Meeting of the International Society for Sexually Transmitted Diseases Research. Denver, Colorado.
15. HTUN, Y., H. BREDELL, D. MARTIN *et al.* 1999. Influence of reproductive tract infections and their treatment on vaginal shedding. Abstr. 056. Thirteenth Meeting of the International Society for Sexually Transmitted Diseases Research. Denver, Colorado.
16. TAHA, T.E., G.A. DALLABETTA & D.R. HOOVER. 1998. Trends of HIV-1 and sexually transmitted diseases among pregnant and postpartum women in urban Malawi. AIDS **16:** 197–203.
17. TAHA, T.E., R.H. GRAY, N.I. KUMWENDA *et al.* 1999. HIV infection and disturbances of vaginal flora during pregnancy. J. Acquired Immune Defic. Syndr. **20:** 52–59.
18. TAHA, T.E., D.R. HOOVER, G.A. DALLABETTA *et al.* Bacterial vaginosis and disturbances of vaginal flora: association with increased acquisition of HIV. AIDS **12:** 1699–1706.
19. TAHA, T.E., G.A. DALLABETTA, J.K. CANNER *et al.* 1995. The effect of human immunodeficiency virus infection on birthweight, and infant and child mortality in urban Malawi. Int. J. Epidemiol. **24:** 1022–1029.
20. BIGGAR, R.J., P.G. MIOTTI, T.E. TAHA *et al.* 1996. Perinatal intervention trial in Africa: effect of a birth canal cleansing intervention to prevent HIV transmission. Lancet **347:** 1647–1650.
21. TAHA, T.E., R.J. BIGGAR, R.L. BROADHEAD *et al.* 1997. Effect of cleansing the birth canal with an antiseptic solution on maternal and newborn morbidity and mortality in Malawi: clinical trial. Br. Med. J. **315:** 216–220.
22. SEMBA, R.D., P.G. MIOTTI, J.D. CHIPHANGWI *et al.* 1994. Maternal vitamin A deficiency and mother-to-infant transmission of HIV-1. Lancet **343:** 1594–1597.
23. SEMBA, R.D., N. KUMWENDA, D.R. HOOVER *et al.* 1999. Human immunodeficiency virus load in breast milk, mastitis, and mother-to-child transmission of human immunodeficiency virus type 1. J. Infect. Dis. **180:** 93–98.
24. WAWER, M.J., N.K. SEWANKAMBO, D. SERWADDA *et al.* 1999. Control of sexually transmitted diseases for AIDS prevention in Uganda: a randomized community trial. Lancet **353:** 525–535.
25. The WORKING GROUP ON MOTHER-TO-CHILD TRANSMISSION OF HIV. 1995. Rates of mother-to-child transmission of HIV-1 in Africa, America, and Europe: results from 13 perinatal studies. J. Acquired Immune Defic. Syndr. **8:** 506–510.
26. FOWLER, M.G. & M.F. ROGERS. 1996. Overview of perinatal HIV infection. J. Nutr. **126:** 2602S–2607S.
27. BERTOLLI, J., M.E. ST. LOUIS, R.J. SIMONDS *et al.* 1996. Estimating the timing of mother-to-child transmission of human immunodeficiency virus in a breast-feeding population in Kinshasa, Zaire. J. Infect. Dis. **174:** 722–726.
28. DUNN, D.T., M.L. NEWELL, A.E. ADES *et al.* 1992. Risk of human immunodeficiency virus type 1 transmission through breastfeeding. Lancet **340:** 585–588.
29. MOCK, P.A., N. SHAFFER, C. BHADRAKOM *et al.* 1999. Maternal viral load and timing of mother-to-child HIV transmission, Bangkok, Thailand. AIDS **13:** 407–414.
30. MANDELBROT, L., M.-J. MAYAUX, A. BONGAIN *et al.* 1996. Obstetric factors and mother-to-child transmission of human immunodeficiency virus type 1: the French perinatal cohorts. Am. J. Obstet. Gynecol. **175:** 661–667.
31. SPERLING, R.S., E.D. SHAPIRO, R.W. COOMBS *et al.* 1996. Maternal viral load, zidovudine treatment, and the risk of transmission of human immunodeficiency virus type 1 from mother to infant. N. Engl. J. Med. **335:** 1621–1629.
32. THE INTERNATIONAL PERINATAL HIV GROUP. 1999. The mode of delivery and the risk of vertical transmission of human immunodeficiency virus type 1. N. Engl. J. Med. **340:** 977–987.
33. FOWLER, M.G. 1997. Update: transmission of HIV-1 from mother to child. Curr. Opin. Obstet. Gynecol. **9:** 343–348.

34. MOFENSON, L.M. 1997. Interaction between timing of perinatal human immunodeficiency virus infection and the design of preventive and therapeutic interventions. Acta Paediatr. (Suppl) **421:** 1–9.
35. VERNAZZA, P.L., J.J. ERON, S.A. FISCUS *et al.* 1999. Sexual transmission of HIV: infectiousness and prevention. AIDS **13:** 155–166.
36. BUCHACZ, K.A., D.A. WILKINSON, J.F. KROWKA *et al.* 1998. Genetic and immunological host factors associated with susceptibility to HIV-1 infection. AIDS **12**(Suppl A): S87–S94.
37. COHEN, M.S. 1998. Sexually transmitted diseases enhance HIV transmission: no longer a hypothesis. Lancet **353** (Suppl III): 5–7.
38. FIORE, J.R., Y.-J. ZHANG, A. BJORNDAL *et al.* 1997. Biological correlates of HIV-1 heterosexual transmission. AIDS **11:** 1089–1094.
39. MOSTAD, S.B. & J.K. KREISS. 1996. Shedding of HIV-1 in the genital tract. AIDS **10:** 1305–1315.
40. LUNARDI-ISKANDAR, Y., J.L. BRYANT, W.A. BLATTNER *et al.* 1998. Effects of a urinary factor from women in early pregnancy on HIV-1, SIV and associated disease. Nat. Med. **4:** 428–434.
41. WATTS, D.H. & R.C. BRUNHAM. 1999. Sexually transmitted diseases, including HIV infection in pregnancy. *In:* Sexually Transmitted Diseases, 3rd Edition. K.K. Holmes *et al.*, Eds. McGraw-Hill. New York.
42. HILLIER, S.L. 1999. Vaginal ecology in pregnancy. *In* Sexually Transmitted Diseases and Adverse Outcomes of Pregnancy. P.J. Hitchcock *et al.*, Eds. ASM Press. Washington, DC.
43. WOLNER-HANSSEN, P. 1999. Trichomoniasis. *In* Sexually Transmitted Diseases and Adverse Outcomes of Pregnancy. P.J. Hitchcock *et al.*, Eds. ASM Press. Washington, DC.
44. HILL, J.A. 1999. Immunology and adverse outcome of pregnancy related to sexually transmitted diseases. *In* Sexually Transmitted Diseases and Adverse Outcomes of Pregnancy. P.J. Hitchcock *et al.*, Eds. ASM Press. Washington, DC.
45. PECKHAM, C. & M.-L. NEWELL. 1997. Human immunodeficiency virus infection and mode of delivery. Acta Paediatr. (Suppl) **421:** 104–106.
46. TEMMERMAN, M., A.O. NYONG'O, J. BWAYO *et al.* 1995. Risk factors for mother-to-child transmission of human immunodeficiency virus-1 infection. Am. J. Obstet. Gynecol. **172:** 700–705.
47. TOVO, P-A., C. GABIANO & S. TULISSO. 1997. Maternal clinical factors influencing HIV-1 transmission. Acta Paediatr. (Suppl) **421:** 52–55.
48. CONSENSUS WORKSHOP. 1992. Maternal factors involved in mother-to-child transmission of HIV-1. J Acquir. Immune Defic. Syndr. **5:** 1019–1029.
49. EUROPEAN COLLABORATIVE STUDY. 1992. Risk factors for mother-to-child transmission of HIV-1. Lancet **339:** 1007–1012.
50. HILLIER, S.L., J.M. MARTIUS, M. KROHN *et al.* 1988. A case-control study of chorioamniotic infection and histologic chorioamnionitis in prematurity. N. Engl. J. Med. **319:** 972–978.
51. WAMBUGO, P., F.A. PLUMMER, R.C. BRUNHAM *et al.* 1991. Are sexually transmitted diseases (STD) opportunistic infections in HIV-1 infected women? Abstract M.C.3061. VII International Conference on AIDS, Florence, Italy.
52. NYONGO, A., P. GICHANGI, M. TEMMERMAN *et al.* 1992. HIV infection as a risk factor for chorioamnionitis in preterm birth. Abstract PoB 3469. VIII International Conference on AIDS-III STD World Congress, Amsterdam, The Netherlands.
53. RYDER, R.W., W. NSA, S.E. HASSIG, *et al.* 1989. Perinatal transmission of the human immunodeficiency virus type 1 to infants of seropositive women in Zaire. N. Engl. J. Med. **320:** 1637–1642.
54. GOEDERT, J., H. MENDEZ, J.E. DRUMMOND *et al.* 1989. Mother-to-infant transmission of human immunodeficiency virus type 1: association with prematurity or low anti-gp120. Lancet **ii:** 1351–1354.
55. SEWANKAMBO, N., R.H. GRAY, M.J. WAWER *et al.*1997. HIV-1 infection associated with abnormal vaginal flora morphology and bacterial vaginosis. Lancet **350:** 546–550.
56. BLOLAND, P. B., J.J. WIRIMA, R.W. STEKETEE *et al.* 1995. Maternal HIV infection and infant mortality in Malawi: evidence for increased mortality due to placental malaria infection. AIDS **9:** 721–726.

57. MOFENSON, L.M. & M.G. FOWLER. 1999. Interruption of materno-fetal transmission. AIDS **13** (Suppl A): S205– S214.
58. MORROW, R.H., R.L. COLEBUNDERS & J. CHIN. 1989. Interaction of HIV infection with endemic tropical diseases. AIDS **3** (Suppl 1): S79–S87.
59. GREENBERG, A.E., W. NSA, R.W. RYDER *et al.* 1991. Plasmodium falciparum malaria and perinatally acquired human immunodeficiency virus type 1 infection in Kinshasa, Zaire. New Engl. J. Med. **325:** 105–109.
60. TAHA, T.E., J.K. CANNER, G.A. DALLABETTA *et al.* 1994. Childhood malaria parasitaemia and human immunodeficiency virus infection in Malawi. Trans. Roy. Soc. Trop. Med. Hyg. **88:** 164–165.
61. CHANDRAMOHAN, D. & B.M. GREENWOOD. 1998. Is there an association between human immunodeficiency virus and plasmodium falciparum? Int. J. Epidemiol. **27:** 296–301.
62. HOFFMAN, I.F., C. JERE, T. TAYLOR *et al.* 1999. The effect of *P. falciparum* malaria on HIV-1 RNA blood plasma concentration. AIDS **13:** 487–494.
63. BULTERYS, M., A. CHOA, A. DUSHIMIMANA *et al.* 1993. Multiple sexual partners and mother-to-child transmission of HIV-1. AIDS **7:** 1639–1645.
64. Lallemant, M., S. Lallemant-Le-Coeur, D. Cheynier *et al.* 1989. Mother-child transmission of HIV-1 and infant survival in Brazzaville, Congo. AIDS **3:** 643–646.
65. MATHESON, P.B., P.A. THOMAS, E.J. ABRAMS *et al.* 1996. Heterosexual behavior during pregnancy and perinatal transmission of HIV-1. AIDS **10:** 1249–1256.
66. BULTERYS, M. & J.J. GOEDERT. 1996. From biology to sexual behavior - towards the prevention of mother-to-child transmission of HIV. AIDS **10:** 1287–1289.
67. NAEYE, R.L. & S. ROSS. 1983. Coitus and chorioamnionitis: a prospective study. Hum. Devel. **6:** 91–94.
68. MOSTAD, S.B., J. OVERBAUGH, D.M. DEVANGE. 1997. Hormonal contraception, vitamin A deficiency, and other risk factors for shedding of HIV-1 infected cells from the cervix and vagina. Lancet **350:** 922–927.
69. JOHN, G.C., R.W. NDUATI, D. MBORI-NGACHA *et al.* 1997. Genital shedding of human immunodeficiency virus type 1 DNA during pregnancy: association with immunosuppression, abnormal cervical or vaginal discharge, and severe vitamin A deficiency. J. Infect. Dis. **175:** 57–62.
70. SEMBA, R.D. 1997. Overview of the potential role of vitamin A in mother-to-child transmission of HIV-1. Acta Paediatr. (Suppl) **421:** 107–112.
71. FAWZI, W.W., G.I. MSAMANGA, D. SPIEGELMAN *et al.* 1998. Randomized trial of effects of vitamin supplements on pregnancy outcomes and T-cell counts in HIV-1-infected women in Tanzania. Lancet **351:** 1477–1482.
72. CLEMETSON, D.B.A., G.B. MOSS, D.M. WILLERFORD *et al.* 1993. Detection of HIV DNA in cervical and vaginal secretions: prevalence and correlates among women in Nairobi, Kenya. J.A.M.A. **269:** 2860–2864.
73. HENIN, Y., L. MANDELBROT, R. HENRION *et al.* 1993. Virus excretion in the cervicovaginal secretions of pregnant and nonpregnant HIV infected women. J. Acquir. Immune Defic. Syndr. **6:** 72–75.
74. GOLDENBERG, R.L., S.H. VERMUND, A.R. GOEPFERT *et al.* 1998. Choriodecidual inflammation: a potentially preventable cause of perinatal HIV-1 transmission. Lancet **352:** 1927–1930.

Nutritional Factors and Vertical Transmission of HIV-1

Epidemiology and Potential Mechanisms

WAFAIE FAWZI[a]

Departments of Nutrition and Epidemiology, Harvard School of Public Health, Boston, Massachusetts 02115, USA

ABSTRACT: Transmission of HIV from mothers to children may occur through the transplacental, intrapartum, or breastfeeding routes. Adequate nutritional status may reduce vertical transmission by affecting several maternal or fetal and child risk factors for transmission including enhancing systemic immune function in the mother or fetus/child; reducing the rate of clinical, immunological, or virological progression in the mother; reducing viral load or the risk of viral shedding in lower genital secretions or breast milk; reducing the risks of low birth weight or prematurity; or by maintaining the integrity of the fetus/child gastrointestinal integrity. In prospective observational studies, low plasma vitamin A levels were associated with higher risks of vertical transmission. However, findings from randomized, controlled trials suggest that supplements of vitamin A or other vitamins are unlikely to have an effect on vertical transmission during pregnancy or the intrapartum period. The effect of other nutrient supplements, such as zinc and selenium, is unknown. Similarly, whether nutrition supplements of mothers during the breastfeeding period has an effect on transmission is unknown. The potential benefits of direct supplementation of children born to HIV-infected women on transmission of HIV, as well as on the risk and severity of childhood infections and mortality, are also important to examine.

INTRODUCTION

As of the end of 1999, more than 33 million people were infected with HIV.[1] About 6 million new infections occur every year worldwide. In several urban centers in sub-Saharan Africa, more than 10% of asymptomatic adults and about 15–30% of women attending prenatal care clinics are infected. HIV infection has also been spreading very fast in parts of Asia and Eastern Europe. Protective relationships between micronutrient status and HIV vertical transmission have been reported in a number of epidemiologic studies. There is interest in the role of micronutrient status in the etiology of HIV transmission and disease progression because improving nutritional status may be a cost-effective prophylactic and treatment modality for HIV-

[a]Address for correspondence: Dr. Wafaie Fawzi, Department of Nutrition, Harvard School of Public Health, 665 Huntington Avenue, Boston, MA 02115. Voice: 617-432-2086; fax: 617-432-2435.

mina@hsph.harvard.edu

seropositive persons, particularly in developing countries where specific anti-retroviral and prophylactic drugs are virtually unavailable.

Adequate nutritional status may reduce vertical transmission by affecting several maternal or fetal and child risk factors for transmission that are mentioned briefly here. The clinical, immunological, or viral stages of HIV disease among pregnant women are important predictors of vertical transmission of infection. Transmission of HIV from mothers to children may occur through the transplacental, intrapartum, or breastfeeding routes; correspondingly, impaired integrity of the epithelial lining of the placenta, lower genital tract, or breast may lead to higher risk of transmission. Prematurity and low birth weight are also risk factors for transmission during labor and during breastfeeding, although they may also be consequences of *in utero* transmission. Integrity of the systemic and gastrointestinal mucosal immune systems in the fetus and child play an important role in reducing the risk of transmission. The role of micronutrients in the etiology of these intermediate maternal and fetal/child risk factors for vertical transmission will be discussed, followed by a presentation of the evidence regarding the direct relationship between micronutrient status (or supplementation) and vertical transmission.

MICRONUTRIENTS, SYSTEMIC IMMUNITY, AND INFECTION

Nutritional deficiencies are associated with impaired immune function and could therefore lead to increased incidence (and severity) of infections. By impairing systemic immunity of the mother, micronutrient deficiency could result in increased risks of opportunistic infections, faster HIV disease progression, and possibly increased risk of vertical transmission of the virus. Micronutrient deficiency in the fetus or child may also play an important role in systemic immune response to infections, including HIV infection.

The relationships between individual and multiple micronutrients, immune function, and non-HIV-related infections have been reported in numerous studies. In a placebo-controlled study among healthy elderly subjects,[2] a daily supplement of vitamins and minerals resulted in higher numbers of natural killer cells and T-cell subsets (including CD4), enhanced proliferation response to mitogen, increased natural killer cell activity and interleukin-2 production, higher antibody response to influenza vaccine, and fewer days of infectious illness. Considerable evidence shows that vitamin A enhances phagocytosis and cell-mediated killing. Vitamin A deficiency is associated with a decrease in the *in vitro* proliferative response of splenic lymphocytes to mitogens as well as a reduction in the delayed-type hypersensitivity. Provitamin A carotenoids such as β-carotene enhance T- and B-cell immunity, either by conversion to vitamin A or by acting as an antioxidant.[3,4] Vitamin A supplementation was associated with improved natural killer cell cytotoxicity in rats[5] and an increased number of natural killer cells in HIV-infected children.[6] Among children whose HIV status was not determined, vitamin A supplementation resulted in significant reductions in the severity of measles and diarrhea, as well as reduced total mortality.[7]

Animal and human studies have shown that vitamin B_6 deficiency affects both humoral and cellular immune function. Vitamin B_6 depletion in healthy elderly significantly reduced total number of lymphocytes, lymphocyte proliferation, and IL-2 production in response to T-cell mitogens; these defects were corrected following vitamin B_6 repletion.[8] Among HIV-positive persons, vitamin B_6 deficiency was associated with reduced natural killer cell cytotoxicity and impaired mitogen-induced lymphocyte proliferation.[9] Riboflavin (B_2) deficiency impairs the ability to generate humoral antibodies in response to test antigens, but research on the effect on cell-mediated immunity is limited.[10] In clinical studies, patients with low levels of serum vitamin B_{12} had impaired neutrophil function, while data from *in-vitro* and animal studies indicate that B_{12} supplements are associated with enhanced antibody function and mitogenic responses.[10]

Vitamin C deficiency in animal models results in depressed cell-mediated immune response. T- and B-lymphocyte proliferative responses are increased following supplementation in some human studies,[11] and enhanced vitamin C status was associated with a lower rate of infections.[12] In a cross-sectional study among patients with cystic fibrosis, vitamin C deficiency was directly related to indices of inflammation including interleukin-6 and tumor necrosis factor-α (TNF-α).[13] Vitamin E deficiency has been shown to impair T-cell-mediated function including DTH, lymphocyte proliferation, and IL-2 production in animal and human studies.[14] Supplementation with vitamin E in healthy elderly significantly improved lymphocyte proliferation, IL-2 production, DTH, and response to T-cell-dependent vaccines and reduced the incidence of self-reported infection.[15,16] In mice infected with murine AIDS, vitamin E supplements was associated with significant improvements in immune response as measured by higher IL-2 production and natural killer cell cytotoxicity as well as reduced production of proinflammatory cytokines TNF-α and IL-6.[17]

Zinc deficiency has adverse effects at multiple points in the immune system and is associated with increased susceptibility to a variety of pathogens.[18] Zinc is crucial for the normal development and function of T lymphocytes, including activation of Th-1 cytokine production, as well the function of macrophages and nonspecific neutrophils. Zinc supplementation resulted in significant reductions in the severity of diarrhea, acute respiratory infections, and malaria among children in several trials.[19] Another important micronutrient is selenium, which is an essential component of the antioxidant enzyme glutathione peroxidase. Data from epidemiologic studies suggest that selenium has a protective effect against certain cancers, particularly in populations where intake is low.[20] Selenium deficiency has been shown in animal studies to inhibit nonspecific immune function, humoral immunity, cellular immunity including cytotoxicity of T-lymphocytes and natural killer cells, and resistance to infection; selenium supplementation, in contrast, enhances these immune functions, as well as resistance to infection.[21] In chronic gut failure patients on total parenteral nutrition, lymphocyte responses to various antigens and mitogens were subnormal on a diet containing 20 µg/day of selenium but improved after two months on a diet containing 200 µg/day of selenium.[22]

MICRONUTRIENTS AND MATERNAL STAGE OF HIV DISEASE

A number of longitudinal studies examined the relationships between micronutrient status and disease progression among adults. In two longitudinal studies among homosexual and bisexual men, the San Francisco Men's Health study[23] and the Multicenter AIDS Cohort Study (MACS),[24,25] higher intake of micronutrients was associated with slower progression of disease. In San Francisco, a significant positive relationship was observed between CD4 counts at baseline and intake of several nutrients including riboflavin, thiamine, and niacin. Multivitamin use, as well as intake of vitamin E, riboflavin, vitamin C, thiamine, and vitamin A, was inversely associated with disease progression. In the MACS study, vitamin A intake had a U-shaped relationship with the risk of progression to AIDS,[24] as well as with risk of death.[25] Higher intakes of niacin, vitamins B_1, B_2, B_6, and vitamin C were associated with slower progression to AIDS, and all of these with the exception of vitamin C were also associated with lower risk of mortality in the same studies. Intake of B vitamins were also associated with a significant protective relationship with disease progression in a study from South Africa.[26]

In two studies among HIV-positive intravenous drug users, serum retinol levels were inversely associated with the risk of mortality.[27,28] In a third study carried out among HIV-positive drug users, subjects who developed biochemical vitamin B_{12} or vitamin A deficiency during an 18-month period experienced a decline in CD4 cell count, while higher cell counts were noted among those whose vitamin B_{12} and vitamin A levels were normalized over the same period.[29] In the MACS study, men with lower serum vitamin E[30] or vitamin B_{12}[31] levels were more likely to progress to AIDS compared with those with higher levels; however, no relationship was observed with serum vitamin A levels.[30]

The relationships between zinc and selenium status and HIV disease progression have also been examined. Low serum selenium levels were associated with significantly higher risks of mortality and the occurrence of AIDS-defining opportunistic infections, even after adjustment for baseline CD4 count and other variables.[32] In the San Francisco Men's Health Study, dietary intake of zinc was positively related to CD4 cell count, but not to progression to AIDS.[23] In the MACS study, dietary zinc intake was associated with an apparent increase in the rate of progression[24] and mortality[25]; in contrast, patients who progressed to AIDS in the same study population had significantly lower serum zinc levels compared with nonprogressors and HIV-negative subjects.[33] In another prospective study, normalization of zinc was associated with higher CD4 cell counts among men.[29] Low plasma zinc concentration was also a significant predictor of AIDS mortality in a study from Miami; however, the relationship was not significant after adjustment for CD4 cell count and other nutrient levels.[32]

The above studies are observational by design. In several of them, the results were adjusted for potential confounding by baseline signs and symptoms and immunological surrogates, such as CD4 cell counts. However, residual confounding is still a possible explanation for the findings. All the studies were carried out among prevalent cohorts of seropositive persons at baseline; hence the duration of infection was not known and therefore not adjusted for in the analyses. The biochemical studies are limited by the fact that low serum vitamin A, zinc, or selenium levels among individuals with infection does not necessarily mean poor status of these nutrients, since low levels may be part of the response to infection.

The relationships between vitamin supplementation and immunological or virological disease progression were examined in a few controlled trials. In a crossover placebo-controlled study among 21 patients, daily β-carotene supplements resulted in a small increase in the total white blood cell count, change in CD4 cell count, and percent change in CD4/CD8 ratio compared to subjects on placebo.[34] In another study by the same investigators, however, this effect was not observed.[35] The lack of effect of vitamin A on immunological endpoints was confirmed in a large placebo-controlled trial among women from Tanzania, but multivitamins excluding A resulted in a significant improvement in CD4, CD8, and CD3 cell counts.[36] Retinol and β-carotene did not result in a change in viral load in a small, placebo-controlled trial among HIV-infected pregnant women from South Africa.[37] There was also no effect of vitamin A supplementation on viral load among intravenous drug users in the United States.[38] In a study from Canada, however, large daily doses of vitamins C and E resulted in a significant reduction in viral load.[39]

MICRONUTRIENTS AND PLACENTAL AND LOWER GENITAL TRACT FACTORS

Poor nutritional status may impair the integrity of placental linings and facilitate transplacental transmission of HIV. The potential relationship between nutrition and placental conditions is suggested by the finding that vitamin A deficiency was associated with reduced placental integrity in rats.[40] Chorioamnionitis also weakens the placental barrier's integrity leading to increased placental permeability to HIV, a higher viral load in amniotic fluid, and possibly an increased risk of transmission.[41] Lower genital tract infection and ascending vaginal infection could result in higher risk of chorioamnionitis, spontaneous premature rupture of membranes, and prematurity, all of which are risk factors for transmission.[42]

The lower genital mucosal barrier probably has an important function in reducing the risk of genital infections, including HIV, and integrity of this barrier may be affected by nutritional status. In early studies among rats, vitamin A deficiency was shown to result in cornification of the epithelium of the lower genital tract.[43,44] A weakened lining may thus lead to a higher risk of injury and bleeding during the process of delivery, and hence a greater risk of the baby becoming exposed to infectious maternal material.

Humoral and cellular mucosal immunity in the lower genital tract may also be associated with vertical transmission. Secretions in the lower genital tract contain anti-HIV antibodies, cytokines, and other immunologic factors.[45] Nutritional deficiency may result in weaker mucosal immunity and a higher risk of viral load and other genital infections. Positive relationships were reported between low serum vitamin A levels among women and the risks of HIV shedding in lower genital tract secretions in two studies from Kenya.[46,47]

MICRONUTRIENTS AND INTEGRITY OF BREAST EPITHELIA

Breast milk contains numerous protective factors, including nonspecific and specific immunoglobulins, lysozymes, lactoferrin, oligosaccharides, glycosaminoglycans, IL-8, RANTES, and secretory leukocyte protease inhibitor (SLPI). Many of these factors have been shown to be associated with inhibition of infections including that of HIV activity *in vitro*. For example, lactoferrin from human milk or colostrum was shown to bind to the V3 loop of the HIV gp120 protein and inhibit HIV-induced cytopathic effects *in vitro*.[48] Similarly, human milk glycosaminoglycans inhibit the binding of HIV gp120 to CD4 cell receptors.[49] SLPI binds to monocytes and may prevent viral infection prior to reverse transcription.[50] Maternal nutritional status is associated with the quality of breast milk, namely the concentrations of macronutrients (including fat), micronutrients (including vitamins and selenium), and immunologic properties.[51] Better maternal micronutrient status may thus result in improved milk quality and, hence, enhanced infant systemic and gastrointestinal mucosal immune response to infections.

Subclinical mastitis, an inflammation of breast tissues defined as a high Na/K ratio in breast milk, was associated with higher viral load in breast milk from HIV-infected women; with higher concentrations of lactoferrin, SLPI, and RANTES; and with a higher risk of transmission of HIV-1 to the baby.[52,53] Evidence from human studies, carried out among persons whose HIV status was not determined, suggest that antioxidants may result in reduced risk of subclinical mastitis. In a study from Tanzania, vitamin E–rich sunflower oil, but not provitamin A–containing palm oil, decreased milk Na/K ratio.[54] In another study from Bangladesh by the same group, vitamin A supplementation was without an effect on subclinical mastitis.[55] Several studies among cattle suggest that supplementation with micronutrients (including selenium and vitamin E) results in significant reduction in risk of mastitis.[56]

The direct relationship between micronutrient status and viral shedding in breast milk was examined in a study from Kenya[57]: low plasma vitamin A concentrations of HIV-infected women during pregnancy were associated with a higher risk of viral shedding in breast milk. However, this was an observation study and shares the limitations reviewed earlier. Similarly, the limitation of serum vitamin A as a marker of vitamin A status applies here. More studies are needed to examine whether nutritional status (or nutritional supplements) have an effect on the risk of viral shedding, viral load, and mucosal immunological factors.

MICRONUTRIENTS AND PREMATURITY AND LOW BIRTH WEIGHT

Inverse relationships between maternal status of individual vitamins and prematurity and low birth weight, two intermediate outcomes on the path to transmission, were reported in a few studies. Among low-income women in Camden, New Jersey, use of nutritional supplements was associated with a 34% reduction in the risk of preterm birth and a 41% reduction of low birth weight[58]; there was no significant relationship between supplement use and the risk of small-for-gestational-age birth. The study was nonrandomized; hence, it is not possible to exclude the possibility of residual confounding by other variables, including socioeconomic status, education, and access and use of prenatal care. In a large, placebo-controlled trial from Nepal, a strong protective effect of about 50% on maternal mortality was found[59] among more than 20,000 pregnancies with a weekly dose of 23,300 IU of vitamin A (equivalent to 7 times the RDA each week). Nevertheless, there were no effects found for either supplement on low-birthweight, prematurity, or small-for-gestational-age birth in a subsample of pregnancies in which birth outcomes were collected.[60] A randomized, double-blind, placebo-controlled trial examined the effects of vitamin supplements on birth outcomes among pregnant women infected with HIV-1 in Dar es Salaam, Tanzania.[36] The study used a 2×2 factorial design to examine the effects of supplements of vitamin A and/or multivitamins (including B_1, B_2, B_6, B_{12}, niacin, B_{12}, folate, C, and E but excluding vitamin A). All women, irrespective of the assigned experimental regimen, were given daily doses of ferrous sulfate, folate, and weekly doses of prophylactic chloroquine phosphate as per standard prenatal care in Tanzania. Multivitamins resulted in a statistically significant reduction of 39% in risk of fetal loss. Multivitamin supplementation also resulted in about 40% reductions in low birth weight, severe preterm birth, and small-for-gestational age birth. The effect of vitamin A supplementation was smaller and not statistically significant. In a placebo-controlled trial among HIV-positive pregnant women in Malawi, daily prenatal vitamin A supplements (10,000 IU) resulted in a 30% reduction in low birth weight but had no effect on prematurity,[61] whereas another trial in South Africa using the same dose of vitamin A that was used in the Tanzania trial (i.e., daily doses of 5,000 IU preformed vitamin A and 30 mg β-carotene), prematurity was reduced by 34% but no effect on low birth weight was noted.[62] Zinc supplements were associated with a significant increase in birth weight among low-income women who participated in a placebo-controlled study in the state of Alabama in the United States,[63] but not among women in another trial among women in Peru.[64]

MICRONUTRIENTS AND FETAL/CHILD GASTROINTESTINAL MUCOSAL IMMUNITY

Integrity of the gastrointestinal mucosal lining of the fetus or child is likely to be essential to preventing transmission of HIV through ingestion of infected amniotic fluid or infected breast milk, respectively. Both the mucosal barrier function and gut immunology are important for combating infections in general. Vitamin A and zinc deficiencies are associated with impaired barrier function of the gastrointestinal tract. Vitamin A deficiency leads to reduced intestinal cell division and differentiation and a reduced number of goblet cells and luminal mucus. In two placebo-controlled trials among infants from India, a large dose of vitamin A resulted in improvement of the barrier function of the gut defined using the lactulose-mannitol dual-sugar intestinal permeability test.[65] Zinc supplements were similarly beneficial in another study from Bangladesh,[66] and both vitamin A and zinc supplements resulted in significant reductions in the severity of diarrhea in several randomized trials among children whose HIV status was not determined.[7,19]

There are humoral and cellular components to gastrointestinal mucosal immunity.[67] Secretory IgA is the major humoral immune response. Cellular components include intraepithelial lymphocytes (mostly CD8 cells) and lamina propria lymphocytes (both CD4 and CD8 cells). IgA and CD8 have a number of cytotoxic capabilities, including antibody-dependent cell-mediated cytotoxicity (ADCC), and probably are important for the defense against viral infections in the gastrointestinal tract.[67,68] Poor nutritional status is associated with impaired mucosal immune response. There is evidence that protein and vitamin A deficiencies are associated with reduced secretory IgA, natural killer cell activity, and intraepithelial lymphocyte count.[69]

MICRONUTRIENTS AND VERTICAL TRANSMISSION OF HIV-1

Findings from the above studies suggest that improved nutritional status may be related to vertical transmission of HIV by enhancing systemic immune function in the mother or fetus/child; reducing the rate of clinical, immunological, or virological progression in the mother; reducing viral load or the risk of viral shedding in lower genital secretions or breast milk; reducing the risks of low birth weight or prematurity; or by maintaining the integrity of the fetus/child gastrointestinal integrity. A number of studies examined the direct relationship between nutritional status and vertical transmission. Prospective observational studies and randomized trials will be reviewed.

A number of observational studies suggest that low serum A levels of vitamin A among HIV-infected pregnant women is associated with a higher risk of vertical transmission of HIV. In a study from Malawi among 474 HIV-infected women, those with higher levels of serum retinol were at a lower risk of transmitting the virus to their babies[70,71] (TABLE 1). Similarly, among HIV-positive women from Rwanda, levels of vitamin A were inversely associated with the risk of having a dead or HIV-positive infant.[72] Results from three studies from the United States were not consistent: low serum vitamin A was associated with a higher risk of vertical transmission in one[73] but not the other two.[74,75] As mentioned earlier for studies that examined the relationships of micronutrients and disease progression, there are alternative explanations to the findings of the association between vitamin A levels and risk of transmission. These include the possibility that serum A levels maybe may be a marker of, rather than a causal factor for, an advanced stage of HIV disease and, hence, transmission. Also, confounding of the results by different lengths of follow-up time or other predictors of transmission among vitamin-deficient and -sufficient groups could explain these findings.

Five randomized placebo-controlled trials are either ongoing or completed with the aim of examining the efficacy of nutritional supplements on the risk of vertical transmission of HIV. In a trial that was carried out in Malawi, HIV-positive pregnant women were randomized to either 10,000 IU or placebo during the prenatal period. The supplements had no effect of transmission at 6 weeks or by 12 months[76] (TABLE 2). In South Africa, pregnant women received either preformed vitamin A and β-carotene or placebo during the prenatal period, and the risks of HIV infection in infants by 3 months of age were similar.[62] However, the authors report that there was a reduction in risk of transmission among premature babies, although the association was not statistically significant. In Tanzania, pregnant women who were infected with HIV-1 were randomized to vitamin A and/or multivitamins (excluding vitamin A) using a two-by-two factorial design. Eligible women were between 12 and 27 weeks of gestation at randomization. Vitamin A and multivitamins did not affect the risk of vertical transmission of HIV *in utero* or during the intrapartum and early breastfeeding periods (up to 6 weeks of age).[77] Women continued to take the supplement throughout the period of breastfeeding, and the effect of vitamin supplements on HIV transmission through breastfeeding and on clinical progression of HIV disease is yet to be ascertained.

Two other trials are being conducted in Zimbabwe to examine the efficacy of nutritional supplements on vertical transmission of HIV. In the first, carried out as a collaboration between the University of Zimbabwe and the Royal Veterinary and Agricultural University in Denmark, 600 HIV-positive women are randomized to placebo or a combination of 14 vitamins and minerals. In the second trial, investigators at the Ministry of Health in Zimbabwe, Johns Hopkins University, and McGill University are enrolling 4000 HIV-positive women in a trial to examine the efficacy

TABLE 1. Prospective cohort studies of micronutrients in relation to vertical transmission of HIV-1

Study site	Population	Exposure: mother serum vitamin A levels	Endpoint and association reported	Association reported[a]	Variables adjusted for
Malawi[70,71]	338 HIV+ women	Increase of 0.45 µmol/L	HIV infection in infants	0.56 (0.37–0.85)	Maternal age, body mass index, CD4 cell count, birth weight and gestational age.
	474 HIV+ women	Increase of 0.40 µmol/L	Infant mortality	0.47 (0.36–0.62)	
Rwanda[72]	302HIV+ women	≥20 vs. <20 µg/dl	Infant death Infant HIV+	0.53 (0.29–0.99) 0.51 (0.29–0.90)	CD4 cell count, hematocrit
U.S. [74]	334 HIV+ pregnant women	≥30 vs. <20 µg/dl	HIV infection in infants	0.56 (0.22–1.45)	Plasma viral RNA, CD4 cell %, birth weight, hard drug use
U.S. [73]	133 HIV+ women	≥1.05 vs. <0.70 µmol/L	HIV infection in infants	0.22 (0.05–0.93)	Percent CD4 cells, mode of delivery, gestational age, duration of membrane rupture, race.
U.S. [75]	95 HIV+ women	Continuous variable	HIV infection in infants	Transmitters: 46.5 µg/dl[b] Non-transmitters: 41.1 µg/dl[b]	None

[a]RR (95% CI).
[b]Mean.

TABLE 2. Randomized, placebo-controlled micronutrient trials in relation to vertical transmission of HIV-1

Study site (reference)	Population	Intervention	Endpoint	Intervention groups		p value
Malawi[76]	700 HIV+ pregnant women	Vitamin A (10,000 IU) or placebo during the antenatal period	HIV infection status at:	Vitamin A[a]	Placebo[a]	
			6 weeks	62 (26.6)	66 (27.8)	0.76
			12 months	65 (27.3)	80 (32.0)	0.25
South Africa[62]	750 HIV+ pregnant women	Preformed vitamin A (5,000 IU) and β-carotene (30 mg) versus placebo;	HIV infection in infants by 3 months of age:	Vitamin A[b] 20.3% (15.7–24.9)	Placebo[b] 22.3% (17.5–27.1)	
Tanzania[77]	1085 HIV+ pregnant women	Placebo-controlled with 2×2 factorial design: preformed vitamin A (5,000 IU) and β-carotene (30 mg); multivitamins (20 mg of B_1, 20 mg of B_2, 25 mg of B_6, 100 mg of niacin, 50 μg of B_{12}, 500 mg of C, 30 mg of vitamin E, and 0.8 mg of folate)		Multivitamins[a]	No multivitamins[a]	
			Fetal loss	31 (5.9)	52 (10.0)	0.02
			HIV + at birth	38 (10.1)	24 (6.6)	0.08
			HIV+ at 6 weeks	53 (21.8)	39 (18.6)	0.39
			HIV+ at 6 weeks among those HIV– at birth	31 (16.2)	28 (15.6)	0.88
				Vitamin A[a]	No vitamin A[a]	
			Fetal loss	37 (7.0)	46 (8.9)	0.25
			HIV + at birth	38 (10.0)	24 (6.7)	0.11
			HIV+ at 6 weeks	53 (22.2)	39 (18.2)	0.30
			HIV+ at 6 weeks among those HIV– at birth	35 (17.9)	24 (13.8)	0.29

[a]Number (n) with percent in parenthesis.
[b]Risk (95% CI).

of a single large dose of vitamin A given to women or their babies at birth on the risks of transmission of HIV and other infant health outcomes.

COMMENTS

Findings from randomized, controlled trials suggest that supplements of vitamin A or other vitamins are unlikely to have an effect on vertical transmission during pregnancy or the intrapartum period. The effect of other nutrient supplements, such as zinc and selenium, is unknown. Similarly, whether nutrition supplements of mothers or babies during the breastfeeding period has an effect on transmission is unknown.

It is not possible to exclude the possibility that doses higher than those used in the above trials may have had a beneficial effect on transmission. However, the doses used in Tanzania and South African studies were already several-fold greater than the recommended dietary allowances.[78] Most women in the trials in Malawi, South Africa, and Tanzania started receiving the supplements at the time of the first prenatal visit, which, as in many countries in subsaharan Africa, is at about 20 weeks of gestation, on average. Another possible explanation for the lack of effect on transmission in these trials may be that supplementation was not provided during the critical period in early fetal life during which programming of the fetal immune system may occur. Evidence that micronutrient deficiencies during early gestation are associated with programming of the immune system was suggested in a study in mice. Zinc deprivation of mice early in gestation resulted in immunodeficiency that persisted for three generations in spite of adequate zinc diets in the second- and third-generation mice.[79]

Research on the role of nutrition in pregnancy outcomes and vertical transmission of HIV has opened the door for examining similar questions among the larger population of HIV-negative women. The beneficial effects of multivitamins on fetal loss, low birth weight, and prematurity obtained in the Tanzania study may be largely mediated through improvements in immune function and/or hematologic status that are unique to HIV-infected women. Hence, while all positive women are likely to benefit from such supplements during pregnancy, the results cannot be automatically generalized to HIV-negative women. Fetal loss and other adverse pregnancy outcomes are major problems in Tanzania and many developing countries, even among HIV-negative women and in settings that provide adequate prenatal care to all women, including iron and folate supplements. Given the much larger size of the HIV-negative population at risk of adverse perinatal outcomes, and the limited resources available to health sectors in most developing countries, it is important to test the efficacy of vitamin supplements among HIV-negative women.

Improvement of nutritional status may also play a role in slowing the progression of HIV disease among children who do become infected, as well as possibly, their infected parent(s). The relationships between vitamin and mineral status and disease progression among adults are reviewed above. Findings from two additional trials from Tanzania and South Africa suggest that vitamin A supplements can reduce morbidity and mortality among infected children. In the trial from South Africa, children born to HIV-infected women were randomized to receive placebo or 50,000 IU of retinol at 1 and 3 months, 100,000 IU at 6 and 9 months, and 200,000 IU at 12 and 15 months. Vitamin A supplements resulted in approximately 50% reduction in diarrheal morbidity among HIV-infected children.[80] In Tanzania, 4-monthly doses of 200,000 IU of vitamin A resulted in large and significant reductions in the risk of total mortality among HIV-positive children and in AIDS-related deaths.[81] The role of other micronutrients among infected children has not been examined.

Many HIV-infected mothers are likely to choose not to breastfeed because of concerns about transmission of the virus. Such babies are likely to be at a higher risk for diarrhea, other childhood infections, and poor growth, all conditions that are associated with higher mortality in developing countries. Uninfected babies are also at a higher risk of morbidity and mortality as their mothers' HIV disease progresses, and that risk is highest among orphans who have little support from the extended family. Micronutrient supplements of children born to infected women, irrespective of their HIV status, may play an important role in reducing infectious mortality and morbidity.

Vertical transmission of HIV ranges from 30 to 45% in many parts of sub-Saharan Africa. In 1999 alone, 470,000 children died of AIDS worldwide,[1] mostly in the developing world, and largely having acquired their infection from their mothers. The findings of significant reductions in transmission with 2 doses of Nevirapine (to the mother at the beginning of labor and to the baby within 72 hours of birth)[82] as well as with a short-course of Zidovudine[83] are encouraging. However, implementing widespread counseling and testing for HIV, providing these drugs to positive women, and the costs of sustaining such a program are major concerns. Prenatal micronutrient supplementation of HIV-infected women is likely to be beneficial in reducing adverse birth outcomes, even if no effect on *in utero* and intrapartum transmission has been reported to date. As attention shifts to finding ways of reducing transmission during pregnancy and the breastfeeding period, the role of nutrition is important to examine. Whether HIV-positive women opt to breastfeed or not, it is important to determine whether provision of micronutrient supplements during breastfeeding to mothers or direct supplementation of their children has an effect on the risk and severity of infections and mortality among mothers and children or on vertical transmission of HIV through breastfeeding.

ACKNOWLEDGMENTS

This work is supported in part by the National Institute of Child Health and Human Development (NICHD R01 32257) and the Fogarty International Center (NIH D43 TW00004).

REFERENCES

1. UNAIDS. 1999. AIDS Epidemic Update. December. Geneva.
2. CHANDRA, R.K. 1992. Effect of vitamin and trace-element supplementation on immune responses and infection in elderly subjects. Lancet **340:** 1124–1127.
3. ROSS, A.C. & C.B. STEPHENSON. 1996. Vitamin A and retinoids in antiviral responses. FASEB J. **10:** 979–985.
4. WATSON, R.R., R.H. PRABHALA, P.M. PLEZIA & D.S. ALBERTS. 1991. Effect of β-carotene on lymphocyte sub-populations in elderly humans: evidence for a dose-response relationship. Am. J. Clin. Nutr. **53:** 90–94.
5. ZHAO, Z. & A.C. ROSS. 1995. Retinoic acid repletion restores the number of leukocytes and their subsets and stimulates natural cytotoxicity in vitamin A-deficient rats. J. Nutr. **125:** 2064–2073.

6. HUSSEY, G., J. HUGHES, S. POTGIETER, *et al.* 1996. Vitamin A status and supplementation and its effects on immunity in children with AIDS. *In* XVII International Vitamin A Consultative Group Meeting, Guatemala City, Guatemala. International Life Sciences Institute, Human Nutrition Institute, p. 81.

7. FAWZI, W.W., T.C. CHALMERS, M.G. HERRERA & F. MOSTELLER. 1993. Vitamin A supplementation and child mortality: a meta-analysis. JAMA **269:** 898–903.

8. MEYDANI, S.N., J.D. RIBAYA-MERCADO, R.M. RUSSELL, *et al.* 1991. Vitamin B-6 deficiency impairs interleukin 2 production and lymphocyte proliferation in elderly adults. Am J. Clin. Nutr. **53:** 1275–1280.

9. BAUM, M.K., E. MANTERO-ATIENZA, G. SHOR-POSNER, *et al.* 1991. Association of vitamin B-6 status with parameters of immune function in early HIV-1 infection. J. Acquir. Immune Defic. Syndr. **4:** 1122–1132.

10. BENDICH, A. & M. COHEN. 1988. B vitamins: effects on specific and nonspecific immune responses. *In* Nutrition and Immunology. R.K. Chandra, Ed.: 101–123. Alan R. Liss, Inc. New York.

11. BENDICH, A. 1988. Antioxidant vitamins and immune responses. *In* Nutrition and Immunology. R.K. Chandra, Ed.: 125–147. Alan R. Liss, Inc. New York.

12. HEMILA, H. 1997. Vitamin C and infectious diseases. *In* Vitamin C in Health and Disease. L. Pacler & J. Fuchs, Eds. Marcel Dekker, Inc. New York.

13. WINKLOHOFER-ROOB, B.M., H. ELLEMUNTER, M. FRÜHWIRTH, *et al.* 1997. Plasma vitamin C concentrations in patients with cystic fibrosis: evidence of associations with lung inflammation. Am. J. Clin. Nutr. **65:** 1858–1866.

14. MEYDANI, S.N., D. WU, M.S. SANTOS & M.G. HAYEK. 1995. Antioxidants and immune response in the aged: overview of present evidence. Am. J. Clin. Nutr. **62**(Suppl.): 1462S–1476S.

15. MEYDANI, S.N., M. MEYDANI, J.B. BLUMBERG, *et al.* 1997. Vitamin E supplementation enhances in vivo immune response in healthy elderly: a dose–response study. JAMA **277:** 1380–1386.

16. MEYDANI, S.N., P.M. BARKLUND, S. LIU, *et al.* 1990. Effect of vitamin E supplementation on immune responsiveness of healthy elderly subjects. Am. J. Clin. Nutr. **52:** 557–563.

17. WANG, Y., D.S. HUANG, B. LIANG & R.R. WATSON. 1994. Nutritional status and immune responses in mice with murine AIDS are normalized by vitamin E supplementation. J. Nutr. **124:** 2024-2032.

18. SHANKAR, A.H. & A.S. PRASAD. 1998. Zinc and immune function: the biological basis of altered resistance to infection. Am. J. Clin. Nutr. **68**(Suppl.): 447S–463S.

19. BLACK, R.E. 1998. Therapeutic and preventive effects of zinc on serious childhood infectious diseases in developing countries. Am. J. Clin. Nutr. **68**(Suppl.): 476S–479S.

20. GARLAND, M., M.J. STAMPFER, W.C. WILLETT & D.J. HUNTER. 1994. The epidemiology of selenium and human cancer. *In* Natural Antioxidants in Human Health and Disease. Academic Press. San Diego, CA. pp. 263–286.

21. KIREMIDJIAN-SCHUMACHER, L. & G. STOTZKY. 1987. Selenium and immune responses. Environ. Res. **42:** 277–303.

22. PERETZ, A., J. NEVE, J. DUCHATEAU, *et al.* 1991. Effects of selenium supplementation on immune parameters in gut failure patients on home parenteral nutrition. Nutrition **7:** 215–221.

23. ABRAMS, B., D. DUNCAN & I. HERTZ-PICCIOTTO. 1993. A prospective study of dietary intake and acquired immune deficiency syndrome in HIV-seropositive homosexual men. J. Acquir. Immune Defic. Syndr. **6:** 949–958.

24. TANG, A.M., N.M.H. GRAHAM, A.J. KIRBY, *et al.* 1993. Dietary micronutrient intake and risk progression to acquired immunodeficiency syndrome (AIDS) in human immunodeficiency virus type 1 (HIV-1)-infected homosexual men. Am. J. Epidemiol. **138:** 1–15.

25. TANG, A.M., N.M.H. GRAHAM & A.J. SAAH. 1996. Effects of micronutrient intake on survival in human immunodeficiency virus type 1 infection. Am. J. Epidemiol. **143:** 1244–1256.

26. KANTER, A.S., D.C. SPENCER, M.H. STEINBERG, *et al.* 1999. Supplemental vitamin B and progression to AIDS and death in black South African patients infected with HIV. J. Acquir. Immune Defic. Syndr. **21:** 252–253.

27. SEMBA, R.D., W.T. CAIAFFA, N.M.H. GRAHAM, *et al.* 1994. Vitamin A deficiency and wasting as predictors of mortality in human immunodeficiency virus-infected injection drug users. J. Infect. Dis. **171:** 1196–1202.
28. SEMBA, R.D., N.M.H. GRAHAM, W.T. CAIAFFA, *et al.* 1993. Increased mortality associated with vitamin A deficiency during human immunodeficiency virus type 1 infection. Arch. Intern. Med. **153:** 2149–2154.
29. BAUM, M.K., G. SHOR-POSNER, Y. LU, *et al.* 1995. Micronutrients and HIV-1 disease progression. AIDS **9:** 1051–1056.
30. TANG, A.M., N.M.H. GRAHAM, R.D. SEMBA & A.J. SAAH. 1997. Association between serum vitamin A and E levels and HIV-1 disease progression. AIDS **11:** 613–620.
31. TANG, A.M., N.M.H. GRAHAM, R.K. CHANDRA & A.J. SAAH. 1997. Low serum vitamin B-12 concentrations are associated with faster human immunodeficiency virus type 1 (HIV-1) disease progression. J. Nutr. **127:** 345–351.
32. BAUM, M.K., G. SHOR-POSNER, S. LAI, *et al.* 1997. High risk of HIV-related mortality is associated with selenium deficiency. J. Acquir. Immune Defic. Syndr. Hum. Retrovirol. **15:** 370–374.
33. GRAHAM, N., D. SORENSEN, N. ODAKA, *et al.* 1991. Relationship of serum copper and zinc levels to HIV-1 seropositivity and progression to AIDS. J. Acquir. Immune Defic. Syndr. **4:** 976–980.
34. COODLEY, G.O., H.D. NELSON, M.O. LOVELESS & C. FOLK. 1993. β-Carotene in HIV infection. J. Acquir. Immune Defic. Syndr. **6:** 272–276.
35. COODLEY, G.O., M.K. COODLEY, R. LUSK, *et al.* 1996. β-Carotene in HIV infection: an extended evaluation. AIDS **10:** 967–973.
36. FAWZI, W.W., G.I. MSAMANGA, D. SPIEGELMAN, *et al.* for the TANZANIA VITAMIN AND HIV INFECTION TRIAL TEAM. 1998. Randomized trial of effects of vitamin supplements on pregnancy outcomes and T cell counts in HIV-1-infected women in Tanzania. Lancet **351:** 1477–1482.
37. COUTSOUDIS, A., D. MOODLEY, K. PILLAY, *et al.* 1997. Effect of vitamin A supplementation on viral load in HIV-1 infected pregnant women. J. Acquir. Immune Defic. Syndr. **15:** 86–87.
38. SEMBA, R.D., C.M. LYLES, J.B. MARGOLICK, *et al.* 1998. Vitamin A supplementation and human immunodeficiency virus load in injection drug users. J. Infect. Dis. **177:** 611–616.
39. ALLARD, J.P., E. AGHDASSI, J. CHAU, *et al.* 1998. Effects of vitamin E and C supplementation on oxidative stress and viral load in HIV-infected subjects. AIDS **12:** 1653–1659.
40. NOBACK, C.R. & Y.I. TAKAHASHI. 1978. Micromorphology of the placenta of rats reared on marginal vitamin-A-deficient diet. Acta Anat. **102:** 195–202.
41. WABWIRE-MANGEN, F., R.H. GRAY, F.A. MMIRO, *et al.* 1999. Placental membrane inflammation and risks of maternal-to-child transmission of HIV-1 in Uganda. J. Acquir. Immune Defic. Syndr. **22:** 379–385.
42. GOLDENBERG, R.L., S.H. VERMUND, A.R. GOEPFERT & W.W. ANDREWS. 1998. Choriodecidual inflammation: a potentially preventable cause of perinatal HIV-1 transmission? Lancet **352:** 1927–1930.
43. WOLBACH, S.B. & R. HOWE PERCY. 1925. Tissue changes following deprivation of fat-soluble A vitamin. J. Exp. Med. **42:** 753–777.
44. KAHN, R.H. 1954. Effect of locally applied vitamin A and estrogen on the rat vagina. Am. J. Anat. **95:** 309–328.
45. ANDERSON, D.J., J.A. POLITCH, L.D. TUCKER, *et al.* 1998. Quantitation of mediators of inflammation and immunity in genital tract secretion and their relevance to HIV type 1 transmission. AIDS Res. Hum. Retrovir. **14**(Suppl.): S43–S49.
46. JOHN, G.C., R.W. NDUATI, D. MBORI-NGACHA, *et al.* 1997. Genital shedding of human immunodeficiency virus type 1 DNA during pregnancy: association with immunosuppression, abnormal cervical or vaginal discharge, and severe vitamin A deficiency. J. Infect. Dis. **175:** 57–62.
47. MOSTAD, S.B., J. OVERBAUGH, D.M. DEVANGE, *et al.* 1997. Hormonal contraception, vitamin A deficiency, and other risk factors for shedding of HIV-1 infected cells from the cervix and vagina. Lancet **350:** 922–927.

48. SWART, P.J., E.M. KUIPERS, C. SMIT, *et al.* 1998. Lactoferrin. Antiviral activity of lactoferrin. Adv. Exp. Med. Biol. **443:** 205–213.
49. NEWBURG, D.S., R.J. LINHARDT, S.A. AMPOFO & R.H. YOLKEN. 1995. Human milk glycosaminoglycans inhibit HIV glycoprotein gp120 binding to its host cell CD4 receptor. J. Nutr. **125:** 419–424.
50. MCNEELY, T.B., D.C. SHUGARS, M. ROSENDAHL, C. TUCKER, *et al.* 1997. Inhibition of human immunodeficiency virus type 1 infectivity by secretory leukocyte protease inhibitor occurs prior to viral reverse transcription. Blood **90:** 1141–1149.
51. EMMETT, P.M. & I.S. ROGERS. 1997. Properties of human milk and their relationship with maternal nutrition. Early Hum. Dev. **49**(Suppl.): S7–S28.
52. SEMBA, R.D., N. KUMWENDA, D.R. HOOVER, *et al.* 1999. Human immunodeficiency virus load in breast milk, mastitis, and mother-to-child transmission of human immunodeficiency virus type 1. J. Infect. Dis. **180:** 93–98.
53. SEMBA, R.D., N. KUMWENDA, T.E. TAHA, *et al.* 1999. Mastitis and immunological factors in breast milk of lactating women in Malawi. Clin. Diagn. Lab. Immunol. **6:** 671–674.
54. FILTEAU, S.M., G. LIETZ, G. MULOKOZI, *et al.* 1999. Milk cytokines and subclinical breast inflammation in Tanzanian women: effects of dietary red palm oil or sunflower oil supplementation. Immunology **97:** 595–600.
55. FILTEAU, S.M., A.L. RICE, J.J. BALL, *et al.* 1999. Breast milk immune factors in Bangladeshi women supplemented postpartum with retinol or β-carotene. Am. J. Clin. Nutr. **69:** 953–958.
56. SEMBA, R.D. & M.C. NEVILLE. 1999. Breast-feeding, mastitis, and HIV transmission: nutritional implications. Nutr. Rev. **57:** 146–153.
57. NDUATI, R.W., G.C. JOHN, B.A. RICHARDSON, *et al.* 1995. Human immunodeficiency virus type-1 infected cells in breast milk: association with immunosuppression and vitamin A deficiency. J. Infect. Dis. **172:** 1461–1468.
58. SCHOLL, T.O., M.L. HEDIGER, A. BENDICH, *et al.* 1997. Use of multivitamin/mineral prenatal supplements: influence on the outcome of pregnancy. Am. J. Epidemiol. **146:** 134–141.
59. WEST, K.P., J. KATZ, S.K. KHATRY, *et al.* 1999. Double blind, cluster randomized trial of low dose supplementation of vitamin A or β-carotene on mortality related to pregnancy in Nepal. Br. Med. J. **318:** 570–575.
60. DREYFUSS, M., K.J. WEST, J. KATZ, *et al.* 1997. Effect of maternal vitamin A or β-carotene supplementation on intrauterine/early infant growth in Nepal. *In* XVIII International Vitamin A Consultative Group Meeting, Cairo, Egypt. International Life Sciences Institute, p. 104.
61. STOLTZFUS, R. & R. KLEMM. 1998. Sustainable control of vitamin A deficiency: Defining progress through assessment, surveillance, evaluation. *In* XVIII International Vitamin A Consultative Group Meeting, Cairo, Egypt. International Life Sciences Institute, pp. 1–139.
62. COUTSOUDIS, A., K. PILLAY, E. SPOONER, *et al.* 1999. Randomized trial testing the effect of vitamin A supplementation on pregnancy outcomes and early mother-to-child HIV-1 transmission in Durban, South Africa. AIDS **13:** 1517–1524.
63. GOLDENBERG, R.L., T. TAMURA, Y. NEGGERS, *et al.* 1995. The effect of zinc supplementation on pregnancy outcome. JAMA **274:** 463–468.
64. CAULFIELD, F.E., N. ZAVALETA, A. FIGUEROA & Z. LEON. 1999. Maternal zinc supplementation does not affect size at birth or pregnancy duration in Peru. J. Nutr. **129:** 1563–1568.
65. MCCULLOUGH, F.S.W., C.A. NORTHROP-CLEWES & D.I. THURNHAM. 1999. The effect of vitamin A on epithelial integrity. Proc. Nutr. Soc. **58:** 289–293.
66. ROY, S.K., R.H. BEHRENS, R. HAIDER, *et al.* 1992. Impact of zinc supplementation on intestinal permeability in Bangladeshi children with acute diarrhoea and persistent diarrhoea syndrome. J. Pediatr. Gastroenterol. Nutr. **15:** 289–296.
67. KEREN, D.F. 1988. Intestinal mucosal immune defense mechanisms. Am. J. Surg. Pathol. **12**(Suppl. 1): 100–105.
68. KAKAI, R., J.J. BWAYO, I.A. WAMOLA, *et al.* 1995. Effect of human immunodeficiency virus on local immunity in children with diarrhoea. E. Afr. Med. J. **72:** 699–702.

69. CHANDRA, R.K. & M. WADHWA. 1989. Nutritional modulation of intestinal mucosal immunity. Immunol. Invest. **18:** 119–126.
70. SEMBA, R.D., P.G. MIOTTI, J.D. CHIPANGWI, *et al.* 1994. Maternal vitamin A deficiency and mother-to-child transmission of HIV-1. Lancet **343:** 1593–1597.
71. SEMBA, R.D., P.G. MIOTTI, J.D. CHIPANGWI, *et al.* 1995. Infant mortality and maternal vitamin A deficiency during human immunodeficiency virus infection. Clin. Infect. Dis. **21:** 966–972.
72. GRAHAM, N., M. BULTERYS, A. CHAO, *et al.* 1993. Effect of maternal vitamin A deficiency on infant mortality and perinatal HIV transmission. National Conference on Human Retroviruses and Related Infection, Baltimore, MD, December 12–16.
73. GREENBERG, B.L., R.D. SEMBA, P.E. VINK, *et al.* 1997. Vitamin A deficiency and maternal–infant transmission of HIV in two metropolitan areas in the United States. AIDS **11:** 325–332.
74. BURNS, D.N. *et al.* 1999. Vitamin A deficiency and other nutritional indices during pregnancy in human immunodeficiency virus infection: prevalence, clinical correlates, and outcome. Women and Infants Transmission Study Group. Clin. Infect. Dis. **29:** 328–334.
75. BURGER, H., A. KOVACS, B. WEISTER, *et al.* 1997. Maternal serum vitamin A levels are not associated with mother-to-child transmission of HIV-1 in the United States. J. Acquir. Immunodef. Syndr. Hum. Retrovirol. **14:** 321–326.
76. SEMBA, R. 1998. Nutritional Interventions: vitamin A and breastfeeding. III International Symposium: Global strategies to Prevent Perinatal HIV Transmission. Valencia, Spain, Nov. 9–10.
77. FAWZI, W., G. MSAMANGA, D. HUNTER, *et al.* 2000. Randomized trial of vitamin supplements in relation to vertical transmission of HIV-1 in Tanzania. J. Aquir. Immune Defic. Syndr. **23:** 246–254.
78. COMMISSION ON LIFE SCIENCES. NATIONAL RESEARCH COUNCIL. 1989. Recommended Dietary Allowances. 10th edit. Subcommittee on the tenth edition of the RDAs. Food and Nutrition Board. National Academy Press. Washington, DC.
79. BEACH, R.S., M.E. GERSHWIN & L.S. HURLEY. 1982. Gestational zinc deprivation in mice: persistence of immunodeficiency for three generations. Science **218:** 469–471.
80. COUTSOUDIS, A., R.A. BOBA, H.M. COOVADIA, *et al.* 1995. The effects of vitamin A supplementation on the morbidity of children born to HIV-infected women. Am. J. Pub. Health **85:** 1076–1081.
81. FAWZI, W.W., R.L. MBISE, E. HERTZMARK, *et al.* 1999. A randomized trial of vitamin A supplements in relation to mortality among HIV infected and uninfected children in Tanzania. Pediatr. Infect. Dis. J. **18:** 127–133.
82. GUAY, L.A., P. MUSOKE, T. FLEMING, *et al.* 1999. Intrapartum and neonatal single-dose nevirapine compared with zidovudine for prevention of mother-to-child transmission of HIV-1 in Kampala, Uganda: HIVNET 012 randomized trial. Lancet **354:** 795–802.
83. MOFENSON, L.M. 1999. Short course zidovudine for prevention of perinatal infection. Lancet **353:** 766–767.

Cesarean Section Delivery to Prevent Vertical Transmission of Human Immunodeficiency Virus Type 1

Associated Risks and Other Considerations

JENNIFER S. READ[a]

Pediatric, Adolescent, and Maternal AIDS Branch, National Institute of Child Health and Human Development, Bethesda, Maryland 20892-7510, USA

ABSTRACT: Delivery by elective cesarean section (ECS), cesarean section prior to labor and rupture of membranes, is associated with a lower rate of vertical transmission of HIV compared with other modes of delivery. The efficacy of ECS among women receiving combination antiretroviral therapy or among women with low viral loads is unknown. In assessing the possible utility of ECS as an intervention to decrease vertical transmission in the United States and other countries, the potential risks associated with operative delivery as well as other considerations should also be addressed. Although cesarean section delivery is associated with an increased rate of postpartum morbidity compared with vaginal delivery in the general population, operative delivery performed emergently carries a higher risk of complications than scheduled or elective procedures. Analyses of the risk of postpartum morbidity according to mode of delivery among HIV-infected women have been performed in the Women and Infants Transmission Study (WITS), the largest database in North America with relevant data, as well as other, smaller databases. These analyses suggest a similar pattern to that observed in the general population. In addition to quantifying the incidence of postpartum morbidity events, it is also important to distinguish between minor and major morbidity. Neonatal morbidity related to ECS is generally due to iatrogenic preterm birth, that is, situations where the gestational age is not accurately assessed prior to delivery. Occupationally acquired HIV infection related to obstetric procedures is a possibility, although risk related to mode of delivery is unknown. The results of economic analyses of ECS compared to vaginal delivery in the US indicate that ECS is a cost-effective intervention in preventing vertical transmission of HIV among women who refrain from breastfeeding. However, more precise estimates of the risk of vertical transmission among women receiving combination antiretroviral therapy and of the potential risks of maternal and pediatric adverse events related to receipt of such therapy are needed. In summary, the benefit of ECS must be weighed against potential risks, and issues such as cost-effectiveness also should be taken into consideration.

[a]Address for correspondence: Jennifer S. Read, MD, MS, MPH, Pediatric, Adolescent, and Maternal AIDS (PAMA) Branch, National Institute of Child Health and Human Development (NICHD), National Institutes of Health (NIH), Executive Building, Room 4B11F, 6100 Executive Boulevard MSC 7510, Bethesda, MD 20892-7510. Fax: 301-496-8678.

jr92o@nih.gov

INTRODUCTION

Cesarean section delivery before the onset of labor and rupture of membranes (elective cesarean section, ECS) is associated with a decreased likelihood of vertical transmission of human immunodeficiency virus type 1 (HIV).[1,2] Based in large part on these findings, the American College of Obstetricians and Gynecologists' Committee on Obstetric Practice recently recommended that HIV-infected women be offered elective, or scheduled, cesarean section delivery to reduce the risk of vertical transmission of HIV.[3] However, the benefit of ECS with regard to mother-infant transmission of HIV must be weighed against possible deleterious effects of surgical delivery.[2,4,5] In addition, the cost-effectiveness of cesarean section to prevent vertical transmission of HIV should be considered.[6]

CESAREAN SECTION DELIVERY AND VERTICAL TRANSMISSION OF HIV

Vertical transmission of HIV occurs in large part during the intrapartum period,[7] through any of several possible mechanisms.[8,9] Thus, it had been postulated that cesarean section performed prior to the onset of labor and rupture of membranes could decrease the risk of vertical transmission. As previously described,[1] initial European studies suggested an association between mode of delivery and vertical transmission of HIV, but such an association was not demonstrated in other studies, and meta-analyses of the literature could neither distinguish between elective and non-elective cesarean section deliveries nor control for potential confounding variables.

In the absence of data from the then uncompleted randomized clinical trial of mode of delivery and vertical transmission of HIV,[2] an international collaborative effort to perform a meta-analysis of individual patient data from prospective cohort studies in order to evaluate the relation between ECS and vertical transmission of HIV was initiated.[1] Prospective cohort studies of at least 100 mother-child pairs, with data on mode of delivery and children's infection status from regions where HIV-infected women are advised not to breastfeed, were eligible for inclusion. Mothers or infants enrolled after the first 7 days of the child's life were excluded, as were mothers not known to be HIV-infected on or before the date of the child's birth, multiple gestation births, and children known to have been breastfed. Cesarean sections performed before rupture of membranes and onset of labor were termed elective, and those performed after rupture of membranes and/or after onset of labor were referred to as non-elective. Instrumented and non-instrumented vaginal deliveries were those performed with and without forceps and/or vacuum suction, respectively.

Individual patient data from 5 European and 10 North American studies were analyzed. The primary analysis dataset was restricted to data regarding those mothers with known subtype of cesarean section (elective or non-elective) or with vaginal delivery, to those children with known HIV infection status (infected or uninfected), and to the older (or oldest) child when there were younger siblings in the dataset; 8,533 mother-child pairs were eligible for inclusion in the primary analysis. The crude odds ratio for the relation between ECS and the infection status of the child were calculated for each study cohort, and these individual odds ratios were then pooled to create a summary estimate of the common odds ratio. This summary odds ratio was 0.45, indicating an approximately 50% lower risk of vertical transmission of HIV with ECS compared to other modes of delivery. Multivariate logistic regression modeling, with adjustment for receipt of antiretroviral therapy, advanced maternal disease, and infant birth weight, continued to demonstrate a significantly lower risk of vertical transmission among women delivering via ECS [adjusted odds ratio = 0.43 (95% confidence interval: 0.33, 0.56)].

In a subanalysis examining the relation between mode of delivery and vertical transmission after stratification according to receipt of antiretroviral therapy, the likelihood of transmission with both ECS and receipt of antiretroviral therapy during the antepartum, intrapartum, and postnatal periods (likely zidovudine prophylaxis) was reduced by approximately 87% compared to other modes of delivery and no receipt of antiretroviral therapy [adjusted odds ratio = 0.13 (95% confidence interval: 0.09, 0.18)]. Transmission rates were decreased with ECS versus other modes of delivery in both groups. Transmission rates (in percent) with 95% confidence intervals were as follows: without antiretroviral therapy [10.4 (7.8, 12.9) versus 19.0 (17.9, 20.0), respectively] and with antiretroviral therapy during the antepartum, intrapartum, and postnatal periods [2.0 (0.0, 4.0) versus 7.3 (5.9, 8.8), respectively].

In the randomized clinical trial of mode of delivery,[2] patients were enrolled in the trial at 34–36 weeks of gestation if HIV infection was confirmed. HIV-infected, pregnant women were ineligible for enrollment if there was an obstetric indication for cesarean section or a contraindication for ECS. If assigned to ECS, surgery was scheduled for 38 weeks' gestation. It was the clinician's decision as to the medical management of patients, including whether or not it was necessary to change the mode of delivery. If the onset of labor occurred before 38 weeks' gestation, cesarean section was undertaken if labor was diagnosed before the second stage. Prophylactic antibiotic therapy was administered for all cesarean section deliveries, with the exact choice of antibiotic the clinician's decision. If assigned to vaginal delivery, spontaneous labor was awaited unless a clinical decision to perform cesarean section was made. Enrollment in the study occurred from 1993–1998. Data regarding 408 women and 370 infants were available for the analyses. None of the women enrolled in this trial breastfed their infants.

Vertical transmission rates according to mode of delivery were determined for both the allocated and the actual modes of delivery. According to the allocated mode of delivery, the transmission rates were significantly higher among women assigned to vaginal delivery rather than ECS (10.5% versus 1.8%, $p < 0.001$). Similar results were obtained when examining actual mode of delivery: 10.2% transmission among vaginal deliveries versus 2.4% among ECS deliveries. Vertical transmission rates according to actual mode of delivery then were stratified by receipt of zidovudine prophylaxis and by maternal CD4+ lymphocyte count. The results of these analyses suggested that the risk of transmission among women undergoing ECS persisted despite zidovudine prophylaxis and in different CD4+ count strata.

Both the individual patient data meta-analysis and the randomized clinical trial indicate the risk of vertical transmission is significantly lower among HIV-infected women who deliver via ECS than among those without such a mode of delivery. Both of these studies evaluated the relation between mode of delivery and vertical transmission in populations of HIV-infected women receiving either no antiretroviral therapy or known or likely zidovudine monotherapy or prophylaxis. HIV-infected women receiving more potent antiretroviral therapy would be expected to have significantly decreased viral loads, and lower maternal viral loads are associated with a lower risk of vertical transmission.[10,11] A question that could not be addressed in either study is whether a lower risk of vertical transmission among women with ECS persists irrespective of maternal viral load. However, more recent data indicate that cesarean section is associated with a lower risk of vertical transmission of HIV even after controlling for viral load.[12] In another study,[13] the lower risk of vertical transmission among women delivering via ECS remained despite stratification according to maternal viral load.

MODE OF DELIVERY AND POSTPARTUM MORBIDITY AMONG HIV-INFECTED WOMEN

Among women without HIV infection, cesarean section delivery has been associated with increased maternal morbidity compared to nonsurgical deliveries.[14–16] However, such associations are subject to confounding by indication, in that often the fetal or maternal indications for cesarean section themselves are associated with postoperative maternal morbidity. Of note, ECS is associated with a lower risk of maternal complications than is emergency cesarean section.[17]

Although HIV-infected women are expected to be at greater risk of postpartum morbidity, especially infectious morbidity, because of the immunosuppression associated with HIV infection, extrapolation of data regarding the risk of postpartum morbidity among women without HIV infection to HIV-infected women must be approached with caution for the following reasons. Many studies of postpartum morbidity among uninfected women were published prior to improvements in medical and obstetric practices over the last several years. Therefore, postpartum morbidity rates reported in such studies are likely to be higher than those observed in current clinical practice. Even in more recent studies, important differences exist in the characteristics of study populations, especially with regard to characteristics associated with the risk of postpartum morbidity aside from HIV infection per se. Also, definitions used for different types of postpartum morbidity vary, sometimes substantially, from study to study, making interstudy comparisons problematic.

Only extremely limited information has been available on the relation between mode of delivery and subsequent maternal morbidity among HIV-infected women. The published literature on postpartum morbidity among HIV-infected women has been sparse, and virtually all analyses published to date have been performed with small study populations. In a study of postpartum morbidity following cesarean section in Italy, 156 HIV-infected and the same number of uninfected women were evaluated.[4] Six major complications were observed (sepsis, severe anemia, pleural effusion, and pneumonia), with HIV-infected women more likely to experience minor complications (fever, endometritis, and wound and urinary tract infections). Among HIV-infected women, a low CD4+ lymphocyte count was the only factor associated with an increased rate of complications. In the randomized clinical trial of mode of delivery,[2] postpartum fever was more common among women who delivered via cesarean section (6.7%) versus vaginal delivery (1.1%) ($p = 0.002$). Postpartum bleeding or intravascular coagulation occurred following one vaginal delivery and one cesarean section delivery. Severe anemia (hemoglobin < 8 g/dL) was reported following six deliveries (two vaginal and four cesarean sections).

The Women and Infants Transmission Study (WITS) is the largest prospective cohort study in North America in which postpartum morbidity data concerning HIV-infected women are routinely collected. WITS is an ongoing, multicenter, prospective cohort study of HIV-infected women and their children. The study began in 1989 and is conducted at pediatric and obstetric outpatient clinics at medical centers in Illinois (Chicago), New York City (Manhattan and Brooklyn), Massachusetts (Boston- Worcester area), Texas (Houston), and Puerto Rico (San Juan). The study's objectives are to describe the natural history of HIV infection among pregnant women and their children and to identify factors associated with both disease progression among mothers and their HIV-infected children and vertical transmission of HIV. Women are enrolled into WITS at any time during pregnancy. Data on the following types of postpartum morbidity are collected in WITS: endometritis, mastitis, urinary tract infection, pneumonia, cesarean section incision or episiotomy infection and dehiscence, clinically significant hemorrhage or severe anemia, and febrile morbidity.

WITS investigators are analyzing the relations between mode of delivery and postpartum morbidity, length of hospitalization following delivery, and rehospitalization within the postpartum period, and preliminary results have been reported.[5] The study population for these analyses will include almost 1,200 HIV-infected women, with data regarding postpartum morbidity collected at two time points: during the delivery hospitalization (primarily through medical record abstraction but also by maternal interview), and at the 8-week postpartum clinic visit (primarily through maternal interview but also via medical record abstraction).

Counseling of HIV-infected pregnant women regarding ECS as a possible intervention to decrease maternal-infant transmission of HIV should include discussion of these results, as well as new data as they become available, regarding the incidence and severity of postpartum morbidity events. Scheduled cesarean section deliveries are generally performed at 39 completed weeks of gestation. However, the American College of Obstetricians and Gynecologists recommends that if cesarean section is performed for prevention of vertical transmission of HIV, delivery be performed at 38 completed weeks of gestation in order to decrease the chances of ruptured membranes or labor onset before delivery.[3] Neonatal morbidity related to ECS generally would be expected to be due to iatrogenic preterm birth, that is, situations where the gestational age is not accurately assessed prior to delivery and delivery occurs earlier than recommended. Finally, as cesarean sections are surgical procedures and more invasive than vaginal delivery, an argument can be made that health care providers would be at higher risk of HIV infection performing cesarean sections than vaginal deliveries. Alternatively, one could postulate that a scheduled, relatively controlled surgical procedure would have a lower risk of accidental transmission of HIV than would a vaginal delivery. However, although occupationally acquired HIV infection related to obstetric procedures is a possibility,[18,19] the risk related to mode of delivery is unknown.

COST-EFFECTIVENESS OF CESAREAN SECTION TO PREVENT VERTICAL TRANSMISSION OF HIV

Estimation of the potential overall costs and the cost per case of pediatric HIV infection avoided with ECS would assist in the development of clinical and public health guidelines regarding the role of cesarean section in preventing vertical transmission of HIV. A cost-effectiveness analysis from the United Kingdom did evaluate cesarean section delivery,[20] but this analysis was performed before completion of recent studies quantifying more precisely than previously possible the relation between mode of delivery and vertical transmission of HIV.[1,2]

Analyses evaluating the cost-effectiveness and cost-benefit of ECS compared to vaginal delivery to prevent vertical transmission of HIV in the US have been performed, and preliminary results have been described.[6] In individual- and population-based analyses, costs and outcomes of cesarean section versus vaginal delivery were assessed among HIV-infected pregnant women receiving no antiretroviral therapy, zidovudine prophylaxis, or combination antiretroviral therapy. Costs of interventions to prevent vertical transmission (mode of delivery and antiretroviral therapy), of postpartum morbidity, and of pediatric care were evaluated. Model outcomes were cases of vertical transmission avoided, years of the child's life saved, and dollars saved by avoiding vertical transmission of HIV.

ECS resulted in fewer HIV cases and decreased costs compared to vaginal delivery among women receiving no antiretroviral therapy during pregnancy. Among women receiving zidovudine prophylaxis or combination antiretroviral therapy, ECS resulted in fewer cases and, despite increased costs, was highly cost-effective. Results of the cost-effectiveness analyses were sensitive to HIV transmission rates according to mode of delivery and to pediatric care costs. Hypothetically, for the entire population of HIV-infected pregnant women in the US, use of ECS instead of vaginal delivery would prevent hundreds of pediatric HIV infections annually and would be cost saving.

The results of this study indicate that ECS is a cost-effective intervention to prevent vertical transmission among HIV-infected women receiving various antiretroviral therapy regimens. To refine and improve upon the economic estimates presented in this analysis, further research is needed. Most importantly, evaluation of the effectiveness of different antiretroviral regimens in preventing vertical transmission and of the possible maternal and pediatric adverse events related to exposure to such therapy is essential. Different antiretroviral therapy regimens could have different effects on vertical transmission as well as types and rates of complications and treatment costs. If vertical transmission rates with antiretroviral therapy were 0%, ECS would only increase costs and not improve outcomes. As more precise data are collected, threshold analyses should be performed to evaluate the conditions under which ECS remains cost-effective. However, based on the findings of this study, ECS is likely to remain a cost-effective intervention over a wide range of possible clinical and economic scenarios.

SUMMARY

Clinical decision-making regarding the management of the HIV-infected pregnant woman must balance the risks and benefits of ECS as well as the risks and benefits of other potential interventions to lower the risk of mother-to-child transmission of HIV. HIV-infected pregnant women should be given the opportunity to make informed decisions regarding all available interventions, including ECS, to prevent transmission of infection to their children.

REFERENCES

1. THE INTERNATIONAL PERINATAL HIV GROUP. 1999. The mode of delivery and the risk of vertical transmission of human immunodeficiency virus type 1: a meta-analysis of 15 prospective cohort studies. N. Engl. J. Med. **340:** 977–987.
2. THE EUROPEAN MODE OF DELIVERY COLLABORATION. 1999. Elective caesarean section versus vaginal delivery in preventing vertical HIV-1 transmission: a randomised clinical trial. Lancet **353:** 1035–1037.
3. AMERICAN COLLEGE OF OBSTETRICIANS AND GYNECOLOGISTS. 1999. Scheduled cesarean delivery and the prevention of vertical transmission of HIV infection. ACOG Committee Opinion Number 219. Washington, DC. ACOG.
4. SEMPRINI, A.E., C. CASTAGNA, M. RAVIZZA *et al.* 1995. The incidence of complications after caesarean section in 156 HIV-positive women. AIDS **9:** 913–917.
5. READ, J., E. KPAMEGAN, R. TUOMALA *et al.* 1999. Mode of delivery and postpartum morbidity among HIV-infected women: The Women and Infants Transmission Study (WITS). Abstracts of the Sixth Conference on Retroviruses and Opportunistic Infections, Chicago, January 31 – February 4, 1999 [abstr. 683].
6. HALPERN, M.T., J.S. READ, D. GANOCZY & D. HARRIS. 2000. Cost-effectiveness of cesarean section delivery to prevent mother-to-child transmission of HIV-1. AIDS **14:** 691–700.
7. ROUZIOUX, C., D. COSTAGLIOLA, M. BURGARD *et al.* 1995. Estimated timing of mother-to-child human immunodeficiency virus type 1 (HIV-1) transmission by use of a Markov model. Am. J. Epidemiol. **142:** 1330–1337.
8. MOFENSON, L.M. 1997. Mother-child HIV-1 transmission: timing and determinants. Obstet. Gynecol. Clin. North Am. **24:** 759–784.
9. KUHN, L. & Z.A. STEIN. 1995. Mother-to-infant HIV transmission: timing, risk factors and prevention. Paediatr. Perinat. Epidemiol. **9:** 1–29.
10. MOFENSON, L.M., J.S. LAMBERT, E.R. STIEHM *et al.* 1999. Risk factors for perinatal transmission of human immunodeficiency virus type 1 in women treated with zidovudine. N. Engl. J. Med. **341:** 385–393.
11. GARCIA, P.M., L.A. KALISH, J. PITT *et al.* 1999. Maternal levels of plasma immunodeficiency virus type 1 RNA and the risk of perinatal transmission. N. Engl. J. Med. **341:** 394–402.
12. SHAFFER, N., A. ROONGPISUTHIPONG, W. SIRIWASIN *et al.* 1999. Maternal viral load and perinatal HIV-1 subtype E transmission, Thailand. J. Infect. Dis. **179:** 590–599.
13. THE EUROPEAN COLLABORATIVE STUDY. 1999. Maternal viral load and vertical transmission of HIV-1: an important factor but not the only one. AIDS **13:** 1377–1385.
14. NATIONAL INSTITUTE OF CHILD HEALTH AND HUMAN DEVELOPMENT (NICHD). 1981. Cesarean Childbirth: Report of a Consensus Development Conference. Bethesda, MD. National Institutes of Health.
15. MILLER, J.M. 1988. Maternal and neonatal morbidity and mortality in cesarean section. Obstet. Gynecol. Clin. North Am. **15:** 629–638.
16. PETITTI, D.B. 1985. Maternal mortality and morbidity in cesarean section. Clin. Obstet. Gynecol. **28:** 763–769.
17. VAN HAM, M., P. VAN DONGEN & J. MULDER. 1997. Maternal consequences of caesarean section: a retrospective study of intra-operative and postoperative maternal complications of caesarean section during a 10-year period. Eur. J. Obstet. Gynecol. Reprod. Biol. **74:** 1–6.
18. IPPOLITO, G., V. PURO, J. HEPTONSTALL *et al.* 1999. Occupational human immunodeficiency virus infection in health care workers: worldwide cases through September 1997. Clin. Infect. Dis. **28:** 365–383.
19. CENTERS FOR DISEASE CONTROL AND PREVENTION. HIV/AIDS Surveillance Report, 1998. **10:** 1–43.
20. RATCLIFFE, J., A.E. ADES, D. GIBB *et al.* 1998. Prevention of mother-to-child transmission of HIV-1 infection: alternative strategies and their cost-effectiveness. AIDS **12:** 1381–1388.

Breast Milk Transmission of HIV-1

Laboratory and Clinical Studies

PHILIPPE VAN DE PERRE[a]

Centre Muraz, Organisation de Coordination et de Coopération pour la lutte contre les Grandes Endémies (OCCGE), Bobo-Dioulasso, Burkina Faso

ABSTRACT: Breast milk transmission of HIV-1 can occur at any time during the entire duration of breastfeeding. The risk of late postnatal transmission (after 2.5 months of age) is 3.2 per 100 child/years of breastfeeding, but early postnatal transmission may be more frequent than previously thought. Exclusive breastfeeding has been suggested to be less risky than mixed feeding. Breast milk contains immunoactive cells, antiinfectious substances, immune globulins, cytokines, and complement factors. HIV-1 has been found in breast milk from HIV-infected mothers as both cell-associated and cell-free particles. Mastitis has been suggested to facilitate transmission of HIV-1. The portal of entry of HIV-1 in the infant mucosae may involve tonsilar lymphoepithelium, M cells, and enterocytes from intestinal surfaces. Anti-HIV-1 SIgA and IgM in breast milk and intestinal fluid may confer some protection. Transmission of HIV-1 by breastfeeding has to be taken into account in designing interventions to reduce/prevent mother-to-child transmission in developing countries.

RISK OF HIV-1 TRANSMISSION BY BREASTFEEDING

Risk of transmission of human immunodeficiency virus type 1 (HIV-1) by breastfeeding has been calculated from studies of sequential polymerase chain reaction (PCR) tests performed in cohorts of HIV-infected children followed from birth.[1,2] In a cohort from Kigali, Rwanda, one- to two-thirds of mother-to-child transmission of HIV-1 was attributed to breastfeeding.[1] The additional risk of mother-to-child transmission (MTCT) of HIV-1 has also been estimated by a meta analysis performed by David Dunn and colleagues at 14% (95% confidence interval [CI]: 7–22%) from prevalent maternal infections and at 26% (95% CI: 13–39%) in incident cases.[3] Transmission can occur at any time during the entire duration of breastfeeding. The risk of late postnatal transmission occurring after 2.5 months of age was 3.2 per hundred children per year of breastfeeding, in an international pooled analysis.[4] Recent studies suggest that the contribution of early postnatal transmission may be more important than previously thought. For example, in a study performed by Paolo Miotti and coworkers in Malawi, the monthly hazard of postnatal transmission dropped from 1% in the first six months of life to 0.5% or less thereafter.[5] Different breastfeeding practices are likely to be associated with different risks of transmission. Anna Coutsoudis and coworkers have measured a lower transmission rate in exclu-

[a]Address for correspondence: Centre Muraz, O.C.C.G.E., B.P. 153, Bobo-Dioulasso, Burkina Faso. Voice: (226) 971341; fax: (226) 970457.
direction.muraz@fasonet.bf

sively breastfed infants (14.6%) compared with mixed-fed infants (24.1%).[6] This difference is plausible because of the protective immunologic painting of infants' mucosal surfaces conferred by exclusive breastfeeding. In this study, however, it is quite difficult to explain why exclusively breastfed infants had a lower transmission rate (14.6%) than children never exposed to HIV by breastfeeding (18.8%).[6]

IMMUNOLOGIC CONTENT OF NORMAL HUMAN MILK

Normal human milk contains not only mammary epithelial cells, which have been shown to replicate HIV-1 *in vitro*,[7] but also immunoactive cells, such as lymphocytes and macrophages. The immunoactive cell content is particularly high in colostrum and transition milk but drops rapidly in mature milk.[8] It also contains antiinfectious substances such as lysozyme, lactoferrin, and secretory IgA (SIgA).[8] It is only recently that human milk has been shown to contain cytokines that are likely to play a major role in modulating the local immune responses.[9]

CONTENT OF BREAST MILK FROM HIV-1-INFECTED WOMEN

HIV can be present in human milk in three potential forms: as cell-free virions that can be measured by RNA PCR or branched DNA technologies; as latent, nonproductive, HIV-infected cells that can be measured by DNA PCR in search or proviral DNA, and as productive HIV-infected cells, which require a technique involving RNA PCR applied on cells after DNA enzymatic destruction. To the best of my knowledge, only the first two forms have been scrutinized so far.

Ruth Nduati and colleagues from Nairobi, Kenya, showed that the proportion of HIV-1-infected cells in total cell content seems to remain constant or even increase slightly over successive lactation stages.[10] Ruth Nduati estimated that ingestion of 100 ml of colostrum or of 800 ml of mature milk from an HIV-infected woman exposes the infant to an average of 25,000 infected cells. In well-described models of retroviral transmission by breast milk in animals, such as bovine leukemia virus, ingestion of milk containing as few as 2,000 BLV-infected cells is sufficient to contaminate calves.[11] In the Nairobi study, shedding of HIV-1-infected cells in breast milk was associated with maternal vitamin A deficiency, in a dose–response manner.[10] This observation has to be linked with the results of another observational study conducted in Malawi, where the rate of MTCT of HIV-1 increased with maternal vitamin A deficiency.[12] The well-known effect of vitamin A on host defenses and integrity of mucosal surfaces may plausibly explain this relationship.

A similar study has shown that cell-free viral load, as measured by quantitative RNA PCR, is detectable in about half the human milk samples from HIV-infected mothers.[13] Viral loads are, however, much lower than in plasma but are slightly higher in mature milk compared with earlier milk samples.

Almost 10 years ago, we reported on transmission by breastfeeding that occurred in a Rwandan child concomitantly with the acquisition of a breast abscess in his mother.[14]

Richard Semba and colleagues recently reported on the impact of mastitis on HIV viral load and transmission.[15] In this study performed in Malawi, 16% of HIV-infected lactating women presented with elevated sodium in milk, suggesting a clinical or subclinical mastitis. HIV viral load was detectable in breast milk in 75% of women with mastitis versus 33% in women without mastitis and was associated with transmission. Mastitis may therefore represent a major risk factor for postnatal transmission of HIV-1 by breastfeeding.

PORTAL OF ENTRY

The portal of entry of HIV-1 in infant mucosal surfaces remains largely unclear. Lymphoepithelial tissue of the tonsils is certainly a reasonable candidate, as it contains antigen-transporting cells in the direct vicinity of dendritic cells and CD4[+] lymphocytes.[16] It has been shown that these cells can support HIV replication *in vitro.*[17]

Intestinal mucosae are also convincing candidates. Conceivably, HIV-1 could be introduced into the submucosae by a breach in the integrity of the epithelial cell layer or by a tiny defect in thigh junctions between epithelial cells as a consequence of a nutritional or infectious stress. Other potential portals of entry for HIV-1 are epithelial cells such as enterocytes and M cells. M cells are highly differentiated epithelial cells of the follicle-associated epithelium, specialized in transport of foreign antigen or infectious agents and priming of mucosa-associated lymphoid tissue consisting of macrophages, T- and B-cells.[18] M cells have no glycocalix nor brush border. After attachment to the apical cell surface, antigens are transported by transcytosis and released on the basolateral surface of the cell in contact with inflammatory cells (macrophages and lymphocytes) protruding from the submucosae. Pioneering studies performed at the laboratory of Marian Neutra in Boston showed attachment, transcytosis, and release of HIV particles in a rabbit M cell.[19] Attachment of HIV virions on the apical cell surface of enterocytes normally does not occur. However, Morgan Bomsel and her colleagues have recently shown that HIV-infected cells get polarized and release HIV particles on contact with human enterocytes.[20] After attachment on the galactosyl ceramide receptor, transcytosis and release of virus in the vicinity of macrophages and lymphocytes of the lamina propria occur exactly as in M cells. Moreover, in elegant experiments she showed that dimeric IgA and IgM could inhibit transcytosis in both extracellular and intracellular compartments, an inhibition that can be prevented by addition of an anti-secretory component.[21,22] Therefore, it is highly likely that the *in vivo* local IgA and IgM immune response is also able to prevent attachment and transcytosis of HIV in the intestinal mucosae.

BREAST MILK FACTORS

Local milk factors such as immune globulins,[23] vitamin A, and nonspecific anti-infectious substances are likely to be important in preventing transmission. In a cohort study performed in Kigali, Rwanda, SIgA and SIgM immune responses were found in breast milk during the entire period of lactation.[24] A specific SIgA response and a persistent specific SIgM response in breast milk were inversely correlated with transmission, suggesting that local maternal defenses against the virus may protect against transmission.[24]

Other substances present in breast milk may also be protective, such as lactoferrin,[25] lyzozyme, mucins, immunocompetent T cells,[26] complement, secretory leukocyte protease inhibitor (SLPI),[27] and other substances that are less clearly characterized.[28–30]

SLPI is a serine protease inhibitor that inhibits HIV-1 entry into host cells *in vitro.*[27] As shown in a study performed by Ed Janoff and collaborators, SLPI is present at potentially active concentrations (above 100 ng/ml) in colostrum and transition milk but decreases rapidly thereafter.[31]

INTERVENTIONS TO PREVENT TRANSMISSION

Recently, in three clinical trials performed in African countries such as the ANRS 049 conducted in Bobo-Dioulasso, Burkina Faso, and Abidjan, Côte d'Ivoire, a short antiretroviral treatment in the mother administered during the last month of pregnancy and during labor/delivery has been shown to reduce significantly the risk of transmission even if breastfeeding is practiced during the first three to six months of life.[32] A follow-up of the children will have to be continued until cessation of exposure by breastfeeding. Indeed, especially if the mechanisms of transmission of HIV-1 from mother to child involve similar mucosal exposure, it is feared that the benefit of maternal antiretroviral treatment on *in utero* and *intra partum* transmission be erased by a "catch-up" effect due to late postnatal transmission if breastfeeding is practiced.[33] In non-breastfed infants, abbreviated antiretroviral regimens, including a simple oral administration of antiretrovirals to the neonate within 48 hours of life, have been suggested to still be effective.[34] All these studies and clinical trials suggest that a simple and short antiretroviral regimen, even with breastfeeding, could be translated into a public health intervention.

CONCLUSIONS

In summary, transmission of HIV-1 by breastfeeding is the result of opposing driving forces such as the presence and forms of the virus, portal of entry, local immune response, lesions of mucosal surfaces, and nonspecific antiinfective substances in breast milk.

We need to learn much more about breast milk transmission of HIV-1, which is involved in at least 30% of newly acquired pediatric HIV infections worldwide, in order to design and implement efficient and applicable interventions. Transmission of HIV-1 by breastfeeding has to be taken into account in designing innovative interventions to reduce/prevent mother-to-child transmission in developing countries, because alternatives to breastfeeding or early cessation of breastfeeding may not be practical in all contexts.

REFERENCES

1. SIMONON, A., P. LEPAGE, E. KARITA, *et al.* 1994. An assessment of the timing of mother-to-child tranmission of human immunodeficiency virus type 1 by means of polymerase chain reaction. J. Acquir. Immune Defic. Syndr. **7:** 952–957.

2. EKPINI, E.R., S.Z. WIKTOR, G.A. SATTEN, *et al.* 1997. Late postnatal mother-to-child transmission of HIV-1 in Abidjan, Côte d'Ivoire. Lancet **349:** 1054–1059.
3. DUNN, D.T., M.L. NEWELL, A.E. ADES & C. PECKHAM. 1992. Risk of human immunodeficiency virus type 1 transmission through breastfeeding. Lancet **340:** 585–588.
4. LEROY, V., M.L. NEWELL, F. DABIS, *et al.*, for the Ghent International Working Group on Mother-to-Child Transmission of HIV. 1998. International multicentre pooled analysis of late postnatal mother-to-child transmission of HIV-1 infection. Lancet **352:** 597–600.
5. MIOTTI, P. 1998. Data presented at the Third International Symposium on Global Strategies to Prevent Perinatal HIV Transmission. Valencia, Spain, November 9–11.
6. COUTSOUDIS, A., K. PILLAY, E. SPOONER, *et al.* for the South African Vitamin A Study Group. 1999. Influence of infant feeding patterns on early mother-to-child transmission of HIV-1 in Durban, South Africa: a prospective cohort study. Lancet **354:** 471–476.
7. TONIOLO, A., C. SERRA, P.G. CONALDI, *et al.* 1995. Productive HIV-1 infection of normal human mammary epithelial cells. AIDS **9:** 859–866.
8. GOLDMAN, A.S., C.G. GARZA, B.L. NICHOLS & R.M. GOLDMAN. 1982. Immunologic factors in human milk during the first year of lactation. J. Pedaitr. **100:** 563–567.
9. GOLDMAN, A.S. 1993. The immune system of human milk: antimicrobial, antiinflammatory and immunomodulating properties. Pediatr. Infect. Dis. J. **12:** 664–671.
10. NDUATI, R.W., G.C. JOHN, B.A. RICHARDSON, *et al.* 1995. Human immunodeficiency virus type 1-infected cells in breast milk: association with immunosuppression and vitamin A deficiency. J. Infect. Dis. **172:** 1461–1468.
11. MAAS-INDERWIESEN, F., A. ALBRECHT, I. BAUSE, *et al.* 1978. Zum Einfluß der Leukosebekämpfung auf die Entwicklung der enzootischen Rinderleukose in Niedersaschsen. Deutsch Tierarztl. Wochenschr. **85:** 309–312.
12. SEMBA, R.D., P.G. MIOTTI, J.D. CHIPHANGWI, *et al.* 1994. Maternal vitamin A deficiency and mother-to-child transmission of HIV-1. Lancet **343:** 1593–1597.
13. LEWIS, P., R. NDUATI, J.K. KREISS, *et al.* 1998. Cell-free human immunodeficiency virus type 1 in breast milk. J. Infect. Dis. **177:** 34–39.
14. VAN DE PERRE, P., D.G. HITIMANA, A. SIMONON, *et al.* 1992. Postnatal transmission of HIV-1 associated with breast abscess. Lancet **339:** 1490–1491.
15. SEMBA, R.D., N. KUMWENDA, D.R. HOOVER, *et al.* 1999. Human immunodeficiency virus load in breast milk, mastitis, and mother-to-child transmission of human immunodeficiency virus type 1. J. Infect. Dis. **180:** 93–98.
16. FRANKEL, S.S., B.M. WENIG, A.P. BURKE, *et al.* 1996. Replication of HIV-1 in dendritic cell-derived syncytia at the mucosal surface of the adenoid. Science **272:** 115–117.
17. FRANKEL, S.S., K. TENNER-RACZ, P. RACZ, *et al.* 1997. Active replication of HIV-1 at the lymphoepithelial surface of the tonsil. Am. J. Pathol. **151:** 89–96.
18. SAVIDGE, T.C. 1996. The life and times of an intestinal M cell. Trends Microbiol. **4:** 301–306.
19. AMERONGEN, H.M., R. WELTZIN, C.M. FARNET, *et al.* 1991. Transepithelial transport of HIV-1 by intestinal M cells: a mechanism for transmission of AIDS. J. Acquir. Immune Defic. Syndr. **4:** 760–765.
20. BOMSEL, M. 1997. Transcytosis of infectious human immunodeficiency virus accross a tight human epithelial cell line barrier. Nat. Med. **3:** 42–47.
21. HOCINI, H., L. BÉLEC, S. ISCAKI, *et al.* 1997. High-level ability of secretory IgA to block HIV type 1 transcytosis: contrasting secretory IgA and IgG responses to glycoprotein 160. AIDS Res. Hum. Retroviruses **13:** 1179–1185.
22. BOMSEL, M., M. HEYMAN, H. HOCINI, *et al.* 1998. Intracellular neutralization of HIV transcytosis across tight epithelial barriers by anti-HIV envelope protein dIgA or IgM. Immunity **9:** 277–287.
23. VAN DE PERRE, P., D.G. HITIMANA & P. LEPAGE. 1988. Human immunodeficiency virus antibodies of the IgG, IgA and IgM sub-classes in the milk of seropositive mothers. J. Pediatr. **113:** 1039–1041.
24. VAN DE PERRE, P., A. SIMONON, D.G. HITIMANA, *et al.* 1993. Infective and anti-infective properties of breast milk from HIV-1 infected women. Lancet **341:** 914–918.

25. HARMSEN, M.C., P.J. SWART, M.P. DE BETHUNE, *et al.* 1995. Antiviral effect of plasma and milk proteins: lactoferrin shows potent activity against both human immunodeficiency virus and cytomegalovirus replication in vitro. J. Infect. Dis. **172:** 380–388.

26. WIRT, D.P., L.T. ADKINS, K.H. PALKOWETZ, *et al.* 1992. Activated and memory T lymphocytes in human milk. Cytometry **13:** 282–290.

27. WAHL, S.M., T.B. MCNEELY, E.N. JANOFF, *et al.* 1997. Secretory leukocyte protease inhibitor (SLPI) in mucosal fluids inhibits HIV-1. Oral Dis. **3(Suppl. 1):** S64–69.

28. NEWBURG, D.S., R.P. VISCIDI, A. RUFF & R.H. YOLKEN. 1992. A human milk factor inhibits binding of human immunodeficiency virus to the CD4 receptor. Pediatr. Res. **31:** 22–28.

29. ISAACS, C.E. & H. THORMAR. 1990. Human milk lipids inactivate enveloped viruses. *In* Breastfeeding, Nutrition, Infection and Infant Growth in Developed and Emerging Countries. S.A. Atkinson, L.A. Hanson & R.K. Chandra, Eds. ARTS Biomedical Publishers and Distributors. St John's, Newfoundland, Canada.

30. SWART, P.J., M.E. KUIPERS, C. SMIT, *et al.* 1996. Antiviral effects of milk proteins: acylation results in polyanionic compounds with potent activity against human immunodeficiency virus types 1 and 2 in vitro. AIDS Res. Hum. Retrovir. **12:** 769–775.

31. JANOFF, E.N., K. EIDMAN, T.B. MCNEELY, *et al.* 1997. Secretory leukocyte protease inhibitor (SLPI), an HIV-1-inhibitory protein and rates of HIV-1 transmission by mucosal fluids. Presented at a Conference on HIV-1 and Mucosal Pathogenesis. NIH, Bethesda, MD, September 11–13.

32. DABIS, F., P. MSELLATI, N. MEDA, *et al.* FOR THE DITRAME STUDY GROUP. 1999. Six-month efficacy, tolerance and acceptability of a short regimen of oral zidovudine in reducing vertical transmission of HIV in breast-fed children. A double-blind placebo controlled multicentre trial, ANRS 049a, Côte d'Ivoire and Burkina Faso. Lancet **353:** 786–792.

33. VAN DE PERRE, P. 1999. Mother-to-child transmission of HIV-1: the "all mucosal" hypothesis as a predominant mechanism of transmission. AIDS **13:** 1133–1138.

34. WADE, N.A., G.S. BIRKHEAD, B.L. WARREN, *et al.* 1998. Abbreviated regimens of zidovudine prophylaxis and perinatal transmission of the human immunodeficiency virus. N. Engl. J. Med. **339:** 1409–1414.

Psychosocial and Community Perspectives on Alternatives to Breastfeeding

MARY T. BASSETT[a]

Department of Community Medicine, University of Zimbabwe Medical School, Avondale, Harare, Zimbabwe

ABSTRACT: In developing countries, what advice to give HIV-positive mothers on infant feeding options remains a vexing public health issue. This paper reviews data on infant feeding practices in sub-Saharan Africa, the cultural context of breastfeeding, and the still meager literature of decision-making by HIV-positive mothers, following impartial counseling. Although prolonged breastfeeding is common, weaning foods typically are introduced early. A minority of women practice the recommended exclusive breastfeeding for 4–6 months. Breastfeeding taboos, expecially regarding colostrum, are common. The usual reason for introduction of weaning foods is to ensure that the baby has enough food. Exclusive formula feeding is perceived as stigmatizing, but acceptable with husband support. The main perceived barrier to formula is cost. Health workers may be less effective in conveying the risk of formula compared to the risk of HIV transmission in breast milk. Studies presently available regarding these issues are few and involve small samples. More studies are planned, and some are under way. By offering actual feeding choices to HIV-positive women, observing what choices they make, and monitoring the outcomes of these choices, we will be better placed to give advice.

INTRODUCTION

Transmission of HIV in breast milk is well established,[1,2] but public health approaches to its prevention in the developing world remain problematic. Present policy recommendations rest decision-making with each individual HIV-positive woman.[3] This uneasy approach to population health, where recommendations usually hold for groups and are not made on a case-by-case basis, reflects the complexity of infant feeding choices.[4,5]

How do women who personally face choices about how to feed their infants view these issues? For an HIV-positive woman, the choice involves an understanding of the risks and benefits of breastfeeding and its alternatives. Assessing the balance of these risks is difficult, even with all the facts. Furthermore, a decision about whether or not to breastfeed does not involve only facts. These choices involve beliefs about mothering and nurturing, and not only the beliefs of the woman, but those of her partner and her community more generally.

[a]Address for correspondence: Department of Community Medicine, University of Zimbabwe Medical School, P.O. Box A-178, Avondale, Harare, Zimbabwe. Voice: (263-4) 791631; fax: (263-4) 795835.

mary@zappuz.co.zw

Although we have been in the clutch of competing risks for years now, largely absent from this discussion has been the view of women themselves regarding these decisions. Many health-care workers, and I would count myself among them, are reluctant to give advice that presupposes choices women do not really have. A person does not simply choose to have money or clean water, and most African women have neither. But it is also true that it is mothers who make the ultimate decision about how to feed their babies. As we all struggle to present HIV-seropositive women with information on the range of feeding choices in a nondirective way, we will learn more about what alternatives are acceptable.

What do I mean by an "acceptable" practice? Research efforts to assess acceptability have focused mainly on adoption of new products (often contraceptive technology).[6] Need for such study of acceptability emerged when researchers learned that simply having a product did not guarantee its use. Both how we define and measure acceptability remains a bit murky. Acceptability clearly is not simply an attribute of a product, although that is part of it. Acceptability has also to do with the context of use, what alternatives exist, what process surrounds adoption, and how the healthcare delivery system presents these decisions. One way to assess acceptability is to ask women what they *think* and what they would do, given a choice. This hypothetical scenario probably is more successful at capturing negative responses. If women do not like something hypothetically, they likely will not use it in practice. But what does it mean when women *say* a product is acceptable. Does this really predict use? Experience suggests that the best way to assess what women will do is to offer them choices and see what they actually choose.

We are just beginning to get some of this information regarding infant feeding choices in the face of HIV/AIDS. Much is still preliminary and not yet published. I will draw on our ongoing experience in southern Africa, especially Zimbabwe, a small country in southern Africa where adult HIV seroprevalence is estimated at 25%.[7] In Zimbabwe, as elsewhere in the developing world, where poverty continues to be the main challenge to raising healthy children, breastfeeding is widely practiced and highly valued.

INFANT FEEDING PRACTICES

A first step toward understanding what is acceptable is to review what we know about practices. What do we know about how women feed their babies? For example, recent work suggests that to consider breastfeeding as "present" or "absent" is misleading with respect to HIV risk. The pattern of breastfeeding, especially mixing with other foods, appears to influence HIV transmission risk.[8,9] What do we know about exclusive breastfeeding? Early weaning is another approach to reducing HIV risk. How widely is this practiced?

The Demographic and Health Surveys,[10] which began about 15 years ago, provide a wealth of data about how infants are fed throughout the developing world. (See TABLE 1.)

These surveys show that in many settings in sub-Saharan Africa, breastfeeding is near universal and of long duration. It is not unusual for mothers to breastfeed infants well into their second year of life. But current recommendations regarding exclusive breastfeeding for the first 4–6 months of life are rarely met in practice. The definition

TABLE 1. Initiation and duration of breastfeeding in selected African countries: data from the Demographic and Health Surveys (DHS)

Country	Year	Ever breastfed	Median duration (months)	Exclusive in <2 months
Kenya	1998	98%	21	28.2%
Eritrea	1998	98%	22	75.5%
Zambia	1996	98%	20	34.5%
Tanzania	1996	97%	22	55.9%
Malawi	1992	97%	20	4.8%
Mali	1995	95%	22	18.7%

of exclusive breastfeeding here is breast milk only, no other liquids or foods. Using this definition, average duration of exclusive breastfeeding is often only 1 or 2 months. Looking at the detailed data for Zimbabwe, even in the first month of life about half of infants receive other food by mouth (see TABLE 2).[11] Water, once permitted in the definition of exclusive breastfeeding, is not the main source of supplement.

Formula milk is not very important in most settings, with under 5% of women reporting its use in most countries. The main weaning foods are traditional weaning foods, based on the dietary staple. Few babies use bottles. These data suggest that prolonged exclusive breastfeeding is rare and supplements are common. This is not to say that there are no groups that successfully practice exclusive breastfeeding for 6 months. Perhaps half do so in Papua New Guinea, for example.[12] In Eritrea, Lesotho, and Uganda, more than half of women exclusively breastfeed to six months.[14]

From these data, we can conclude that in many African settings giving non–breast milk foods, generally not formula, is acceptable and widely practiced. Exclusive breastfeeding is the best nutritional choice. Why do women not rely on their milk supply for longer periods? Insight into motivations for observed behavior come from studies with more depth than surveys. Anthropologists have repeatedly described cultural taboos surrounding both colostrum and mature milk.[14] Often mentioned are the mother's concern that the baby needs more food and the mother's own work demands, which may limit the time she has to breastfeed.

Colostrum taboos are not important in Zimbabwe, but worldwide belief that colostrum should be discarded is widespread and ancient. Colostrum may be viewed as stale, unclean, and insufficient. There are also taboos regarding mature milk. It is believed that a mother's emotional state or sexual behavior can cause "bad milk" or that milk can be "spoiled" by a mother's grief, anger, or fear. Sexual activity, especially with a nonspousal partner, may contaminate breast milk. If a mother is ill, her milk may not be good. Also, a new pregnancy makes improper and unsafe the further suckling of an infant.

But most often a mother reports that supplements are meant to make the baby healthier and that breast milk is insufficient. Intertwined with concerns that breast milk is inadequate are the demands exclusive feeding place on a woman's time. Exclusive breastfeeding is time consuming. A study in Sweden where mothers fed on demand exclusively for at least 4 months showed that mothers fed babies up to 10

TABLE 2. Feeding patterns by age (in months) among Zimbabwean infants, Zimbabwe Demographic and Health Survey 1994[11]

Age (months)	Not breastfeeding (%)	Exclusively breastfeeding	Breast milk and:	
			Plain water	Supplements
<2	0.4	18.6	29.0	51.9
2–3	2.1	13.7	18.9	65.2
4–5	0.5	0.9	9.0	89.6
6–7	0.8	0.8	3.8	94.7
8–9	1.4	0.0	1.9	96.7
10–11	5.0	1.3	0.0	93.7

times a day and 5 times a night.[15] Some babies suckled for up to 2 hours and 45 minutes. In a setting where women's labor is central to the household economy, alternative feedings release the mother from her feeding role and allow her to attend to other roles as peasant farmers, informal sector traders, or wage earners.

Demands on women's time are substantial and relentless. A decade and a half ago, a study showed that for the average rural Zimbabwean woman, the workday began at 5 A.M. and ended at 9 P.M.[16] Since 1992, when Zimbabwe began its economic reform program, households have come under growing financial pressure and the demands on women's time probably have increased. A full two-thirds of Zimbabweans live below the poverty datum line, and about one-third earn too little to ensure food security.[17] Households have responded by greatly expanding the ways in which they earn money.[18] As women strive to earn money in more ways, they have to consider how they allocate their time to these many roles, all of which contribute to the well-being of their children. Although breast milk production may be a woman's responsibility, the purchase and preparation of other foods can involve other household members. Women frequently do not have access to household income. Purchase of supplemental foods usually means her husband shifts cash to infant feeding.[21,22]

In summary, early mixed feeding is the most common infant feeding regimen. But foregoing breastfeeding altogether is extremely rare, far less common than prolonged exclusive breastfeeding. If an HIV-positive woman chooses not to breastfeed *at all*, she makes a dramatic departure from accepted behavior.

HIV-POSITIVE WOMEN: DECISIONS BASED ON INFORMATION OFFERED

This brings us to how women use information about the competing risks of formula feeding and breastfeeding. At present, the UNAIDS/WHO/UNICEF recommendations are as follows.[21] First, for all women who are HIV-negative or who do not know their status, breastfeeding is the best choice, with exclusive breastfeeding for the first six months of life. For the HIV-positive woman, a choice of either breastfeeding or replacement feeding should be made after balanced counseling. Replacement feeding may be with infant formula or modified animal milks. Heat-treated expressed breast milk is an additional alternative.

Our data on how women view these options are very limited. A few small studies suggest that, if they could, most HIV-infected women would choose formula feeding, with cost viewed as the major obstacle. Take for example a questionnaire survey in Cape Town among 88 women known to be HIV-positive, many identified because of a sick baby.[22,23] After receiving information about the competing risks of breastfeeding and formula feeding, 83% of the women would prefer to formula-feed their next child, although only half believed they could afford formula.

Additional data come from our survey now under way in an urban township outside Harare. Based on the first 50 women interviewed by Danielle Gottlieb and Ratidzai Mapfungautsi, all women with babies under 6 months of age, 45 women agreed that a mother with HIV should not breastfeed (none agreed that a mother who worked should not breastfeed). The Cape Town study also suggested that women were already changing their behavior based on their serostatus. Of the minority of women (15 of 88) who knew their status at the time of delivery, about half breastfed, compared to nearly all mothers who did not know their status.

In our study setting, an urban township, formula is generally viewed quite negatively. We asked some 200 mothers of infants attending an urban well-baby clinic what they knew about infant formula. None used formula, about half reported that they knew someone who had been formula fed, but only 20% thought that a formula-fed baby could be healthy.[24] These findings seem to be confirmed in the preliminary findings of the ongoing in-depth questionnaire. Although 90% of women agreed that HIV-positive mothers should not breastfeed, only 14% thought that a formula-fed baby could be healthy.

Few studies have examined how effective health workers are at conveying these complex issues. The Cape Town study suggested that healthworkers might be less effective in conveying the risk of formula feeding than breastfeeding. Only 47% of formula-feeding mothers could give risks of formula compared to 72% of breastfeeding mothers.

Formula is expensive, as are other replacement options. The commitment to formula feeding extends beyond the financial planning horizon of many—probably most—families that now live week to week, day to day, or even meal to meal. In Zimbabwe, where the minimum wage for the lowest paid workers is less than ZWD 1000 per month, infant formula costs nearly ZWD 500 per month, and lower cost alternatives using home modification of animal milk cost about ZWD 300 per month.[25] Many families derive income solely from the "informal sector" and do not receive a paycheck. It is very worrying to think about a mother suppressing lactation only to find herself unable to buy replacement food after a month or two. That HIV-positive women appreciate this is suggested by some other comments in an ongoing study by ZVITAMBO: "It's very disturbing, *pachivanhu*. We have to breastfeed most of the time. We cannot afford replacement feeding costs. If not breastfed the baby will die because of lack of food."[26]

A study in Ndola, Zambia is looking at just such real-life issues in preparation of replacement feeding.[27] How will mothers boil water "for 5 minutes" without a clock? How will water be stored? How will they measure proportions without standard measuring containers? How will leftover formula be stored? Can mothers manage cup- and spoon-feeding babies, even at night? What will happen if there is no food or no money? The logistical issues were substantial. Learning to measure will require attention to locally available containers. But these obstacles seemed possible to overcome. Water could be boiled and babies fed by cup and spoon. But the problem of "no food and no money" was more intractable.

While endorsing formula, most anticipated family disapproval and little social support. Women in Cape Town noted that failure to breastfeed would be interpreted as either selfish or a sign of promiscuity. This statement of the views of a father in an ongoing study by ZVITAMBO echoes this attitude: "... not breastfeeding meant that the wife is confirming that the child is not his or she is promiscuous."

From these discussions, which included fathers and lactating women with different serostatus, emerged a uniform expectation that not breastfeeding would meet with disapproval. But the economic barrier appeared the more important barrier, especially if the couple agreed that the child should not be breastfed. In our preliminary data women also noted that not breastfeeding was a clear signal that a woman was either unfaithful or had HIV, but that a woman could still make this decision with her husband's agreement. Failure to involve husbands, however, might lead to beatings or the return of the women to her natal home. Although traditional culture leaves decisions about weaning to female relatives, men felt strongly that the decision was the couple's to make. The data, albeit scant, suggest a critical need to involve men in the decision-making process.

CONCLUSIONS

What can be concluded about community perspectives on breastfeeding? In Africa, breastfeeding initiation is near universal, and early mixed feeding patterns are deeply entrenched. Prolonging exclusive breastfeeding or adopting exclusive replacement feeding both represent departures from the social norms. Offered information on risks and benefits of formula and breastfeeding by HIV-infected women, the preference appears to be for formula feeding. This may reflect the difficulty in adequately conveying risks of replacement feeding, or it may reflect a mother's response to the simple calculus of certain death with HIV infection versus "higher risk" with replacement feeding. After all, formula feeding has for years been recommended to HIV-infected mothers in rich countries. Perhaps also not surprisingly, both men and women place a high value on infant survival, even in face of social stigma. Adoption of replacement feeding in the absence of the husband's approval is risky, but with the husband's support, tradition may be set aside.

But most of these data are based on hypothetical scenarios. We need to know a lot more, not only what women and men *say* they would do but what they actually do in practice. This research is under way. I have cited current work in Ndola by Ellen Piwoz and colleagues. The International Center for Research on Women (ICRW) is also collaborating on similar work in Africa. In Zimbabwe, Dr. Wendy Holmes and colleagues in Batsirai will be examining the feasibility of the whole range of choices being presented to women. The only way we will know what choices women will make in the real world and how well they will cope with these choices is to offer them and assess them. By learning from those who must make and live with these hard choices, public health workers will be in a better position to offer advice.

ACKNOWLEDGMENTS

My thanks to Naume Tavengwa, Lorrie Gavin, Peter Iliff, and the team at the Zvitambo Project for sharing unpublished data.

NOTES AND REFERENCES

1. DUNN, D.T. *et al.* 1992. Risk of human immunodeficiency virus 1 transmission through breastfeeding. Lancet **340:** 585–588.
2. BOBAT, R. *et al.* 1997. Breastfeeding by HIV-1 infected women and the outcome in their infants: a cohort study from Durban, South Africa. AIDS **11:** 1627–1633.
3. UNAIDS, WHO & UNICEF. 1997. HIV and infant feeding: a joint policy statement. 1998. Reproduced in Annex 1, HIV and Infant: Guidelines for Decision-makers. WHO/FRH/NUT/CHD 98.1 UNAIDS.98.3 UNICEF/PDNUT/CJ 98-1. Geneva.
4. MORRISON, P. 1999. HIV and infant feeding: to breastfeed of not to breastfeed. The dilemma of competing risks. Part 1. Breastfeeding Rev. **7:** 5–13.
5. PREBLE, E.A. & E.G. PIWOZ. 1995. HIV and infant feeding: a chronology of research and policy advances and their implications for programs. The LINKAGES project. Washington, DC. Support for Analysis and Research in Africa (SARA) project. September, 1995.
6. HEISE, L. 1996. Acceptability research in reproductive health. Unpublished manuscript. Centre for Health and Gender Equality (CHANGE). Washington, DC.
7. JOINT UNITED NATIONS PROGRAM ON HIV/AIDS (UNAIDS). 1998. AIDS epidemic update: December 1998. UNAIDS. Geneva.
8. COUTSOUDIS, A. *et al.* 1999. Influence of infant feeding patterns on early mother-to-child transmission of HIV-1 in Durban, South Africa. Lancet **354:** 471–476.
9. TESS, B.H. *et al.* 1998. Infant feeding and risk of mother-to-child transmission of HIV-1 in Sao Paolo State, Brazil. Sao Paolo Collaborative study for vertical transmission of HIV-1. J. Acquir. Immune Defic. Syndr. Hum. Retrovirol. **19:** 188–194.
10. The Demographic Health Surveys programs are conducted worldwide in collaboration with the appropriate host ministry by Macro International, Calverton, Maryland.
11. CENTRAL STATISTICAL OFFICE (ZIMBABWE) AND MACRO INTERNATIONAL INC. 1995. Zimbabwe Demographic and Health Survey, 1994. Central Statistical Office and Macro International Inc. Calverton, Maryland.
12. FRIESEN, P. *et al.* 1998. Infant feeding practices in Papua New Guinea. Ann. Trop. Paediatr. **18:** 209–215.
13. POPULATION REFERENCE BUREAU. Breastfeeding patterns in the developing world. Measure communication, 1875 Connecticut Ave., NW, Suite 520, Washington, DC 20009, USA.
14. GUNNLAUGSSON, G. & J. EINARSDOTTIR. 1993. Colostrum and ideas about bad milk: a case study from Guinea Bissau. Soc. Sci. Med. **36:** 283–288.
15. HORNELL, A. *et al.* 1999. Breastfeeding patterns in exclusively breastfed infants I: a longitudinal prospective study in Uppsala, Sweden. Acta Paediatr. **88:** 203–211.
16. UNICEF. 1992. Children in Zimbabwe: A Situation Analysis. UNICEF: Zimbabwe, P.O. Box 1250, Harare, Zimbabwe.
17. CENTRAL STATISTICAL OFFICE. 1998. Poverty survey in Zimbabwe. CSO: Zimbabwe P.O. Box CY342, Harare, Zimbabwe.
18. BIJLMAKERS, L.A., M.T. BASSETT & D.M. SANDERS. 1998. Socio-economic stress, health and child nutritional status at a time of economic structural adjustment. A three-year longtudinal study. Research Report No. 105. Nordiska Afrikainstitutet. Uppsala, Sweden.
19. MAHER, V. 1992. Breast feeding and maternal depletion: natural law or cultural arrangements. *In* The Anthropology of Breastfeeding: Natural Law or Social Contract? V. Maher, Ed. St. Martins Press. New York.
20. RAPHAEL, D. & F. DAVIS. 1985. Only Mothers Know: Patterns of Infant Feeding in Traditional Cultures. Greenwood Press. London.

21. WHO, JOINT UNITED NATIONS PROGRAMMES ON HIV/AIDS (UNAIDS) & UNICEF. 1998. HIV and infant feeding: guidelines for decision makers 1998. (UNAIDS/98.4, WHO/FRH/NUT/98.2, UNICEF/PD/NUT(J)98.2).

22. KUHN, L. *et al.* 2000. Child feeding practices of HIV-positive mothers in Cape Town, South Africa. AIDS **13:** 144–146.

23. KUHN, L. *et al.* Child feeding practices and attitudes on HIV seropositive mothers in Cape Town, South Africa. Unpublished manuscript.

24. MAPONGA, C.C. *et al.* 1999. Readiness for HIV counselling and testing in the antenatal care setting in urban Zimbabwe. Abstract No. 0425. Second Conference on Global Strategies for the Prevention of HIV Transmission to the Infant. September 1–5. Montreal, Canada.

25. MINISTRY OF HEALTH AND CHILD WELFARE. 1999. Department of Nutrition Mimeo. Draft guidelines on infant feeding. July. P.O. Box CY1144, Causeway, Harare, Zimbabwe.

26. GAVIN, L. *et al.* 1999. The development of an intervention to counsel women in Zimbabwe about HIV and infant feeding. Abstract No. 269. Second Conference on Global Strategies for the Prevention of HIV Transmission to the Infant. September 1–5. Montreal, Canada.

27. PIWOZ, E.G. 1999. Replacement feeding for HIV+ African women: how we learned what women and men think about mother-to-child transmission, breastfeeding and the alternatives. Paper presented to the CRHCS Woorkshop for Nutrition and HIV/AIDS. Maputo, Mozambique, February 8–12.

Influence of Infant Feeding Patterns on Early Mother-to-Child Transmission of HIV-1 in Durban, South Africa

A. COUTSOUDIS[a]

Department of Paediatrics and Child Health, University of Natal, Congella, South Africa

ABSTRACT: Previous studies on the effect of breastfeeding on mother-to-child transmission (MTCT) of HIV have not attempted to examine the influence of different types of breastfeeding practice. To attempt to address some of these inadequacies, infant feeding practices of 549 HIV-infected women involved in a trial in Durban, South Africa were documented prospectively. Women were counseled on infant feeding choices according to UNAIDS guidelines, and those who chose to breastfeed were encouraged to practice exclusive breastfeeding. The MTCT rates of HIV-1 at 3 months were compared in the three different feeding groups (never breastfed, exclusive breastfeeding, and mixed breastfeeding). At 3 months, 18.8% of 156 never-breastfed children were infected compared to 21.3% of 393 breastfed children ($p = 0.50$). Children exclusively breastfed to at least 3 months ($n = 103$) were less likely to be infected (14.3%) than those receiving mixed feeding before 3 months (24.1%) ($p = 0.03$). After adjustment for potential confounders (maternal CD4:CD8 ratio, syphilis screening test results, and preterm delivery), exclusive breastfeeding carried a significantly lower risk of HIV-1 transmission than mixed feeding (hazard ratio [HR] 0.52, 95% CI: 0.28–0.98) and an equivalent risk to no breastfeeding (HR 0.85, 95% CI: 0.51–1.42). Our findings have important implications for HIV and infant feeding policies in developing countries, and it is critical that further research be undertaken. In the meantime, breastfeeding policies for HIV-infected women require urgent review. If confirmed, exclusive breastfeeding may offer HIV-infected women in developing countries an affordable, culturally acceptable, and effective means of reducing MTCT of HIV-1 while maintaining the overwhelming benefits of breastfeeding.

INTRODUCTION

Most studies on breast milk transmission (including those in Dunn's meta-analysis[1]) are flawed because they have failed to account for the effects of different types of breastfeeding practices, that is, exclusive or mixed breastfeeding. According to demographic and health surveys, most women in the developed world practice mixed breastfeeding—that is, addition of water, herbal teas, cereals, and so forth early on in the infant's life. Therefore, the majority of studies on which policy recommendations have been made were in fact reporting the effect of mixed breastfeeding on

[a]Address for correspondence: Dr. A. Coutsoudis, Dept. Paediatrics and Child Health, University of Natal, Private Bag 7, Congella 4013, South Africa. Voice: 27-31-2604489; fax: 27-31-2604388.

coutsoud@med.und.ac.za

MTCT of HIV. Two reports have attempted to examine the effect of different breast-feeding patterns on MTCT, but both of these had limitations. An earlier study in South Africa[2] used an arbitrary definition of exclusive breastfeeding. The practice described as exclusive breastfeeding was in fact, according to the WHO definition, mixed breast-feeding. The other study in Brazil[3] was a retrospective study. We have conducted for the first time a prospective study examining the impact of infant feeding practices on MTCT of HIV. This study on the effect of infant feeding patterns on MTCT of HIV was nested within a vitamin A intervention trial to reduce MTCT of HIV.[4]

METHODS

The breastfeeding study involved HIV-infected women who, during the antenatal period, received counseling about the disadvantages and advantages of breastfeeding for HIV-infected women and were asked to make a choice about how they would feed their infants. Women were recruited at antenatal clinics at two hospitals in Durban, South Africa, King Edward VIIIth Hospital, and McCords Hospital. All research staff were supportive of whatever method of feeding women had chosen. Those women choosing to formula feed were not supplied with free formula; however, they were given the opportunity to purchase subsidized formula from the hospital stores. Those opting to breastfeed were encouraged to exclusively breastfeed according to the strict WHO definitions (namely, no water, herbal teas, etc.). Mothers were asked to attend a follow-up clinic when their infants were 1 week, 6 weeks, and 3 months of age and thereafter every 3 months. At each visit mothers were asked about feeding of the infant and breastfeeding practices. Specific questions were asked about feeding of any fluid or solids, and the responses were recorded on a data sheet, which allowed for a record of the date at which each item was introduced to the infant. Venous blood was drawn from the mothers on entry to the study for baseline differential count and lymphocyte subset analysis. The CD4 T-cell subset was enumerated by flow cytometry on a Coulter EPICS Profile 2 Flow Cytometer (Coulter Electronics, Miami, Fl) using specific monoclonal antibodies. Baseline serum vitamin A concentrations were determined by reverse-phase, high-pressure liquid chromatography.[5] In a subsample of women, a quantitative assay of HIV viral RNA was determined.

Infant venous blood was drawn on the first day after birth and again at 1 week, 6 weeks, and 3 months of age and at three-month intervals thereafter until 15 months of age. If the mother was still breastfeeding, infant venous blood was drawn at 3 months after cessation of breastfeeding. Plasma was separated within 5 hours and stored at $-70°C$ for possible subsequent quantitative assay of HIV viral RNA using polymerase chain reaction (PCR, Roche Molecular Systems, Branchburg, NJ, USA).[6] RNA was extracted from 200 µl of plasma in the presence of an internal RNA standard, and an aliquot was subjected to reverse transcription–PCR amplification with *Thermus thermophilus* HB8 (Tth) DNA polymerase in the presence of dUTP and UNG. The relative amounts of the internal standard and HIV-1-specific PCR products were quantified after PCR with a microtiter format enzyme-linked immunosorbent-like assay. The analytic limit of detection of the assay is about 10 RNA copies (about 400 copies/ml), with a linear dynamic range of at least 4 log units and a coefficient of variation of generally 25%. RNA tests were performed among children who had two positive ELISA tests at 9 and 15 months, starting with the earliest sample and tested sequentially until the first positive test. In children who had not yet reached 15 months of age but who had reached 9 months, an ELISA test (Abbott Laboratories, Chicago) was performed at 9 months as well as a 6-month RNA-PCR test. If these were positive, the RNA test was measured in the stored plasma samples starting with the earliest sample until the first positive test. Children who had not yet reached 9 months had an RNA-PCR test performed on each of their last two samples, and, if these were positive, samples were tested from the earliest sample, as described above.

The study was approved by the Ethics Committee of the University of Natal. Written informed consent was obtained from all women who participated in the trial.

Statistical Methods

The analysis was restricted to singleton infants for simplicity because twins may be more difficult to breastfeed and may be more vulnerable to early mortality. Breastfeeding duration was estimated using Kaplan-Meier life-table methods. Among mothers known to have stopped breastfeeding, the mother's reported age of the child when breastfeeding stopped was used as the endpoint. Among mothers lost to follow-up or who had not yet stopped breastfeeding when this analysis was undertaken, the child was censored at the age they were last seen.

The proportions of children in each feeding group infected by 3 months of age were estimated using Kaplan-Meier life-table methods as used in the analysis of the ACTG 076 trial.[7] This statistical method, which takes into account the prospective nature of the data, estimates the cumulative probability of testing positive at each sequential time point. A single PCR positive result was considered evidence of infection. Children with no positive results were retained in the analysis as uninfected until the age of their last negative test, at which time they were censored. Children with later negative results but who were missing earlier test results were assumed to be negative at earlier time-points. Differences between the feeding groups were tested using a Z statistic calculated as the difference in the probabilities of infection by 3 months in the two groups divided by the square root of the sum of their variances from the Kaplan-Meier life-table model. These probabilities estimate transmission detectable by specific ages but may underestimate true transmission occurring by the specific age since there is a delay between actual and detectable infection and variable intervals between testing. This underestimation is greater for postnatal than for perinatal transmission because it occurs closer in time to the endpoint of the analysis. Cox Proportional Hazards models using follow-up data to 3 months were used for multivariable analysis to adjust for potential confounders.

RESULTS

Study Sample

Six hundred sixty-one women recruited into the vitamin A clinical trial were known to have had a live birth at one of the two study hospitals (631 women had singletons, 28 women had twins, and 2 women delivered a single live birth following fetal death of the co-twin). Among the 631 singletons, 79 (12.5%) were not followed

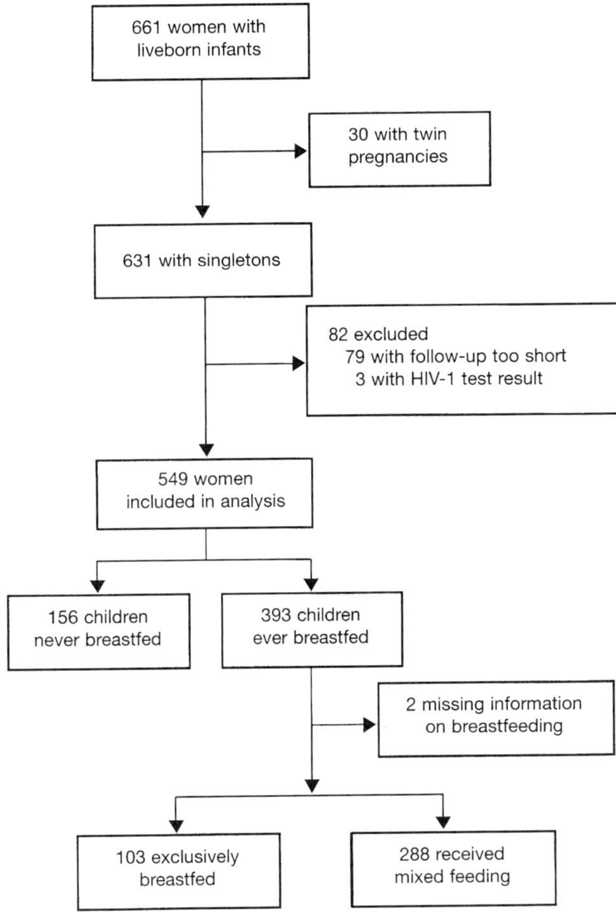

FIGURE 1. Cohort profile.

for long enough to establish their feeding practices, and 3 were followed but had no HIV test results available. The remaining 549 singletons were included in the analysis (see trial profile, FIG. 1). Those included did not differ significantly from those excluded in assigned treatment group (vitamin A or placebo), maternal CD4[+] T-lymphocyte counts, CD4:CD8 ratio, hemoglobin, serum retinol, parity, syphilis screening test results, infant gender, birth weight, or preterm delivery; but those included were less likely to have had a cesarean delivery.

Feeding Practices

Of the 549, 71.6% initiated at least some breastfeeding. Among the 393 who elected to breastfeed, 78.6% were still breastfeeding at one month, and 59.4% at three months. The median duration of all breastfeeding was 6 months (interquartile range [IQR] 1–10 months). Among the 393 breastfeeders, 43.2% breastfed exclusively to one month and 21.7% breastfed exclusively to 3 months. The median duration of exclusive breastfeeding was one month (IQR 0–3 months).

The proportions of women electing to initiate at least some breastfeeding and its duration did not differ by most maternal or child characteristics potentially associated with mother-to-child HIV transmission. The choice to initiate at least some breastfeeding was more common among women with less education, who lived in homes without electricity, and who had no water source in their home or on their property. Among breastfeeders, duration of exclusive breastfeeding was not as consistently related to these socioeconomic indicators.

Probability of Early HIV Transmission by Feeding Practices

Vitamin A supplementation had no effect on MTCT of HIV; therefore, the two groups (placebo and vitamin A supplemented) were treated as one group. The transmission rate at 3 months in 156 children who were never breastfed was 18.8% compared to 24.1% in the 288 infants who had received breast milk together with other feeds. However, among the 103 infants who were exclusively breastfed, 14.6% were infected, which is significantly different from the rate in those receiving mixed breastfeeding ($p = 0.03$) and not very different from those who had never been breastfed. There were no differences between exclusive breastfeeders and mixed breastfeeders in terms of all the risk factors for transmission, for example, maternal viral load, CD4 counts, positive syphilis, and preterm deliveries. At one day of age, the estimated proportion infected was 6.4% in the never-breastfed group compared to 6.8% in the exclusively breastfed group and 5.2% in the nonexclusively breastfed group. The fact that these transmission rates, which are measuring *in utero* infection, were similar in the three feeding groups lends further support for the fact that the groups did not differ initially in their risk of HIV transmission. After adjusting for

TABLE 1. Associations between feeding practices and the risk of HIV infection by 3 months of age adjusting for other transmission risk factors

Characteristic	n	Percent HIV-infected by 3 months	Adjusted hazard ratios[a] (95% CI)	p value
Never breastfed	156	18.8	0.85 (0.51–1.42)	
Exclusively breastfed ≥3 months	103	14.6	0.52 (0.28–0.98)	0.53
Breastfed + other food < 3 months	288	24.1		0.04
Maternal CD4:CD8 ratio at enrollment				
< 0.5	207	29.3		
≥ 0.5	285	14.8	2.08 (1.34–3.25)	0.001
Syphilis screening test				
Positive	63	29.5		
Negative	379	20.7	1.78 (1.03–3.07)	0.04
Preterm delivery	53	23.4		
Term delivery	461	20.1	1.96 (0.99–3.86)	0.05

[a]Adjusted hazard ratios are derived from a Cox Proportional Hazards model with all of the characteristics shown in the Table as independent variables .

potential confounders (*viz.*, maternal CD4/CD8 ratio; preterm delivery, and syphilis screening test results) exclusive breastfeeding carried a 48% lower risk for HIV-1 transmission than mixed feeding (Hazard Ratio 0.52; CI 0.28-0.98) (TABLE 1). Adjustment for treatment assignment (vitamin A or placebo) or maternal serum retinol level at enrollment (presupplementation), either alone or in combination with the other variables, did not change the magnitude of the associations between the risk of HIV infection by 3 months of age and feeding practices.

DISCUSSION

In conclusion, our study has shown that exclusive breastfeeding for 3 months substantially lowers risk of MTCT of HIV compared to mixed breastfeeding. Are the results biologically plausible? In the last few years several large studies have documented the benefits of exclusive breastfeeding in comparison with mixed breastfeeding in non-HIV-infected women. Apart from immune factors, which may inhibit HIV infection, breast milk contains growth factors such as epidermal growth factor and transforming growth factor-β, which may enhance the maturation of the gut epithelial barrier thus maintaining its integrity and hindering passage of the virus through this barrier.[8–11] Ingestion of contaminated water, fluids, and food or food allergens may lead to gut mucosal injury and disruption of immunological barriers in the gut. HIV-1 may be less likely to penetrate intact and healthy gastrointestinal mucosa of infants. A recent study in Guatemala[12] using the lactulose/mannitol permeability test to test intestinal function showed that a significantly larger number of infants receiving mixed breastfeeding had impaired gut function when compared to those receiving exclusive breastfeeding.

Our study was the first to collect, prospectively, detailed information on feeding practices and to advocate exclusive breastfeeding for women who elected to breastfeed, thus providing an opportunity to have a large enough group of truly exclusively breastfed children to examine. It may be argued that our study was not a randomized, controlled trial, and therefore there were characteristics of the mothers that resulted in self-selection to the exclusive breastfeeding, mixed, and formula-fed groups. Most maternal or child characteristics potentially associated with MTCT of HIV were not different among the three groups. However, positive syphilis tests and some indicators of socioeconomic status (*viz.*, absence of electricity or water in the house, less maternal education, and unemployment) were more frequent among women who chose to breastfeed. There were no consistent differences in these characteristics among mothers who exclusively breastfed compared to those who gave mixed feeds. Nevertheless, a limitation of this study is the fact that there may be variables among the different feeding groups that we were unable to measure and that may have accounted for feeding choices made. Additionally, women with healthier children may have been able to continue breastfeeding for longer; however, our own experience in interacting with the mothers suggests that those who introduced other food despite our advice tended to do so because of social pressure rather than because of their child's health. An analysis of the infant morbidity data collected in the study is planned to control for the possibility that sick/HIV-infected infants were more likely to have received mixed breastfeeding.

Since publication of our study in the *Lancet,*[13] there has been considerable discussion about our findings. One of the concerns has been that the Malawian study published recently by Miotti *et al.*[14] is at variance with our findings. We do not believe that our results are at odds with the findings of Miotti *et al.* In our study at 3 months, the rate of transmission attributable to all breastfeeding (calculated as the difference between transmission in the breastfeeding group [21.3%] and in the formula feeding group [18.8%]) was 2.5%. This rate of transmission attributable to breastfeeding to 3 months is almost exactly the same as that predicted by the Malawi study, which calculated the hazard rate of all breastfeeding to be 0.7% per month in the first 6 months of life. The Malawi study reported only rates of all breastfeeding transmission; it did not distinguish between exclusive and mixed breastfeeding, as we did in our study. Our study may help explain their observation that risks of breastfeeding transmission are greater in the first 6 months, because mixed breastfeeding is a common practice in the first 6 months at a time when the infant's gut is still immature and most likely to be at risk for HIV infection.

A second point of concern that has been raised is our finding that the transmission rate in those exclusively breastfed was lower than in those never breastfed. Although this difference was not statistically significant, we suggested in our *Lancet* paper[13] that there is a possibility that the virus, in the infant who acquired it during delivery, could have been neutralized by immune factors present in breast milk but not in formula feeds. Breast milk contains nonspecific immune factors, and these have been shown to have anti-viral and anti-HIV effects *in vitro*; these factors include secretory leukocyte protease inhibitor,[8] lactoferrin, complement, and a glycosaminoglycan.[9] In addition we have recent data that show that if the early deaths are excluded, the nonsignificant differences between the exclusive breastfeeding and formula feeding groups disappear, whereas the risk of transmission in the mixed-feeding group remains higher than in the exclusive breastfeeding group.

A final concern is that the mothers who did not exclusively breastfeed were those who were sicker and therefore more likely to transmit the virus to their infants. After publication of our findings, we have determined the HIV viral load in a subsample of mothers who exclusively breastfed and compared it to those who did not. We found no difference in the viral load between the two ($\log_{10}$ 4.42 vs. 4.54, respectively). This together with the fact that the CD4 counts were also similar (499 vs, 463, respectively) suggests that the mothers' health was not related to the choice to breastfeed exclusively.

The most important limitation of our study is the fact that we were unable to validate mothers' reports of feeding practices. However, we did check that the information given at a visit was consistent with that given at previous visits. Mothers did not benefit by misrepresenting their feeding method, and individuals who counseled women on feeding choices were different from those collecting follow-up information. Specific care was taken not to pass judgment on choices made by the mother.

RECOMMENDATIONS

HIV-infected women who choose to breastfeed, or who have no other choice open to them but breastfeeding, should be informed about the advantages of exclusive breastfeeding and encouraged and actively supported to breastfeed exclusively. Although exclusive breastfeeding is not the norm in most cultures where HIV prevalence is high, a recent study has shown that behavior change is possible[15] given sufficient active support.

ACKNOWLEDGMENTS

For their invaluable assistance we wish to thank the following persons, groups, and organizations: The South African Vitamin A Study Group—Gill Sinclair, Anne Mburu, Nolwandle Mngqundaniso, Kerry Uebel, Ingrid Coetzee, Ken Annamalai, Trevor Doorasamy, Ugene Govender, Juana Willumsen, Nigel Rollins, Jagidesa Moodley, and Daya Moodley; Dr. H. Holst, superintendent, McCord Hospital, for valuable cooperation and for allowing us access to patients in the antenatal clinic; Dr. L. Dwarkapersad, chief medical superintendent, King Edward Hospital for permission to conduct the study at King Edward VIIIth Hospital; the nursing staff at McCord and King Edward Hospitals for their assistance and cooperation; Ms. T. Ngubane, Ms. T. Buthelezi, and Ms. J. Sibanyoni for providing counseling to the women in the study; Ms. D. Naicker, Ms. A. Mngadi, and Ms. J. Mshenshela for assistance with the follow-up clinics; Ms. I. Elson, Analytical Unit, University of Natal, for vitamin A analysis; Prof. A. Smith, Dr. D. York, and Ms. S. Madurai, Department of Virology, University of Natal for HIV testing; and Dr. Z. Stein, Gertrude H. Sergievsky Center, Columbia University, New York, for valuable discussions about study design and interpretation of data. Finally we thank the mothers and their children for participating in the study.

REFERENCES

1. DUNN, T.D.T. *et al.* 1992. Risk of human immunodeficiency virus type 1 transmission through breastfeeding. Lancet **340:** 585–588.
2. BOBAT, R. *et al.* 1997. Breastfeeding by HIV-1 infected women and outcome in their infants: a cohort study from Durban, South Africa. AIDS **11:** 1627–1633.
3. TESS, B.H. *et al.* 1998. Infant feeding and risk of mother-to-child transmission of HIV-1 in Sao Paulo State, Brazil. J. Acquir. Immune Defic. Syndr. Hum. Retrovirol. **19:** 189–194.
4. COUTSOUDIS, A., *et al.* 1999. Randomized trial testing the effect of vitamin A supplementation on pregnancy outcomes and early mother-to-child HIV-1 transmission in Durban, South Africa. AIDS **13:** 1517–1524.
5. CATIGNIANI, G.L. *et al.* 1983. Simultaneous determination of retinol and alpha-tocopherol in serum or plasma by liquid chromatography. Clin. Chem. **29:** 708–712.
6. MULDER, J. *et al.* 1994. Rapid and simple PCR assay for a quantitation of human immunodeficiency virus type 1 RNA in plasma. J. Clin. Microbiol. **32:** 292–300.
7. CONNOR, E.M. *et al.* 1994. Reduction of maternal–infant transmission of human immunodeficiency virus type 1 with zidovudine treatment. N. Engl. J. Med. **331:** 1173–1180.
8. WAHL, S.M. *et al.* 1997. Secretory leucocyte protease inhibitor (SLPI) in mucosal fluids inhibits HIV-1. Oral Dis. **3:** S64–69.
9. NEWBURG, D.S. *et al.* 1992. A human milk factor inhibits binding of the human immunodeficiency virus to the CD4 receptor. Paediatr. Res. **31:** 22–28.
10. UDALL, J.N. *et al.* 1981. Development of the gastrointestinal mucosal barrier: the effect of natural versus artificial feeding on intestinal permeability to macromolecules. Pediatr. Res. **15:** 245–249.
11. PLANCHON, S.M. *et al.* 1994. Regulation of intestinal epithelial barrier function. J. Immunol. **153:** 5730–5739.

12. GOTO, K. *et al. 1999.* Epidemiology of altered intestinal permeability to lactulose and mannitol in Guatemalan infants. J. Pediatr. Gastroenterol. Nutr. **28:** 282–290.
13. COUTSOUDIS, A. *et al.* 1999. Influence of infant-feeding patterns on early mother-to-child transmission of HIV-1 in Durban, South Africa. Lancet **354:** 471–476.
14. MIOTTI, P.G. *et al.* 1999. HIV transmission through breastfeeding—a study in Malawi. JAMA **282:** 744–749.
15. MORROW, A.L. *et al.* 1999. Efficacy of home-based peer counselling to promote exclusive breastfeeding: a randomised controlled trial. Lancet **353:** 1226–1231.

Future Directions

LUDMILA LHOTSKA[a] AND HELEN ARMSTRONG

Nutrition Section, UNICEF, New York, New York 10017, USA

ABSTRACT: Despite progress in promotion and support of breastfeeding over the past decade, the HIV pandemic necessitates new actions based on human rights, such as voluntary and confidential testing and counseling, offering HIV-positive women objective information on the risks and costs of all infant feeding options, and providing appropriate support for their decisions. Implementation of the Baby-Friendly Hospital Initiative and the International Code of Marketing are essential components of a rights-based policy response to HIV and will lessen spillover of replacement feeding among HIV-negative women. Protective effects of nevirapine and exclusive breastfeeding, as well as the listed additional topics, require further research. We have yet to make exclusive breastfeeding easy and common when mothers choose to breastfeed.

HISTORICAL CONTEXT

Since the 1980s, UNICEF has worked with colleague agencies, governments, and nongovernmental organizations to reverse the global decline in breastfeeding that has been closely associated with high rates of needless infant and young child morbidity and mortality. It has often been proposed that improving conditions for women so that breastfeeding could be easier and longer would save approximately one and a half million children's lives per year. This estimate is derived from epidemiological studies that show high rates of mortality from diarrheal diseases and acute respiratory infections in infants who are not breastfed.

Optimal child health cannot be achieved without the foundation of exclusive breastfeeding for about six months followed by continued breastfeeding with appropriate complementary foods well into the second year or beyond.[1] Fulfillment of each child's right to the highest attainable standard of health, in conformity with the Convention on the Rights of the Child, thus depends on programs that promote, protect, and support breastfeeding.[2]

Considerable progress in increasing rates of initiation and prevalence of breastfeeding has been made through the past decade.[3] Yet the HIV pandemic poses a threat to this progress. In some countries, breastfeeding practices and policies have been negatively affected by the fear of mother-to-child transmission of HIV, while programs to identify infected mothers and offer them treatment and viable infant feeding options have yet to be widely available in most countries of high HIV prevalence. If breastfeeding cultures—already vulnerable to commercial undermining and to other pressures on mothers—needlessly deteriorate further, the impact on infants and young children will be devastating.

How, then, can we best move forward?

[a]Address for correspondence: Nutrition Section TA 24 A, UNICEF, 3 UN Plaza, New York, NY 10017, USA. Voice: 212-824-6371; fax 212-824-6465.
llhotska@unicef.org

FOUR OPERATIONAL TARGETS FOR INCREASED BREASTFEEDING

Effective actions to maintain and increase breastfeeding rates have been implemented widely and could be applied in all settings. The International Code of Marketing of Breastmilk Substitutes, developed through consultations with all stakeholders during the late 1970s and adopted as a recommendation by the World Health Assembly in 1981, when fully implemented, protects all women from commercial influences on how they choose to feed their infants.[4] Subsequent Resolutions of the World Health Assembly have clarified provisions of the Code, particularly with regard to provision of free and low-cost supplies of formula, bottles, and teats (that is, bottle nipples and pacifiers).[5]

Implementation of the Code of Marketing has been slow but steady, and at present 21 countries have passed legislation or binding regulations that embody all of its provisions. Another 27 have many provisions as law, and 29 have drafted a law that awaits final approval.[6] Where no national code has yet been adopted, all parties including manufacturers and distributors are expected to abide by the provisions of the International Code itself. However, compliance with the Code has been inconsistent on the part of manufacturers, with particular disregard for the universal nature of the Code in industrialized and newly independent states, as well as continued violations of the Code in many developing countries. Stronger enforcement of Code provisions is needed to ensure that its articles are universally upheld.

Regulation of marketing is necessary to create the climate for increased breastfeeding, but it is not sufficient. Women also need to be empowered through promotion of breastfeeding by appropriate national policies, improvements in maternity care, and ongoing access to support through any doubts and difficulties. The challenges faced by employed women, and the millions more who support their families through unpaid or casual labor, must also be addressed. To this end, three operational targets defined by the Innocenti Declaration of 1990 offer tested routes:

- the establishment of breastfeeding committees and coordinators with due authority in many nations,

- the implementation in all countries of the International Code of Marketing of Breastmilk Substitutes, and

- the provision of maternity leaves and other entitlements for all working women.[1]

A fourth Innocenti Declaration operational target was the transformation of maternity practices known as the Baby-Friendly Hospital Initiative, which makes the care given to women perinatally more supportive of both breastfeeding and of mother–infant bonding. Currently there are 14,654 Baby-Friendly Hospitals designated according to international criteria in 132 countries,[7] ensuring that mothers and infants can get off to the best start for exclusive breastfeeding.

It must be understood that any mother in a Baby-Friendly Hospital may choose not to breastfeed. The BFHI has always been a program that restores choice to mothers, offering help to breastfeed and the conditions that make breastfeeding simple, but not refusing the Baby-Friendly designation where some women choose not to breastfeed for reasons outside the control of the hospital. Because Baby-Friendly Hospitals protect all mothers from commercial promotion of artificial feeding products, each woman can make free choices about replacement feeding on a basis of objective information from professional staff. Supplies of infant formula, in accord with the Code of Marketing, are purchased through normal procurement channels.[8]

HIV AND INFANT FEEDING POLICIES, 1992 AND 1997

In 1992, a technical consultation among UN agencies and experts weighed the risks of mother-to-child transmission of HIV (MTCT) through breastfeeding against the known risks of artificial feeding in suboptimal conditions. On epidemiological grounds, it was concluded that where infectious disease was the commonest cause of infant deaths, women should be advised to breastfeed even if they were HIV positive.[9] Although the intention had been to express a balanced judgment to be applied case by case, this statement was widely misinterpreted as recommending that all HIV-positive women in developing countries should breastfeed, while all in industrialized countries should not.

Development of new recommendations became possible with the increase in understanding of MTCT risks between 1992 and 1996 and was in accord with growing international emphasis on human rights. Following renewed technical consultations, the 1997 joint UNAIDS/WHO/UNICEF statement emphasized individualized counseling and fully informed decision-making for women in all countries.[10] Women would not be instructed what to do, nor would policies require them to feed their infants in specified ways. Each tested HIV-positive mother would be given counseling on all options and enabled to make a decision appropriate to her own situation. *Guidelines for Decision Makers* and *A Guide for Health Care Managers and Supervisors* were published in 1998, along with a review of the evidence for breastmilk transmission of HIV, in order to assist governments in developing appropriate responses to the HIV epidemic.[11]

RIGHTS AS A BASIS FOR PROGRAMS

The basis for an adequate program to reduce MTCT is to fulfill every woman's rights to obtain full information, to make her own decision, and to receive support in carrying out that decision. Being female, pregnant, illiterate, sick, young, or HIV-positive does not remove these universal human rights.

The right to voluntary and confidential counseling and testing (VCCT) is the foundation of the woman's right to know (or choose not to know) her HIV status. UNICEF advocates greatly increasing women's access to pretest counseling, voluntary testing, and voluntary return for results in the context of further post-test counseling. UNICEF also urges that the information be kept strictly confidential, recognizing that in some circumstances this means that the information about a woman's HIV status should not be written into her medical record, and that in many settings mandatory notification of partners may endanger women's safety, livelihoods, and access to their children.

Recognizing that there are a range of infant feeding options for HIV-positive women who choose not to breastfeed, or to switch from breastfeeding to an alternative before they would otherwise have done so, UNICEF works to provide affordable options. The UNICEF Supply Division will be able to provide inexpensive generic formula, meeting Codex Alimentarius standards, from a manufacturer that has never violated the International Code of Marketing of Breastmilk Substitutes, specifically for the use of HIV-positive women. UNICEF will also be able to supply daily packets of a micronutrient mix bringing home-prepared formula up to Codex Alimentarius standards, for use in those countries where fresh milk or dried full cream milk are more affordable than tinned formula.

Throughout WHO and UNICEF materials, feeding of any fluids including breastmilk substitutes is encouraged from an open cup, not a feeding bottle. Feeding bottles entail needless additional risks of contamination, infant infections, dental problems, and inattentive care, as well as requiring more resources of fuel, water, and caregiver time.[12] Open cups may be used from birth, as pioneered in eastern Africa and now increasingly a part of up-to-date infant care.[13]

Protection, promotion and support of breastfeeding for the majority of infants who would benefit from it is even more vital than previously, due to the danger of spillover—needless abandonment of breastfeeding among women of negative or unknown HIV status who react with fear to the possibility of HIV transmitted through breastmilk. When the right to information through VCCT is fulfilled, and all women have access to testing and to treatment and full unbiased information on their infant feeding options if HIV-positive, spillover can be minimized.

To the danger that women might abandon breastfeeding needlessly, one must add a complementary concern—that HIV-positive women may choose to breastfeed for fear of stigmatization if they do not. Protection of HIV-positive women from stigma and violence and support for their free choices will be intrinsic to effective programs for prevention of MTCT.

KEY ACTIONS

Implementation of the International Code of Marketing of Breastmilk Substitutes

As promotion of breastmilk substitutes can undermine women's confidence in their ability to breastfeed, implementation of the International Code is fundamental to protection of mothers and children. It has, in fact, been recommended by the Commission on the Rights of the Child as a component of fulfilling children's rights. (For example, the Commission on the Rights of the Child recommended to Luxembourg, that implementation of the Code was a needed step in meeting the rights of children in that nation.)

The Code makes full provision for mothers who choose not to breastfeed. It does not restrict the availability of products on the market and ensures that appropriate, objective information will be provided by the health-care system. Women's choice among products is not skewed by free samples or other maternity center promotion of certain brands, nor by advertising and public information campaigns sponsored by particular companies. Health professionals too are protected from commercial gifts, biased information, and other inducements to promote products under the scope of the Code. Implementation of the Code is one of the most important means of addressing the spillover already affecting breastfeeding rates and public attitudes in many countries.

The Baby-Friendly Hospital Initiative

The prevalence of HIV in the population served by a hospital should not change its Baby-Friendly practices. However, its antenatal services should be strengthened, to provide information about prevention of HIV infection, VCCT, and interventions to reduce MTCT including changes in obstetric routines. If a mother is HIV-positive and chooses not to breastfeed at all, this is an acceptable medical indication for her to give complete replacement feeding from birth, but not for the infant to be taken away from her, deprived of skin-to-skin contact and rooming in, or fed on a timetable. Baby-Friendly practices enhance care for all infants and mothers and may increase the bonding of those who do not breastfeed.

In a Baby-Friendly Hospital, there are no free or subsidized supplies of formula, bottles, or teats from manufacturers, regardless of the number of women who choose not to breastfeed. All supplies will be paid for at the published wholesale price, or at a price not lower than 80% of what parents must pay on the retail market. If necessary, the infant's family can bring in their chosen breastmilk substitute, and ideally the mother will prepare and give cup feeds herself while in hospital so as to learn good and consistent practices under helpful supervision. Further details are given in *HIV and Infant Feeding: A Guide for Health Care Managers and Supervisors.*[11]

Some special conditions may exist where supplies are already paid for in full by the government or by another agency. In these cases, compliance with the Code requires that the supply given to the mother be continued for as long as the need exists, a minimum of 20 kg for six months being the usual amount needed by each infant. In view of the danger that a few free tins given to a nonbreastfeeding family will create dependency that then obliges them to purchase products, this Code provision is especially necessary for the protection of the mothers who choose not to breastfeed.[4,11]

Training in Counseling of HIV-Positive Mothers

WHO and UNICEF are finalizing a three-day HIV and Infant Feeding Counselling course[14] to be given in conjunction with their existing Breastfeeding Counselling course.[15] These will prepare health workers to counsel mothers on all options—including exclusive breastfeeding, breastmilk feeding, and all forms of replacement feeding—to help tested HIV-positive mothers weigh the relative risks and costs of those options in a realistic way and to support them in whatever decisions they make as their infant grows or circumstances change.

PILOT PROJECTS

Eleven high-prevalence countries (Botswana, Burkina Faso, Cambodia, Côte d'Ivoire, Honduras, Kenya, Rwanda, Tanzania, Uganda, Zambia, and Zimbabwe) are currently engaged in pilot projects on MTCT that will tell us, from a variety of settings and nationally determined programs, the feasibility and effects of:

- voluntary and confidential counseling and testing;
- appropriate infant feeding counseling and follow-up of the child and the family, including provision of support for mother's infant feeding decisions; and
- the best practical measures for preventing spillover.

With recent advances in antiretroviral therapy (ART), the effects of these new drugs on MTCT with varying patterns of infant feeding will be explored. Our current state of knowledge suggests that if HIV-positive women choose to breastfeed, they should be supported to do so exclusively for about the first six months. If they decide at any point to switch to replacement feeding, the transition should perhaps be rapid due to the elevated risks of MTCT that may be faced by infants who are partially breastfed and also given breastmilk substitutes.[16]

NEW DIRECTIONS FOR RESEARCH

Recent findings now hold out hope for reductions in MTCT even where many women choose to breastfeed. The recent Uganda studies showing a reduction when mother and infant are treated with single dose nevirapine suggests that effective treatment will no longer be prohibitively expensive.[17] Previously, studies of ARV therapy had been linked to avoidance of breastfeeding, as in the valuable northern Thailand research on the short course of zidovudine.[18]

Ongoing work in South Africa suggests that we have greatly underestimated the extent to which the gut damage associated with formula and perhaps with other supplementation of breastfeeding may increase risks of transmission.[16] If exclusive breastfeeding can be well supported in HIV-positive women, as was shown to be possible in Durban despite a culture of partial breastfeeding, risks of transmission may be further reduced. Repetition of these studies combining the drug therapy with an emphasis on exclusive breastfeeding during the early months will help to answer the many outstanding questions raised by these encouraging findings.

Many previous studies have aggregated exclusive and partial breastfeeding into a single category. New research methods will be needed in order to collect adequate detail about infant feeding patterns in new studies. We need to distinguish and analyze data on exclusive breastfeeding; partial breastfeeding with any other milk, fluid, or food; and no breastfeeding—using standard international indicators.[19]

WHO and UNICEF are working on a paper that will specify research techniques permitting exclusive breastfeeding to be distinguished from partial breastfeeding in design, data collection, analysis, and reporting of results. Quantification of breastmilk intakes may also permit determination of dose–response relationships. More specific data on the nature and amounts of supplementary feeds are also needed, as it may be hypothesized that water, tea, milk, and food supplements have differentiable effects on infant gut permeability and so potentially on MTCT of HIV.

It has also become clear that researchers should follow all infants for at least two years, with particular attention to morbidity and mortality in both breastfed and artificially fed cohorts. A report by Nduati[20] shows no significant difference in survival at age two years between such cohorts of infants born to HIV-positive mothers. Even with safe piped water, care from nearby health centers and a major hospital, free infant formula, and a maternal education level averaging eight years, the artificially fed group in Nairobi were not significantly protected from death compared to the breastfed infants up to 24 months. Yet more of the surviving breastfed infants were HIV-positive; and to determine eventual outcomes, it is clearly necessary to follow both cohorts well beyond two years.

THE CURRENT CONSENSUS REGARDING INFANT FEEDING

At the second global conference on MTCT in Montreal, September 1999, presentations and discussions made it clear that there were some encouraging developments on which participants generally agreed:

- Based on the results of the Uganda nevirapine trial among breastfeeding women,[17] nevirapine is an appropriate alternative to zidovudine therapy to prevent MTCT through breastfeeding.

- The 1997 joint HIV and Infant Feeding policy, and the subsequent joint documents issued by UNAIDS, WHO, and UNICEF, continue to be appropriate, as they include the option of exclusive breastfeeding with or without early cessation among the choices to be offered to mothers. These documents were reaffirmed by the appended WHO/UNICEF statement of 3 September 1999 (APPENDIX 1).

- There is an urgent need to explore the feasibility at the household level of various forms of replacement feeding, so as to improve the effectiveness of household procedures recommended to mothers who choose not to breastfeed and to determine whether those recommendations are realistic. Among these are means of hand-expressing milk and treating it before feeding it by cup, means of cooling heat-treated breastmilk or home-prepared formula, and safe means of storing various milks under home conditions (TABLE 1).

- There is a need to learn whether MTCT may be affected by management of breastfeeding that leads toward higher sodium levels in breastmilk or even causes clinical mastitis. Some early evidence suggests that such conditions, to which supplementation may contribute, could be associated with higher rates of MTCT, presumably through the opening of intracellular junctions that would normally be closed in full lactation.

- Additional studies of exclusive breastfeeding by HIV-positive mothers who choose this option should be undertaken, with modified methods and with the addition of nevirapine therapy where appropriate, in order to confirm findings associating MTCT with particular infant feeding patterns—exclusive breastfeeding, partial breastfeeding, and none.

THE IMMEDIATE CHALLENGE—MAKING EXCLUSIVE BREASTFEEDING EASY AND COMMON

Throughout the world, although widely recommended as the foundation of infant health and cognitive development, exclusive breastfeeding is not yet the predominant pattern of infant feeding even where HIV prevalence is very low. With a few exceptions, neither industrialized nor developing countries demonstrate rising prevalence of exclusive breastfeeding at about six months.[21] Even in countries with high rates of breastfeeding initiation and long average durations, customs of early supplementation are deeply embedded. Step 10 of the BFHI, the fostering of community mother-to-mother support for exclusive and sustained breastfeeding, has proven the most difficult to implement yet may be key to increasing exclusive breastfeeding rates.

TABLE 1. Some pressing research questions proposed by WHO and UNICEF

What is the risk of transmission of HIV through exclusive breastfeeding compared to mixed feeding? (Additional evidence is urgently needed to confirm or refute the early reports.)

What is the acceptability and feasibility of the modified breastfeeding options?

How effectively does ensuring a good breastfeeding technique prevent mastitis and elevated sodium levels in breastmilk?

What is the feasibility of replacement feeding in resource-poor settings? How can a mother measure and prepare feedings accurately and hygienically?

What instruction and help are necessary to ensure that women can give adequate replacement feedings?

How can mothers overcome practical difficulties such as management of replacement feedings at night, for example, in village settings?

What is the infant mortality and morbidity associated with replacement feeding?

NOTE: Implementation of interventions is urgently needed and must proceed on the basis of what we know now. Presented here are a number of important research questions, relating to both breastfeeding and replacement feeding, answers to which must be sought to guide implementation in the future.

Making exclusive breastfeeding the commonest infant feeding pattern to about six months challenges health and social systems in every country. While we wait to know more about whether exclusive breastfeeding really lessens or even prevents mother-to-child transmission of HIV through breastfeeding, it is most urgent that we learn how to make exclusive breastfeeding and fulfillment of women's rights a reality wherever we work and live.

REFERENCES

1. UNICEF. 1990. Innocenti Declaration on the Protection, Promotion and Support of Breastfeeding. Florence, Italy, August 1.
2. 1989. Convention on the Rights of the Child. Adopted by the General Assembly of the United Nations on 20 November 1989. Article 24.
3. UNICEF. 1999. Progress of Nations. UNICEF. New York. p 7.
4. WHO. 1981. International Code of Marketing of Breast-milk Substitutes. WHO. Geneva.
5. WHO. 1986. World Health Assembly Resolution 39.28 of May 1986; World Health Assembly Resolution 47.5 of 1994. WHO. Geneva.
6. INTERNATIONAL CODE DOCUMENTATION CENTRE. 1998. State of the Code by Country. ICDC. Penang, Malaysia.
7. UNICEF. 1999. BFHI database figures, 1 November 1999. UNICEF. New York. Nutrition Section (unpublished).
8. UNICEF & WHO. 1992. BFHI Part III: External Assessors' Manual. UNICEF. New York.
9. WHO. 1992. Consensus statement from the WHO/UNICEF consultation on HIV transmission and breastfeeding. Wkly. Epidem. Rec. **24:** 177–179.
10. UNAIDS, WHO & UNICEF. 1997. HIV and Breastfeeding: A Policy Statement. UNAIDS. Geneva.
11. UNAIDS, UNICEF & WHO. 1998. HIV and Infant Feeding: (a) A Review of HIV Ttransmission through Breastfeeding UNAIDS 98.5. (b) Guidelines for Decision

Makers. UNAIDS 98.3. (c) A Guide for Health Care Managers and Supervisors. UNAIDS. 98.4. WHO. Geneva.

12. UNICEF NUTRITION SECTION. 1998. Research in Action: Techniques of Feeding Infants: The Case for Cup Feeding. UNICEF. New York. (informal publication)
13. WHO & UNICEF. 1995. Management of Childhood Illness: Counsel the Mother. WHO/CDR/95.14. WHO. Geneva.
14. WHO & UNICEF. 2000. HIV and Infant Feeding Counselling: A Training Course. WHO. Geneva.
15. WHO & UNICEF. 1993. Breastfeeding Counselling: A Training Course. WHO/CDR/ 93.4 UNICEF/PD/NUT/93.2. WHO. Geneva.
16. COUTSOUDIS, A. *et al.* 1999. Influence of infant-feeding patterns on early mother-to-child transmission of HIV-1 in Durban, South Africa: a prospective cohort study. Lancet **354:** 471–476.
17. GUAY, L. 1999 A randomized trial of single-dose nevirapine to mother and infant versus azidothymidine in Kampala, Uganda for prevention of mother-to-infant transmission of HIV-1 (HIVNET 012). Presentation at the Second Conference on Global Strategies for the Prevention of HIV transmission from Mothers to Infants. Montreal, Canada, September 5–6.
18. CENTERS FOR DISEASE CONTROL. 1998. Administration of zidovudine during late pregnancy and delivery to prevent perinatal HIV transmission—Thailand 1996–98. Morbid. Mortal. Wkly. Rpt. **47(8).**
19. WORLD HEALTH ORGANIZATION. 1991. Indicators for assessing breast-feeding practices. WHO/CDD/SER/91.14. WHO. Geneva.
20. NDUATI, R. 1999. Clinical studies of breast vs. formula feeding. Presentation at the Second Conference on Global Strategies for the Prevention of HIV transmission from Mothers to Infants. Montreal, Canada, September 5–6.
21. POPULATION REFERENCE BUREAU. 1999. Breastfeeding patterns in the developing world with selected maternal and child health indicators. PRB Washington [chart].

Appendix I

INFANT FEEDING AND MOTHER-TO-CHILD TRANSMISSION OF HIV

WHO/UNICEF/UNAIDS STATEMENT ON CURRENT STATUS OF WHO/UNICEF/UNAIDS POLICY GUIDELINES

3 September 1999

A recent early report of evidence that HIV is less likely to be transmitted through exclusive breastfeeding does not warrant a change in existing WHO/ UNICEF/UNAIDS policy.

In the last ten years, evidence has accumulated that HIV can be transmitted through breastmilk. WHO and UNAIDS currently estimate that a child breastfeeding from a mother who is HIV positive has a 15% risk of infection by this route. Every year 200,000 infants may acquire HIV in this way. Where resources permit, many HIV-positive mothers now choose to feed their babies artificially, and to avoid breastfeeding altogether. In resource-poor settings, where the risks of artificial feeding may be particularly high, the decision for both individual mothers and policy-makers is more difficult. The situation has led in some settings to a loss of support for initiatives to promote breastfeeding, and to some women avoiding breastfeeding even if they do not know their HIV status.

In 1997, UNAIDS, WHO and UNICEF issued a joint policy statement on HIV and infant feeding, which stated that

> As a general principle, in all populations, irrespective of HIV infection rates, breastfeeding should continue to be protected, promoted and supported.

> Counselling for women who are aware of their HIV status should include the best available information on the benefits of breastfeeding, on the risk of HIV transmission through breastfeeding, and on the risks and possible advantages associated with other methods of infant feeding.

> It is therefore important that women be empowered to make fully informed decisions about infant feeding, and that they be suitably supported in carrying them out.

In 1998, WHO, UNICEF and UNAIDS held a technical consultation on HIV and Infant Feeding, and issued guidelines with a human rights perspective, based on the joint policy statement.[1] These guidelines call for a strengthening of initiatives to protect, promote and support breastfeeding among mothers who are HIV-negative or of unknown HIV status, and they describe several infant feeding options for consideration by HIV-positive mothers. These include the following:

- replacement feeding with commercial formula or home prepared formula,
- breastfeeding in the way generally recommended,
- breastfeeding exclusively and stopping early,
- use of heat-treated, expressed breastmilk, and
- wet-nursing.

The options should be exercised in all cases with timely and adequate complementary feeding. There is no attempt to favor any one of these options over the others, as the principal recommendation is for mothers to receive counselling that will enable them to make a fully informed decision appropriate to their situation and resources. The responsibility of the policy-maker and health care manager is to provide the necessary support to enable mothers to make and carry out their choice, whether to breastfeed or to use replacement feeds. Some policy-makers consider that it is necessary to make infant formula available to mothers who choose the latter option. This has led to widespread public misunderstanding of the WHO/UNAIDS/UNICEF policy statement, and an inaccurate belief that the guidelines promote replacement feeding for all HIV infected mothers.

The studies on which existing estimates of transmission are based do not distinguish between infants who are exclusively breastfed and those, usually the majority, who are both breastfed and receive other foods or drinks. A recently published early report[2] suggests that exclusive breastfeeding, that is, when an infant is given no other food or drink of any sort, may be less likely to transmit infection than mixed feeding, possibly because other foods can damage the infant's gut, and make it easier for the virus to cross the intestinal mucosa. This report has raised the hopes of many health workers, who are concerned about the adverse effects on child health of decreasing rates of breastfeeding. The question has been raised as to whether or not WHO/UNICEF/UNAIDS should revise its HIV and infant feeding recommendation.

The information contained in this early report is interesting and important. However, because of limitations of the study size and design, firm conclusions cannot be drawn without further research. That such research should be conducted as a matter of urgency is clear, and has been identified by WHO as a priority.

The current guidelines clearly indicate that for HIV-positive mothers who choose to breastfeed, the safest option is to breastfeed exclusively to minimise the risk of other childhood infections such as diarrhoea, using a good technique to reduce the risk of mastitis and nipple damage which could increase transmission of HIV. Stopping breastfeeding when the infant is 3–6 months old is an option to avoid late post-natal transmission, and at this older age the health hazards for the child, and the social difficulties for the mother associated with not breastfeeding are fewer.

Short-term exclusive breastfeeding is already included in the WHO/UNICEF/UNAIDS guidelines as one of the feeding options. The information in the early report, if confirmed, would strengthen the case for choosing it as both feasible and effective. However, there can be no justification for dropping replacement feeding as one of the options, for mothers who wish to use it, while there is any possibility of transmission of HIV through breastmilk.

The existing WHO/UNICEF/UNAIDS policy and guidelines remain appropriate according to existing scientific evidence, and there is no present indication that they should be changed. The guidelines accommodate all reasonable infant feeding options for mothers with HIV, and support a fully informed choice, which will allow mothers to be provided with better information as it becomes available.

(1) UNAIDS, UNICEF & WHO. 1998. HIV and Infant Feeding: (a) A Review of HIV Ttransmission through Breastfeeding UNAIDS 98.5. (b) Guidelines for Decision Makers. UNAIDS 98.3. (c) A Guide for Health Care Managers and Supervisors. UNAIDS. 98.4. WHO. Geneva.

(2) COUTSOUDIS, A. *et al.* 1999. Influence of infant-feeding patterns on early mother-to-child transmission of HIV-1 in Durban, South Africa: a prospective cohort study. Lancet **354:** 471–476.

Mastitis and Transmission of Human Immunodeficiency Virus through Breast Milk

RICHARD D. SEMBA[a]

Ocular Immunology Service, Johns Hopkins University School of Medicine, Baltimore, Maryland, USA

ABSTRACT: Mastitis, an inflammation in the breast, has recently been linked with higher human immunodeficiency virus (HIV) load in breast milk and higher risk of mother-to-child transmission of HIV. Among 334 HIV-infected women in Malawi who were breastfeeding, the prevalence of mastitis, as indicated by elevated breast milk sodium, was 16.4% at six weeks and 2.8% at six months postpartum. Mastitis is associated with significantly higher concentrations of immunological and inflammatory mediators in breast milk, including lactoferrin, lysozyme, secretory leukocyte protease inhibitor, interleukin-8, and RANTES. Mastitis is potentially preventable by improving micronutrient status of breastfeeding women and can be treated with antibiotics and clinical management. These studies in Malawi suggest that mastitis may contribute to transmission of HIV through breast milk.

INTRODUCTION

Mastitis is an inflammation of the breast that is often characterized by tenderness and erythema and sometimes fever. During mastitis, the tight junctions of mammary alveolar cells open up, and this process is accompanied by an increase in sodium, inflammatory cells, and inflammatory and immunological mediators in breast milk.[1] Mastitis is usually unilateral, and the highest incidence is in the first several weeks of breastfeeding. In industrialized countries, mastitis has generally been considered a problem of low morbidity, as affected women are often treated by midwives and nurse practitioners, and sometimes over the telephone.[2] Mastitis appears to be more common than previously believed, as large, longitudinal studies that have followed lactating women in the USA,[3] Finland,[4] and Australia[5,6] suggest that 20–33% of women may develop clinically apparent mastitis. There are several known risk factors for mastitis (TABLE 1).

Over the last decade, mastitis has been hypothesized to be a potential risk factor for higher human immunodeficiency virus (HIV) load in breast milk and higher mother-to-child transmission of HIV.[7–9] Breast abscess, a complication of mastitis, has been associated with postnatal transmission of HIV.[10] Nipple cracks, which predispose to mastitis, have also been examined as a possible risk factor for vertical transmission.[7] Immunological and inflammatory mediators in breast milk have been thought to influence mother-to-child transmission of HIV, both through direct effects against HIV in milk and through passive immunological protection of milk factors

[a]Address for correspondence: Richard D. Semba, M.D., M.P.H., Associate Professor, Ocular Immunology Service, 550 N. Broadway, Suite 700, Baltimore, MD 21205.

TABLE 1. Risk factors for mastitis

Risk factor
Nipple cracks
Other nipple abnormalities
Poorly feeding infant
Increased oxidative stress
Systemic inflammation
Poor vitamin A status
Poor vitamin D status
Poor vitamin E status
Poor selenium status

for the breastfeeding infant.[11,12] About 5–15% of infants may become infected with HIV through breast milk,[13-15] and higher transmission seems to occur during the early months of breastfeeding.[15] Breast milk of HIV-infected women has been shown to contain HIV,[16–18] although factors that might influence HIV load in breast milk are not clear.

STUDIES OF MASTITIS IN MALAWI

We began investigation of mastitis in both HIV-positive and HIV-negative breast-feeding women seen at Queen Elizabeth Central Hospital in Blantyre, Malawi in 1995 and 1996.[19–21] The three aims of the study were to determine the prevalence of mastitis at 6 weeks and 6 months postpartum in breastfeeding women, to examine the relationship between laboratory indicators of mastitis and breast milk HIV load, and to determine whether mastitis and breast milk HIV load are associated with vertical transmission of HIV. Universal breastfeeding is the policy recommendation of the Ministry of Health of Malawi, given conditions of hygiene and access to clean water. Breastfeeding seems prudent because of the frequent cholera epidemics that occur in the study population. Women were followed from the second trimester of pregnancy through delivery and until their child was 12 months of age.

Mastitis was assessed by measuring several laboratory indicators in human milk, including sodium, lactoferrin, lysozyme, and other immunological and inflammatory mediators. Elevated breast milk sodium was first proposed as an indicator of mastitis by Linzell and Peaker in 1972,[22] and it has been used in human studies of mastitis.[23,24] Mastitis was defined on the basis of a breast milk sodium >12 mmol/l, which is greater than three standard deviations above sodium concentrations in normal human milk as measured by ion-selective electrodes.[19] In methodology from the older literature, atomic absorption spectroscopy has generally reported higher values for sodium in normal human milk than ion-selective electrodes, and caution should be used in making comparisons of human milk sodium concentrations obtained by these two different methods.

The point prevalence of mastitis, as defined by elevated breast milk sodium concentrations, was 16.4% among 334 HIV-positive women at six weeks postpartum and 2.8% at six months postpartum. Among 96 HIV-negative women, 15.6% had elevated breast milk sodium concentrations at six weeks postpartum. The similar prevalence of mastitis in both groups suggests that HIV infection itself does not cause mastitis. Mothers with mastitis had higher plasma HIV load than mothers with without mastitis, suggesting that more advanced HIV disease and/or factors associated with more advanced HIV disease may increase the risk of mastitis. Median cell-free HIV load in breast milk was significantly higher among women with mastitis than women without mastitis, 920 copies/ml compared with <200 copies/mL, or undetectable ($p < 0.0001$), respectively.[19]

Women with mastitis had significantly higher concentrations of lysozyme, lactoferrin, and secretory leukocyte protease inhibitor in breast milk compared to women without mastitis.[19,21] Lysozyme, a 12-kDa single chain protein, lyses certain bacteria by cleaving peptidoglycans of bacterial cell walls,[25] and elevated lysozyme concentrations have been reported in milk during mastitis.[26] Lactoferrin, a 703-amino acid glycoprotein, has reported bacteriostatic, bactericidal, and antiviral properties,[27,28] and also increases in milk during mastitis.[29] Secretory leukocyte protease inhibitor (SLPI), an 11.7-kDa serine protease inhibitor, protects host tissues from degradation by proteases which are released by polymorphonuclear leukocytes, and SLPI appears to inhibit the infectivity of HIV.[30,31]

Mastitis, as measured by elevated breast milk sodium concentrations, was associated with significantly higher mother-to-child transmission of HIV at both 6 weeks and 12 months of age. HIV transmission can occur *in utero*, during delivery, and through breastfeeding; and this study could not distinguish how much transmission occurred via these three mechanisms. However, these data suggest that more HIV transmission occurred between 6 weeks and 12 months of age among women who had mastitis compared with women who did not have mastitis at 6 weeks postpartum. Longitudinal studies suggest that transmission of HIV through breast milk occurs at the highest rate in the first three months following delivery.[15] The prevalence of mastitis of 16.4% at six weeks and 2.8% at six months postpartum is consistent with a higher rate of transmission of HIV through breast milk in the first three months postpartum.

In 96 HIV-negative women, breast milk lactoferrin, lysozyme, SLPI, IL-8, and RANTES were measured; and correlation was made with breast milk sodium levels.[20] For all factors except lysozyme, there was a high and significant degree of correlation between breast milk sodium levels and each factor. There was also high correlation between the individual factors in breast milk. These observations support the idea that elevated sodium levels in breast milk are an indicator of inflammation in the breast, or mastitis. Human milk contains high concentrations of IL-8 and RANTES, two chemokines that may be produced in milk primarily by mammary epithelial cells.[32] IL-8 is produced after inflammatory stimuli and is thought to play a role in the recruitment and activation of neutrophils.[33] RANTES, a chemokine produced by CD8$^+$ lymphocytes and natural killer cells, has been shown to inhibit HIV infection *in vitro* by interacting with the HIV-1 coreceptor CCR-5 on CD4$^+$ lymphocytes.[34]

LIMITATIONS OF THE STUDIES

The studies in Malawi examined the relationship between mastitis, HIV load in breast milk, and vertical transmission. Although these studies provide some early insight into mastitis, there are several limitations that deserve discussion. First, the study was based on breast milk samples that had been archived. No clinical correlation with a careful breast exam was possible, and future studies need to address this issue. Thus, whether mastitis in this study is "subclinical" or "clinical" is an unsettled issue. Second, because this was a retrospective analysis, leukocyte counts and microbiological cultures of breast milk were not conducted. It is not known whether this mastitis is sterile or associated with a low-grade infection. Lactation failure and the termination of weaning can also contribute to a mastitis-like picture; however, none of the women appeared to have lactation failure and none were weaning at six weeks postpartum. The finding of point prevalences of mastitis at six weeks and six months postpartum of 16.4% and 2.8%, respectively, are inconsistent with the idea that lactation failure, mixed feeding, or termination of weaning accounted for the elevation of breast milk sodium in this study. Third, breast milk was taken from one breast only, thus, any measurement of the point prevalence of mastitis at any particular time from the study in Malawi is likely to be an underestimation. Finally, the measurement of cell-free HIV load does not measure HIV associated with leukocytes in milk or the possible presence of HIV in the lipid layer of milk. The quantitation of HIV-infected cells in breast milk or in lipid still remains a methodological challenge.

OTHER RECENT OBSERVATIONS OF MASTITIS

A recent prospective study of over 400 HIV-infected women in Nairobi, Kenya suggests that nipple lesions, clinically apparent mastitis, maternal CD4[+] lymphocyte count, and maternal seroconversion while breastfeeding were risk factors for postnatal mother-to-child transmission of HIV.[35] These maternal risk factors were independently associated with HIV transmission in multivariate logistic regression models. The association between mastitis, as indicated by elevated sodium/potassium ratio in breast milk, and elevated breast milk HIV load has been observed among HIV-infected lactating women in Durban, South Africa.[36] In this study, breast milk was collected from both breasts at different time points, and mastitis, as indicated by elevated sodium/potassium ratio in breast milk, was usually unilateral.

CAN TREATMENT OF MASTITIS REDUCE HIV TRANSMISSION?

It is unclear from our current state of knowledge whether mastitis, as shown by these different laboratory indicators in breast milk, is a sterile inflammation or a low-grade microbial infection. It is a reasonable hypothesis that a low-grade, recurrent, or chronic microbial infection may be involved. Few microbiological investigations of mastitis have ever been done, and all have been conducted in industrialized countries.[1] The principle pathogen implicated in mastitis has been *Staphylococcus au-*

reus. Should future studies demonstrate that mastitis, as indicated by elevated breast milk sodium, is largely an infectious process, this raises the question whether antibiotic treatment of mastitis could reduce HIV load in breast milk. Mastitis is usually unilateral, which suggests that clinical management during the period of antibiotic treatment might consist of breastfeeding from the uninvolved breast, with instructions to the mother on periodic emptying of the involved breast.

CAN MASTITIS BE PREVENTED?

Mastitis is a major problem for the dairy industry worldwide, and most data regarding the prevention of mastitis come from the veterinary literature, which has been reviewed in part elsewhere.[1,37] Mastitis or subclinical mastitis in animals has been associated with low or deficient status of vitamin and minerals, including vitamins A, D, and E, and selenium.[38–41] Supplementation with vitamins A, D, and E has been shown to lower the incidence of mastitis in dairy herds.[42,43]

A recent study suggests that supplementation with vitamin A or beta-carotene did not influence the incidence of mastitis, as indicated by an elevated sodium/potassium ratio, among breastfeeding women in Bangladesh.[44] Supplementation with vitamin E–rich sunflower oil reduced subclinical mastitis among breastfeeding women in Tanzania,[45] and this study was the first demonstration that a micronutrient intervention might reduce mastitis in humans. Both animal and human studies suggest that micronutrient supplementation may be a potential intervention to prevent mastitis among HIV-infected women who are breastfeeding, and such an intervention might influence transmission of HIV through breast milk.

ACKNOWLEDGMENTS

We thank the mothers who participated in this study; the staff of the Johns Hopkins Project; the Malawi Health Sciences Research Committee; and Anne Willoughby, Robert Nugent, and Kenneth Bridbord of the National Institutes of Health. This research was supported in part by the National Institutes of Health (HD32247, HD30042, HIVNET contract N01-AI-35173-117), the Fogarty International Center, and the United States Agency for International Development (Cooperative Agreement HRN-A-00-97-00015-00).

REFERENCES

1. SEMBA, R.D. & M.C. NEVILLE. 1999. Breast-feeding, mastitis, and HIV transmission: nutritional implications. Nutr. Rev. **57:** 146–153.
2. LAWRENCE, R.A. 1994. Breastfeeding: A Guide for the Medical Profession. Mosby. St. Louis, MO.
3. RIORDAN, J. & F. NICHOLS. 1990. A descriptive study of lactation mastitis in long-term breastfeeding women. J. Hum. Lact. **6:** 53–58.
4. KINLAY, J.R., D.L. O'CONNELL & S. KINLAY. 1998. Incidence of mastitis in breastfeeding women during the first six months after delivery: a prospective cohort study. Med. J. Aust. **169:** 310–312.

5. JONSSON, S. & M.O. PULKKINEN. 1994. Mastitis today: incidence, prevention and treatment. Ann. Chir. Gynaecol. Suppl. **208:** 84–87.

6. FETHERSTON, C. 1997. Characteristics of lactation mastitis in a Western Australian cohort. Breastfeed. Rev. **5:** 5–11.

7. NDUATI, R.W., G.C. JOHN, B.A. RICHARDSON, *et al.* 1995. Human immunodeficiency virus type-1-infected cells in breast milk: association with immunosuppression and vitamin A deficiency. J. Infect. Dis. **172:** 1461–1468.

8. NAGELKERKE, N.J.D., S. MOSES, J.E. EMBREE, *et al.* 1995. The duration of breastfeeding by HIV-1-infected mothers in developing countries: balancing benefits and risks. J. Acquir. Immune Defic. Syndr. Hum. Retrovirol. **8:** 176–181.

9. KREISS, J. 1997. Breastfeeding and vertical transmission of HIV-1. Acta Paediatr. Suppl. **421:** 113–117.

10. VAN DE PERRE, P., D.G. HITIMANA, A. SIMONON, *et al.* 1992. Postnatal transmission of HIV-1 associated with breast abscess. Lancet **339:** 1490–1491.

11. VAN DE PERRE, P., A. SIMONON, D.G. HITIMANA, *et al.* 1993. Infective and anti-infective properties of breastmilk from HIV-1-infected women. Lancet **341:** 914–918.

12. VAN DE PERRE, P. 1995. Postnatal transmission of human immunodeficiency virus type 1: the breast-feeding dilemma. Am. J. Obstet. Gynecol. **173:** 483–487.

13. DUNN, D.T., M.L. NEWELL, A.E. ADES, *et al.* 1992. Risk of human immunodeficiency virus type 1 transmission through breastfeeding. Lancet **340:** 585–588.

14. LEROY, V., M.L. NEWELL, F. DABIS, *et al.* 1998. International multicentre pooled analysis of late postnatal mother-to-child transmission of HIV-1. Ghent International Working Group on Mother-to-Child Transmission of HIV. Lancet **352:** 597–600.

15. MIOTTI, P.G., T.E.T. TAHA, N.I. KUMWENDA, *et al.* 1999. HIV transmission through breastfeeding: a study in Malawi. JAMA **282:** 744–749.

16. THIRY, L., S. SPRECHER-GOLDBERGER, T. JONCKHEER, *et al.* 1985. Isolation of AIDS virus from cell-free breast milk of three healthy virus carriers. Lancet **2:** 891–892.

17. RUFF, A.J., J. COBERLY, N.A. HALSEY, *et al.* 1994. Prevalence of HIV-1 DNA and p24 antigen in breast milk and correlation with maternal factors. J. Acquir. Immune Defic. Syndr. **7:** 68–73.

18. LEWIS, P., NDUATI, R., J.K. KREISS, *et al.* 1998. Cell-free human immunodeficiency virus type 1 in breast milk. J. Infect. Dis. **177:** 34–39.

19. SEMBA, R.D., N. KUMWENDA, D.R. HOOVER, *et al.* 1999. Human immunodeficiency virus load in breast milk, mastitis, and mother-to-child transmission of human immunodeficiency virus type 1. J. Infect. Dis. **180:** 93–98.

20. SEMBA, R.D., N. KUMWENDA, T.E. TAHA, *et al.* 1999. Mastitis and immunological factors in breast milk of lactating women in Malawi. Clin. Diagn. Lab. Immunol. **6(5):** 671–674.

21. SEMBA, R.D., N. KUMWENDA, T.E. TAHA, *et al.* 1999. Mastitis and immunological factors in breast milk of human immunodeficiency virus-infected women. J. Hum. Lact. **15(4):** 301–306.

22. LINZELL, J.L. & M. PEAKER. 1972. Day-to-day variations in breast milk composition in the goat and cow as a guide to subclinical mastitis. Br. Vet. J. **128:** 284–295.

23. CONNOR, A.E. 1979. Elevated levels of sodium and chloride in milk from mastitic breast. Pediatrics **63:** 910–911.

24. NEVILLE, M.C., R.P. KELLER, J. SEACAT, *et al.* 1984. Studies on human lactation. I. With-in feed and between-breast variation in selected components of human milk. Am. J. Clin. Nutr. **40:** 635-636.

25. CHIPMAN, D.M. & N. SHARON. 1969. Mechanism of lysozyme action. Science **165:** 454–465.

26. FARID, A., S.A. SELIM, M. ABDEL-GHANI, *et al.* 1984. Diagnosis of bovine subclinical mastitis by determination of lysozyme level in milk. Arch. Exp. Vet. Med. **38:** 857–862.

27. NUIJENS, J.H., P.II. C. VAN BERKEL & FL. SCHANBACHER. Structure and biological actions of lactoferrin. J. Mammary Gland Biol. Neoplasia **1:** 285–295.

28. HARMSEN, M.C., P.J. SWART, M.P. DE BÉTHUNE, *et al.* 1995. Antiviral effects of plasma and milk proteins: lactoferrin shows potent activity against both human immunodeficiency virus and human cytomegalovirus replication in vitro. J. Infect. Dis. **172:** 380–388.

29. HARMON, R.J., F.L. SCHANBACHER, L.C. FERGUSON, *et al.* 1976. Changes in lactoferrin, immunoglobulin G, bovine serum albumin, and α-lactalbumin during acute experimental and natural coliform mastitis in cows. Infect. Immun. **13:** 533–542.
30. THOMPSSON, R.C. & K. OHLSSON. 1986. Isolation, properties and complete amino acid sequence of human secretory leukocyte protease inhibitor, a potent inhibitor of leukocyte protease. Proc. Natl. Acad. Sci. U.S.A. **83:** 6692–6696.
31. MCNEELY, T.B., D.C. SHUGARS, M. ROSENDAHL, *et al.* 1997. Inhibition of human immunodeficiency virus type 1 infectivity by secretory leukocyte protease inhibitor occurs prior to viral reverse transcription. Blood **90:** 1141–1149.
32. MICHIE, C.A., E. TANTSCHER, T. SCHALL, *et al.* 1998. Physiological secretion of chemokines in human breast milk. Eur. Cytokine Netw. **9:** 123–129.
33. BAGGIOLINI, M., P. LOETSCHER & B. MOSER. 1995. Interleukin-8 and the chemokine family. Int. J. Immunopharmacol. **17:** 103–108.
34. DRAGIC, T., V. LITWIN, G.P. ALLAWAY, *et al.* 1996. HIV-1 entry into $CD4^+$ cells is mediated by the chemokine receptor CC-CKR-5. Nature **381:** 667–673.
35. EMBREE, J.E., S. NJENGA, P. DATTA, *et al.* 1999. Risk factors for postnatal mother-to-child transmission of HIV-1 [Abstract]. Final Program and Abstracts of the Second Conference on Global Strategies for the Prevention of HIV Transmission from Mothers to Infants, September 1–6, Montreal, Canada, p. 62.
36. WILLUMSEN, J., S.M. FILTEAU, A. COUTSOUDIS, *et al.* 1999. Subclinical mastitis and breastmilk viral load among lactating women infected with HIV-1 in South Africa [Abstract]. Final Program and Abstracts of the Second Conference on Global Strategies for the Prevention of HIV Transmission from Mothers to Infants, September 1–6, Montreal, Canada, p. 67.
37. MILLER, G.Y., P.C. BARTLETT, S.E. LANCE, *et al.* 1993. Costs of clinical mastitis and mastitis prevention in dairy herds. J. Am. Vet. Med. Assoc. **202:** 1230–1236.
38. GERLOFF, B.J. 1992. Effect of selenium supplementation on dairy cattle. J. Anim. Sci. **70:** 3934–3940.
39. SMITH, K.L., J.S. HOGAN & W.P. WEISS. 1997. Dietary vitamin E and selenium affect mastitis and milk quality. J. Anim. Sci. **75:** 1659–1665.
40. WEISS, W.P., J.S. HOGAN, K.L. SMITH, *et al.* 1990. Relationships among selenium, vitamin E, and mammary gland health in commercial dairy herds. J. Dairy Sci. **73:** 381–390.
41. NDIWENI, N., T.R. FIELD, M.R. WILLIAMS, *et al.* 1991. Studies of the incidence of clinical mastitis and blood levels of vitamin E and selenium in dairy herds in England. Vet. Rec. **129:** 86–88.
42. NAGASHIMA, M., M. OTSUKA, T. SINSEKI, *et al.* 1995. Effects of a vitamin A, D, E premix of the water soluble granule type on somatic cell counts in the milk of dairy cows. J. Vet. Med. Jpn. **48:** 977–981.
43. BARNOUIN, J. & M. CHASSAGNE. 1998. Factors associated with clinical mastitis incidence in French dairy herds during late gestation and early lactation. Vet. Res. **29:** 159–171.
44. FILTEAU, S.M., A.L. RICE, J.J. BALL, *et al.* 1999. Breast milk immune factors in Bangladeshi women supplemented postpartum with retinol or β-carotene. Am. J. Clin. Nutr. **69:** 953–958.
45. FILTEAU, S.M., G. LIETZ, G. MULOKOZI, *et al.* 1999. Milk cytokines and subclinical breast inflammation in Tanzanian women: effects of dietary red palm oil or sunflower oil supplementation. Immunology **97:** 595–600.

Orphans and HIV

The Second Wave of the HIV Epidemic

ALBINA DU BOISROUVRAY[a]

Association François-Xavier Bagnoud, New York, New York 10020, USA

In our global world today, women and children do not come first. If they are poor, they come last. Orphans lose the advocacy of their parents for their rights, which have been specified in the United Nations Convention on the Rights of the Child. Society as a whole has a poor record acting as an advocate for the rights of orphaned children.

In 1988, I read an interview given by the late Jonathan Mann in the *Herald Tribune* in which he said that by the year 2000, AIDS was going to create "cohorts of orphans," many of whom would be infected with the disease. At that time, I was just beginning to get my life together after the death of my son and was establishing the Association François-Xavier Bagnoud (FXB). I wanted to use my resources to rescue children not cared for by others. Jonathan's declaration made me choose to put the focus on those children affected by AIDS. Children don't vote; they cannot lobby for themselves. And at FXB, we are committed to forgotten people in forgotten places.

In the very early stage of the AIDS pandemic, I established François-Xavier Bagnoud houses where a small number of children without parents and suffering from AIDS could live in a family setting and receive tender loving care until they died. The Association allocated significant resources to these houses to show the world how important it was to take care of these children in need and give them the best love possible during their short lives. Quality, the best, where there was a limited quantity of time. These houses are living statements against discrimination.

Fear and prejudice were not the only characteristics of the early stages of the pandemic. Ignorance and denial were also prevalent. In the early 1990s, the Association supported Jonathan Mann's effort to provide an accurate description of the AIDS pandemic after he left WHO. When he released his findings in mid-1992, explaining how widespread AIDS would become by the year 2000, it made the front pages of newspapers worldwide, but brought denials by WHO, which still refused to acknowledge the extent of the pandemic.

It is ironic and sad that last July (1999), *The New York Times* published an interview with Peter Piot of UNAIDS saying that the criticism aimed at Mann in the early 1990s had come full circle. Then, WHO criticized Mann's figures as excessive. Now, UNAIDS and WHO, whom Jonathan had inspired to change, were being criticized by academic scientists for again exaggerating the extent of AIDS in Africa. "When we look at the figures today, they are worse than Jonathan published," said Dr. Piot.

[a]Address for correspondence: Countess Albina du Boisrouvray, c/o Suzi Peel, Executive Director, FXB US Foundation, 651 Huntington Ave., Suite 711C, Boston, MA 02115. Voice: 617-432-3511; Fax: 617-432-3578.
suzi@fxb.org

I think that we are making similar mistakes today, especially in India, a country I have been working in for 10 years. Two years ago, the infection rate in that country was estimated to be under 1%. But taking estimates of the rate of the spread of the epidemic from "AIDS in the World," which the FXB Center published in the early 1990s, I am suggesting that the rate is at least 4%. That would be 40 million people already infected. What surfaced in sub-Saharan Africa will soon produce the same cruel picture in India, when country-wide testing starts there.

UNICEF itself admits that for 10 years it didn't or couldn't collect data on orphans. Meanwhile, In 35 countries, the rate at which children are orphaned doubled, tripled, and even quadrupled between 1994 and 1997. In 1997 alone, 1.6 million children were newly orphaned by AIDS.

- Worldwide, a very conservative figure from UNAIDS says that more than 8.2 million children have lost their parents to AIDS. Over 90% of those orphaned live in Africa.

- According to other serious sources, in sub-Saharan Africa by the year 2000 the number of orphans will reach 13 million, 10.4 million of whom will be under the age of 15.

- The fear is that Asia will see its orphan population triple by the year 2000.

- One in every three children orphaned by HIV/AIDS is under the age of 5.

- Sometime between the year 2010 and 2020, the global number of infants and children under 15 who have lost their mother or both parents to AIDS will reach 40 million, the size of the population of a country like Colombia.

There is no "second wave" of AIDS orphans as such. We are still fully immersed in the first wave, which spreads silently and has become a tidal wave, increasing with devastating force. The second wave is the shocking fact that, while rich countries have mastered the epidemic mostly by means of drugs, in the poor countries death is spreading like bad weeds thriving in an environment of financial and political neglect. On our shrinking planet, in our global family at the end of this millennium, the children are awash in misery.

- 12 million children under 5 years of age die each year.

- 30% of all these deaths are linked to starvation and malnutrition.

- Nearly 160 million children are malnourished.

- More than 250 million children are working as child laborers.

- Next year, there will be 120 million orphaned or abandoned children. And 100 million will be struggling to survive on the streets of our mega-cities.

- 650 million children, at a minimum, live in abject poverty, on less than one dollar a day.

How can we begin to protect the orphans of the first wave and confront the so-called "second wave of the epidemic" unless we begin to respect the right of these children to have the basic necessities for existence: clean water, food, shelter, health care, and education? The powerful tools developed by Jonathan Mann and his team at the François-Xavier Bagnoud Center for Health and Human Rights at the Harvard School of Public Health are essential here. It was the AIDS pandemic that led us to see the inextricable connection between health and human rights. Families deprived of their rights—the right to food, clean water, medical care, education, training, and to protect themselves from violence and sexual abuse and to vote for their leaders—were the people most likely to be struck hardest by HIV and AIDS. The people stigmatized and discriminated against because of AIDS demonstrated the validity of the Health and Human Rights paradigm. By implementing human rights, we take the first essential steps to promoting the health of the poorest populations in the world, and attacking the roots of poverty. Health is by itself one of the governmental obligations signed and ratified by countries at the Convention on the Rights of the Child, Article 24.

To see how visible this is, one need only look at sub-Saharan Africa. It is the poorest region of the world, and it is the most devastated by AIDS. Of the 14 million persons who have died of AIDS worldwide, more than 11 million have been Africans. This region of the world represents about 60% of the world's total HIV infections and almost 90% of the current HIV infections in adults and adolescents in Africa itself. AIDS killed 1.4 million people in eastern and sub-Saharan Africa last year, surpassing armed conflict as the number one killer. It is not surprising that, according to UNDP, these countries have the lowest standards of living in the world. And life is getting shorter and shorter in the subregion, with life expectancy decreasing by 5 to 10 years over the next 10 years in countries like Malawi and Zambia. Men and women are dying at the ripe old age of 40.

Children orphaned by AIDS bear another burden as they watch their parents grow weaker and weaker from the disease until they waste away and die. Often they alone care for their parents and suffer because they do not have simple medications to ease their loved ones' pain.

Often, after the death of their parents, these children face prejudice and neglect at the hands of their guardians or communities, or they are shunned by their community because of fears that they have the virus too. Experience tells us that orphans have frighteningly higher rates of malnutrition, stunted growth, and illiteracy. Sometimes relatives exploit them by taking their meager inheritances.

These children often have to bear heavier workloads and may be treated more harshly than their foster family's own children. They are less likely to go to school and more likely to be depressed. Young girls are especially vulnerable to sexual exploitation and abuse and lack of equal access to education. And the orphans of the HIV/AIDS pandemic are all too often much more vulnerable to HIV infection itself, which expands the impact of HIV/AIDS on families and fuels the epidemic.

As I traveled the world this past decade developing the programs of the FXB Association, I confronted many sad situations. I also became aware that in some cultures, the way I was rescuing a few of these children through setting up FXB houses was not always an adequate solution for all children orphaned by AIDS—whether or not they themselves were suffering from the disease. That was obvious in Africa where the acknowledged numbers were far too great for the houses to accommodate, and the culture has a deep-rooted tradition of extended family. In Uganda, for example, child orphans were frequently cared for by members of their extended families, often grandparents. So in that country, the Association took a different approach to providing care for thousands of such children.

We started a modest program to provide the necessities for children orphaned by AIDS. We helped families who had taken in orphaned children to set up small businesses to support the additional burdens that they had assumed. This enabled them to barter goods and services to local schools to pay the children's school fees. This took place in three communities in Luwero, Uganda, where there were about 7800 orphans, 51% of whom had lost their parents to AIDS. We helped set up more than 800 income-generating projects for these guardian families and extended the project schools. To date, 3200 children have been enrolled in 51 schools. Thirty-four schools have added classrooms, teachers, and supplies from the proceeds of these micro-enterprises. One school constructed a new tin roof from the funds made available, giving students, teachers, and the local community another way to secure precious water from the rains. These children are not depressed; they are not violated sexually; and they are learning the tools for a productive human life. And the families who have taken them in have been rewarded by the smiles of the youngsters and additional secure income for themselves.

I mention this effort because it can be replicated worldwide wherever there are orphans, from the 1.1 million in Uganda, to the 520,000 in Tanzania, to who knows how many in India, to the unknown number that there will be when the extent of the epidemic is acknowledged. Large sums of money are needed to help these young children, as well as the sensitivity to approach the task in the proper manner, getting the input of concerned communities about the best ways of implementing and reevaluating projects by means of a continuing dialogue.

The basic necessities for these children—a roof over their heads, sufficient food to nourish them, clothing that is suitable to their communities, and education—should be taken care of.

Programs must also address the psychological traumas and stress that these children have experienced upon the death of a parent or that come from their living alone for long periods of time. The highest priority is to treat any catastrophic illnesses affecting these children. They should receive the best health care available to treat chronic diseases that have gone unattended. Finally, they should have access to the simple joys of childhood and love.

To help communities provide for the increasing numbers of orphans, new approaches are needed. Normally, the extended or immediate family is the most appropriate environment for the child. When that is not available, other families can care for the child, supported actively by community involvement.

Nevertheless, neither the extended family, itself often severely affected by AIDS, nor existing institutions are the complete answer for the growing numbers of children surviving after the death of one or both parents. Other options should be developed by the wider community. For example, in our FXB House in Barranquilla, Colombia, neighboring families devised their own ways to structure the care of children with HIV/AIDS where previously there were fear and ignorance. And in South Africa, the government subsidizes the training of foster parents to care for children and infants infected with HIV.

Innovative orphan care programs in Zimbabwe, South Africa, Tanzania, and Uganda show that community visiting, involvement, and responsibility for these children work well if organized by community peers or opinion leaders. In some places, village heads have designated land to be cultivated by all villagers to feed orphans and families of those suffering from AIDS-related illness.

Church groups have begun orphan-visiting programs in which women are trained to identify the neediest orphan households in their area, visit them on a regular basis, provide guidance and emotional support, and help with necessities.

In Southeast Asia, the African approach will soon be needed because cohorts of orphans will start to appear, as they have in Africa. It is worthwhile pointing out that in Thailand, FXB spends $5,000 per child a year in FXB houses, providing jobs for numerous women at the same time. Yet, a child in a public health environment such as the Suriraj Hospital in Bangkok, without any particular effort made toward providing tender loving care, costs $4800 a year—pretty much the same. We spend the same amount in Africa for 100 times more children, not including food or medicine. These children have the best basic survival structures, but no access to the best possible care on all the multiple and complex levels that children in the family-type care houses do, for there are no public health-care structures to deliver it.

We must also involve orphaned children as active participants in their lives and look to them to help us find the best solution. AIDS orphans in Zimbabwe were asked about their needs in an initiative called "let the children speak." As the community became more aware of the children's real needs, plans were made to implement the children's suggestions.

For many children who are orphaned by HIV/AIDS, opportunities to receive information about health, sexuality, and HIV/AIDS may be even more remote than for their peers. They become isolated because of discrimination or because they leave school and become less visible in the community. Additional efforts need to be made to include them. These children have knowledge and experience that can provide valuable insights about the actual conditions, concerns, difficulties, and needs of children most affected by HIV/AIDS. Many have demonstrated their courage and abilities while caring for themselves and often for siblings and other family members. They are credible as peer educators because of this first-hand knowledge of HIV/AIDS. For all these reasons, they must be included as partners.

As we confront this bleak landscape, we do see signs of action. In July 1999, the United States government committed $10 million for AIDS orphans programs and the following September convened a leadership meeting to chart the outlines of an African Leaders Summit on orphans. On World AIDS Day, December 1, 1999, the United Nations, with support from NGOS and governments, hosted a conference on children orphaned by AIDS. Business and religious leaders are also beginning to take hopeful initiatives. South Africa has decided to manufacture much needed but expensive drugs for its people, although international patent law prohibits it. Four women who are development ministers in Europe have linked together and pledged to fight against poverty. By implementing human rights conventions, governments can attack the roots of poverty and effectively fight the AIDS epidemic, which, as Peter Piot of UNAIDS states, is spreading three times faster than rates of funding to control it. The International AIDS Vaccine Initiative (IAVI) stuns us with the following figures:

- $20 billion spent annually on the prevention, research, and treatment of AIDS.

- $300 million spent on vaccine research, of which only $50–70 million was spent on vaccine products.

- Of that, only \$10–15 million was spent for the strains that affect 95% of people infected by AIDS. Meanwhile, Kenya can spend only \$8 per capita per year on heath care and Ethiopia, \$3.

Even when a vaccine is found, the 40 million orphans of the pandemic in 2010 will remain orphans, and in this global world, they are a global responsibility. Dr. Kituuka of Uganda put this well at this conference when she said: "The orphan we care for today might be the leader of our country tomorrow."

A global rise of civil society is beginning to stir. It is scattered and needs knitting together. More and more young people under 30 want to be volunteers. At this conference, we have heard about an initiative in India by Dr. Solomon to network buddies in the developed world to fund medicines for children with AIDS and other diseases. On the ninth of October, the UNDP, together with Cisco Systems, will launch Netaid, connecting millions of people through rock concerts and on the Internet to match donors with projects. In France, Jacques Attali has devised a network to provide grass roots organizations all over Africa with income-generating projects. The efforts now coalescing to alleviate poverty must give priority to care for children and focus on the orphans of the epidemic in order to give the best quality of care to those infected. One type of model will not be enough: a whole palette of models must be tried. Meanwhile, we must all work to prevent worldwide maternal–infant transmission. Health-care structures must be set up to make medicine available and help IAVI fund a cheap vaccine for the strains that affect 95% of current cases. FXB is supporting the development of a cheap, autogenous, therapeutic vaccine developed by Dr. Jim Oleske.

What is needed is money and the means to channel it directly to trustworthy recipients supported by community-based organizations and committed grassroots leaders. This should be possible, even on a planet where, according to Jeff Sachs of the Center for International Development (CID) at Harvard, the three richest people in the world own assets that exceed the combined GDP of the planet's poorest 48 countries.

The following may sound like a provocative and unrealistic dream, but many of the new relationships that we see budding today and those just mentioned, such as the South African initiative between haves and have-nots, seemed totally provocative and unrealistic 10 years ago.

So, what if the world's richest people as compiled by Forbes magazine—almost 500 people worth more than 2 trillion dollars—gave 2% of their wealth to the orphans affected and infected by AIDS. That sum would make an endowment of \$40 billion. If it were to be invested at 5% a year, as we do at FXB, it would yield \$2 billion annually for efforts to implement Article 24 of the Convention on the Rights of the Child; \$2 billion could provide programs like the one the FXB has established in Uganda for the 40 million orphans estimated to be affected by 2010. What about corporations that are not signatories to the U.N. Convention and are not accountable for respecting these rights? They should also be made to pay their dues to these children.

This demand must be made to these people and corporations. If they fail to respond, we will remind them of what Martin Luther King, Jr. said: that in this generation "we will have to repent not so much for the evil deeds of wicked people, but for the appalling silence of good people."

Forgotten issues of forgotten people in forgotten places have to be pushed forward with the support of the media. At this juncture of our history, sharing has become mandatory and unavoidable. AIDS is the single greatest threat to global development and economic sustainability for both the rich and poor.

Using the World Wide Web and its technology to bypass bureaucracy and corruption and involving the international accounting companies and international volunteer lawyers, the Association Francois-Xavier Bagnoud and I will undertake a realistic plan in the coming year to challenge and mobilize The Forbes 500 richest people and corporations to give 2% of their wealth to programs to provide basic human rights to children, giving first priority to these AIDS orphans. These orphans urgently need our solidarity and help; we must not allow the rich areas of the world to forget them.

"We are one world, and these children are our children," said Archbishop Desmond Tutu. "Their destiny is our destiny. *Each one of us can make a difference*. Each can help save lives."

Some Recent Developments in the International Guidelines on the Ethics of Research Involving Human Subjects[a]

ROBERT J. LEVINE[b]

Departments of Medicine and Pharmacology, Yale University School of Medicine, New Haven, Connecticut 06520, USA

ABSTRACT: We are in a period of reconsideration and revision of international ethical guidelines for the conduct of biomedical research involving human subjects. The proximate cause of much of this activity is the recent controversy over the ethics of the use of a placebo control in the clinical trials of the short-duration regimen of zidovudine for prevention of perinatal transmission of HIV infection, trials that were carried out in several so-called technologically developing countries. Critics of these trials claimed that they were in violation of Article II.3 of the Declaration of Helsinki, which states: "In any medical study, every patient—including those of a control group, if any—should be assured of the best proven diagnostic and therapeutic method. This does not exclude the use of inert placebo in studies where no proven diagnostic or therapeutic method exists." The critics claimed that since the "best proven . . . method" is the 076 regimen, this is what must be provided to members of the control groups. Failure to do so, they asserted, was a serious breach of ethics. In response to this allegation, several major international and national agencies convened multidisciplinary groups to consider the ethics of multinational clinical research. The first thing they realized was that Article II.3 was in error in that it did not reflect contemporary ethical thinking. Moreover, it was routinely violated in research conducted in developed as well as in developing countries. What replaces this standard? The 1993 CIOMS International Ethical Guidelines for Biomedical Research Involving Human Subjects include several criteria for justification of research carried out in developing countries. Most importantly, the research must be responsive to the health needs and priorities of the host country. They also require that any therapeutic products developed in such research must be made "reasonably available" to residents of the host country. A new standard is emerging for selecting therapies to be administered to participants in multinational clinical trials and for use as the control "treatment" in such trials. It is called the "highest attainable and sustainable" therapeutic method. Application of this standard differs from application of the "best proven method" standard in that it permits the evaluation of new therapies that are responsive to the health needs and priorities of resource-poor countries. It has long been recognized that the Declaration of Helsinki is a flawed document in that it relies on the illogical distinction between therapeutic and nontherapeutic research. This distinction has been removed from the most recent draft revisions of the Helsinki and the CIOMS documents.

[a]This article is based on a paper presented to The Second Conference on Global Strategies for the Prevention of HIV Transmission from Mothers to Infants in Montreal, Quebec on September 3, 1999. Portions of this paper are excerpted or adapted from previous publications by the author.

[b]Address for correspondence: Dr. Robert J. Levine, Departments of Medicine and Pharmacology, Yale University School of Medicine, 333 Cedar Street, New Haven, CT 06520.

In the 1990s there has been a striking increase in interest in conducting multinational clinical trials. Most of this interest has been connected directly to the AIDS pandemic. Effective methods are needed urgently to treat patients who are already infected with HIV and to reduce the incidence of new infections.

Most of the clinical trials designed to deal with the AIDS problems in resource-poor countries are at least partially supported and carried out by sponsors and investigators from the industrialized countries. These trials necessarily are conducted in the resource-poor countries, with the inhabitants of these countries serving as research subjects.

Research involving human subjects must be conducted in compliance with legal and ethical standards. The recent increase in multinational collaborations has forced us to recognize that standards developed in the industrialized nations may not be applicable in the resource-poor nations. This recognition, in turn, has generated a high level of interest in developing international codes of ethics that are applicable to all regions in the world. A by-product of this project has been a growing recognition that the existing documents each have serious flaws that limit their applicability even in the countries in which they were developed.

It is often said that the AIDS pandemic has presented us with novel ethical problems that make it necessary to revise ethical codes and regulations for the protection of the rights and welfare of human research subjects. I disagree. I believe that most of the "novel" problems presented by AIDS have been there all along. Social and political features particular to the AIDS pandemic have forced us to pay attention to problems that should have been addressed long ago.[1]

Since World War II, three major international codes of research ethics have been developed: these are the Nuremberg Code, the World Medical Association's Declaration of Helsinki, and the International Ethical Guidelines for Biomedical Research Involving Human Subjects of the Council of International Organizations of Medical Sciences. A full discussion of each of these documents and their relation to each other is beyond the scope of this paper. (For a more complete discussion, see Levine.[2]) In this article I will concentrate on the Declaration of Helsinki because most critics of multinational clinical trials base their criticism on interpretations of this document.

THE DECLARATION OF HELSINKI

The Declaration of Helsinki was first promulgated by the World Medical Association at its meeting in Helsinki, Finland in 1964; subsequently, it has been amended several times.[2] I believe that the Declaration urgently requires revision.[3] I shall discuss the two most important reasons for my holding this belief: First, the Declaration is an illogical document. It categorizes all research as either "therapeutic" or "nontherapeutic"; every document that relies on this distinction contains errors — errors that are not intended by their authors and that, when exposed, often embarrass their authors. I shall provide some examples of such errors. Secondly, the Declaration is seriously out of touch with contemporary ethical thinking. For example, it takes an unnecessarily rigid stance against placebo-controlled clinical trials. Because of such errors, the Declaration is widely disregarded. Investigators in every academic medical center in the United States routinely do research that violates the standards established by the Declaration. This widespread and routine disregard for the Declaration undermines its authority and credibility.

Therapeutic and Nontherapeutic Research

First, let us consider the distinction between therapeutic and nontherapeutic research. Section II of the Declaration sets forth the guidelines developed for therapeutic research; Section III is concerned with nontherapeutic research. Putting one article from Section II in immediate proximity with one from Section III helps elucidate the logical flaw:

> **II.6** The doctor can combine medical research with professional care...only to the extent that...research is justified by its potential diagnostic or therapeutic value for the patient.

> **III.2** The subjects should be volunteers—either healthy persons or patients for whom the experimental design is not related to the patient's illness.

Let us consider what is ruled out by this pair of articles. They rule out all research in the field of pathogenesis, in the field of pathophysiology, and the entire field of epidemiology. Consider, for example, a recently published study that examines the role of neurotransmitters in the pathogenesis of mental depression. This study was nontherapeutic. It certainly could not be justified in terms of its potential diagnostic or therapeutic benefit to the patient. Therefore, according to the Declaration, it could only be done on normal volunteers or on patients who have some disease other than depression. This is what I mean by illogical and embarrassing.

The problems in the category of therapeutic research are equally troubling. The concept of therapeutic research is incoherent. At least some of the components of every research protocol are nontherapeutic; when they are all nontherapeutic, use of the term "nontherapeutic research" might be justified. When we evaluate entire protocols as either therapeutic or nontherapeutic, as required by the Declaration of Helsinki, we end up with what I call the "fallacy of the package deal." Those who use this distinction typically classify as "therapeutic research" any protocol that includes one or more components that are intended to be therapeutic; therefore, the nontherapeutic components of the protocol are justified improperly according to the more permissive standards developed for therapeutic research.

Such erroneous justifications in the recent past have included the following: in trials of thrombolytic therapy, repeated coronary angiograms on patients who had clinical indications for only one; liver biopsies performed for no reason other than to disguise treatment assignments in a double-blind, placebo-controlled trial; repeated endoscopies in a population of patients with peptic ulcers who had clinical indications for no more than one; and administration of placebo by way of a catheter inserted into the coronary artery. I do not want to be misunderstood as saying that any of these procedures was unethical. I am simply arguing that they should not be justified according to standards developed for "therapeutic research."

These examples illustrate the necessity for a vocabulary that enables the evaluation of these components of research. The United States and Canada, each recognizing the problems caused by the distinction between therapeutic and nontherapeutic research, purged these concepts from their regulations and guidelines in the 1970s. In the United States, in response to the recommendations of the National Commission for the Protection of Human Subjects of Biomedical and Behavioral Research

(National Commission), federal regulations were revised in the early 1980s to classify interventions and procedures—not entire protocols—as either beneficial or not.[4,5] In the language of the regulations for research involving children, interventions or procedures are classified as either those that hold out the prospect of direct benefit, or those that do not hold out such a prospect. They are referred to in the regulations as either beneficial or nonbeneficial. The justification of beneficial procedures is similar in principle to that employed in the practice of medicine. The intervention or procedure must hold out the prospect for the individual patient/subject of an improvement in his or her health. Moreover, in most cases there should be no other therapeutic procedure known to be superior to the one(s) being evaluated. There is no ceiling imposed on the degree of risk that may be imposed in the pursuit of therapeutic benefit—only that it must be reasonable in relation to the anticipated benefits.[5]

Obviously, nontherapeutic procedures cannot be justified in terms of their expected benefit for the patient/subject. They must be justified instead by the benefits one hopes to produce for society. The amount of risk that may be presented to vulnerable subjects by nonbeneficial procedures is limited by the so-called threshold standards in the regulations. For example, for research involving children, nonbeneficial interventions or procedures that present no more than minimal risk may be employed without special justification. Interventions and procedures that present only "a minor increase over minimal risk" must be justified on the grounds that the procedure itself "is likely to yield...knowledge...which is of vital importance for the understanding or amelioration of the subjects' disorder or condition," and "the intervention or procedure presents experiences to subjects that are reasonably commensurate with those inherent in [the subjects'] actual or expected medical...situations." Interventions or procedures that present more than a minor increase over minimal risk must be reviewed and approved at the national level.

Best Proven Therapeutic Method Standard

As I mentioned at the outset, the Declaration of Helsinki not only has logical flaws, but it is also out of touch with contemporary ethical thinking. This will be illustrated by considering Article II.3.

> In any medical study, every patient—including those of a control group, if any—should be assured of the best proven diagnostic and therapeutic method. This does not exclude the use of inert placebo in studies where no proven diagnostic or therapeutic method exists.

Let us consider the implications of this article. This article would rule out the development of all new therapies for conditions for which there are already existing "proven" therapies. One cannot evaluate a new therapy unless you withhold those that have already been demonstrated safe and effective for the same indication. Strict application of this standard would have prevented the evaluation of the effectiveness of cimetidine and other H2 receptor antagonists for the treatment of peptic ulcer because the withholding of belladonna and its derivatives would have been considered an unethical withholding of the "best proven therapeutic method." Similarly, the development of new and improved antihypertensive drugs would have ceased with the establishment of the ganglionic blockers. This is also an illustration of what I mean by embarrassing.

Article II.3 also forbids placebo controls in clinical trials in which there is virtually no risk from withholding proven therapy. Consider research in the field of analgesics and antihistamines. No experienced person would ever recommend that you are required to have an active control in the evaluation of a new analgesic. Article II.3 also rules out the use of placebo controls in clinical trials in which there is a very remote possibility of an adverse consequence of withholding the active drug, such as trials of new antihypertensives and of new oral hypoglycemic agents. Insisting on active controls in these areas would introduce major inefficiencies in the research enterprise without much compensating benefit; the amount of injury to research subjects that would be prevented by requiring active controls is so small that it can be and generally is considered negligible.

Placebo-controlled trials of analgesics, antihypertensives, and oral hypoglycemics are conducted commonly, and the results are published in medical journals. Parenthetically, it is worth noticing that such publication is yet another routine violation of Helsinki; Article I.8 holds that "reports of experimentation not in accordance with the principles laid down in this Declaration should not be accepted for publication."

Now let us turn to the most controversial interpretation of Article II.3, that this Article requires the provision of the best proven therapeutic method that is available in the industrialized countries even when conducting research in countries in which such therapy is not available. This interpretation has provoked the most acrimonious debate in in the field of research ethics since the 1970s. The debate was begun with the publication in *The New England Journal of Medicine* of an article that denounced as unethical the clinical trials that were being carried out in certain developing countries to evaluate the effectiveness of the short-duration regimen of AZT in preventing perinatal transmission of HIV infection.[6] The editor of the *New England Journal* opined that these trials were, in certain respects, reminiscent of the notorious Tuskegee syphilis studies[7]; this is, in contemporary American culture, one of the most powerful metaphors for symbolizing evil in the field of research ethics. The other side of the controversy is exemplified by a statement of a physician-researcher from Uganda, one of the countries in which the trials were conducted. He accused the editor of a form of "ethical imperialism" that asserts that the Western vision of research ethics must dominate the conduct of research everywhere in the world.

Let us consider this clinical trial in some detail as a case study. At the time the trial began, and indeed to this day the standard in industrialized countries like the United States, is the so-called 076 regimen. The name comes from ACTG protocol number 76, the AIDS Clinical Trial Group protocol that established its safety and efficacy. The 076 regimen reduces perinatal transmission of HIV infection by about 67%; the cost of the chemicals alone for treating each infected pregnant woman was, in 1997, about $800. Why can't we just provide the 076 regimen to women infected with HIV in the developing countries? First and foremost is the cost. Eight hundred dollars per woman is approximately 80 times the annual per capita health expenditure in many of the sub-Saharan African countries in which these trials were carried out. The cost of the chemicals is not the only problem; there are several other obstacles, most of which are also related to finances. I shall name some of the others. (For a more complete discussion of these problems, see Ref. 8.)

Provision of the 076 regimen would also have required a revision of the customs within the host countries for seeking prenatal care. In most of these countries, women simply do not consult a health-care professional early enough in pregnancy to begin the regular 076 regimen. It would also have required intravenous administration of AZT during delivery; in most regions of the host countries, no facilities exist for the intravenous administration of anything. And finally, in the host countries for these trials, with the exception of Thailand, women breastfeed their newborn babies even when they know they have HIV. The risk to the babies of providing them with any available alternatives to breastfeeding may be even greater than the risk of exposing them to infection with HIV through breastfeeding. The transmission rate of HIV infection by way of breastfeeding is about 14%. But in the regions in which the "short-duration" regimen of AZT was evaluated, particularly in sub-Saharan Africa, the death rate from infant diarrheal syndromes is about 4 million per year. In these countries, there is no infant formula. We could make the infant formula available in these countries, but that would not help. One cannot mix the formula with the local water supply because it is contaminated with, among other things, the pathogens that cause the deadly infant diarrheal syndrome.

To sum up: It is clear that the 076 regimen of AZT cannot be made available to most HIV-infected pregnant women in the resource-poor countries now or in the forseeable future. This is the main reason that it is essential to find methods to reduce the rate of perinatal transmission of HIV that are within the financial reach of the resource-poor countries. That was the primary justification for conducting the clinical trials of the short-duration regimen of AZT. The cost of the AZT in this regimen was about 10% of that of the 076 regimen. Moreover, there was no need for intravenous therapy or administration of the drug to the babies. At the time the trials began, it seemed likely that two of the countries could afford to provide the short-duration regimen if it proved effective; there was also a commitment from international agencies to assist the other resource-poor countries in securing and providing the drug.

Now let us consider whether the best proven therapeutic method standard for a clinical trial should be construed to mean the best therapy available anywhere in the world or the standard that prevails in the host country. Guidance on this point can be found in another document—the International Ethical Guidelines for Biomedical Research Involving Human Subjects—a document prepared by the Council of International Organizations of Medical Sciences (CIOMS) in collaboration with the World Health Organization (WHO). This document, which (unlike any other international document) explicitly addresses the problems of multinational research, offers some guidelines that I believe are far superior to informed consent and other traditional protections in preventing the exploitation of people in developing countries. First, for any research that is sponsored by an agency in an industrialized country and carried out in a developing country: the research goals must be responsive to the health needs and the priorities of the host country or community. Secondly, it requires that any product developed in the course of such research must be made reasonably available to the inhabitants of the host country. This then focuses multinational research on the needs of the country in which the research is carried out. No more conducting phase I drug studies in Africa simply because it's less expensive and less vigorously regulated.

CIOMS also provides some commentary on the problem with the Declaration of Helsinki: "[T]he Declaration does not provide for controlled clinical trials. Rather, it assures the freedom of the physician 'to use a new diagnostic and therapeutic measure, if in his or her judgment it offers hope of saving life, reestablishing health or alleviating suffering' (Article II.1). Also in regard to Phase II and Phase III drug trials, there are customary and ethically justified exceptions to the requirements of the Declaration of Helsinki. A placebo given to a control group, for example, cannot be justified by its 'potential diagnostic or therapeutic value for the patient,' as Article II.6 prescribes."

In my analysis, the initiation of a research program cannot be considered the same as the establishment of an entitlement to the best therapy that is available anywhere in the world.[8] Secondly, the relevant standard is the one that prevails in the host country.[8] I think it would be improper to withhold anything that is generally available in the host country in order to do research designed to evaluate something else.

THE HIGHEST ATTAINABLE AND SUSTAINABLE THERAPEUTIC METHOD

A new ethical standard is now emerging on the international research ethics scene. This standard is called the "highest attainable and sustainable therapeutic method" standard. This ungainly name requires some explanation: "highest attainable" means that under the circumstances of the clinical trial, the level of therapy one should provide should be the best one can do. The level of therapy that is generally available in the host country should not necessarily be considered sufficient; rather, it should be considered a minimum—the least that might be considered ethically acceptable.

"Sustainable" means a level of treatment that one can reasonably expect to be continued in the host country after the research program has been completed. It is a level of treatment that the host country can reasonably be expected to maintain relying only on its own resources when the extra resources provided by sponsors from industrialized countries are no longer available.

"Sustainability," then, serves as a constraint on "highest attainable." One should provide the highest level of therapy that one can under the circumstances of the clinical trial; however, one should keep in mind that if the level of therapy is not sustainable, the results of the trial may not be responsive to the needs and priorities of the host country and the therapeutic product developed in the research program may not be reasonably available to inhabitants of the host country. A very important consideration is that provision of a therapy that is not sustainable may distort the research setting to the extent that the results may not be applicable in the host country.

The "highest attainable and sustainable therapeutic method" standard is reflected in the near-final draft of the UNAIDS Guidance Document for the conduct of multinational trials of HIV prevention vaccine and in the current draft of the revision of the CIOMS International Ethical Guidelines. A closely related standard is reflected in the current draft revision of the Declaration of Helsinki.

The "highest attainable and sustainable therapeutic method" standard applies to selecting therapies that are to be evaluated in resource-poor countries and also to selecting some of the treatments that would be made available to subjects in the course of conducting the clinical trials. To illustrate the latter application, let us consider a clinical trial of a new HIV-preventive vaccine that is to be carried out in a resource-poor country. It is assumed that such a vaccine will not prevent infection. Rather, one hopes that it will prevent or retard the progression from infection to the development of clinical disease. Thus, in a field trial of such a vaccine, the primary outcome measure is likely to be some manifestation of disease resulting from HIV infection.

Now let us further suppose that at the time this trial is initiated, the standard of care in industrialized countries is to administer a course of antiretroviral drugs to health-care workers who have occupational exposures to HIV—a treatment known as post-exposure prophylaxis (PEP). And let us further suppose that in the context of the vaccine trial one could use antiretroviral drugs for the purpose of PEP. However, the cost of such PEP would ensure that it could not be sustained after the vaccine trial was concluded. Is it morally obligatory to provide PEP to participants in the vaccine trial?

PEP could be required ethically if the criterion were only "highest attainable." However, because PEP is not sustainable, it would appear that it is not ethically required. The practical implications should also be mentioned. If PEP were provided to subjects in the vaccine trial and if it were highly effective in preventing progression of HIV infection to disease, there would be so few "primary outcomes" that one might never learn whether the vaccine is effective. Or if it were merely moderately effective in delaying progression to disease, it would be highly questionable whether the data derived from the vaccine trial were truly relevant to disease prevention in the country in which the trial was conducted.[9]

The reason that provision of antiretroviral PEP is not morally obligatory is related primarily to its lack of sustainability and not merely because it might reduce the efficiency of the trial by decreasing the number of outcome events. Counseling research subjects about reducing behaviors that increase their risk of HIV infection would similarly, if effective, reduce the efficiency of vaccine trials by decreasing the number of outcome events. However, because counseling can be sustained even in resource-poor countries after the vaccine trials have been completed, it is generally required ethically to provide counseling during the course of vaccine trials.

Those who insist that Helsinki Article II.3 must be interpreted as requiring the provision of the best proven therapeutic method that is available in industrialized countries even when research is carried out to address the needs of resource-poor countries must understand the implications of this position. To consider once again our case study—the trials of the "short-duration AZT regimen" in preventing perinatal transmission of HIV—most resource-poor countries cannot even afford to purchase sufficient AZT to implement the best therapeutic method (the 076 regimen). In order to truly provide the "best," it is also necessary to provide all of the other advantages that exist in industrialized countries that enable the 076 regimen to be effective. These include, among other things, infant formula as an alternative to breast-feeding, a water supply that is safe for infants, and the facilities for intravenous administration of drugs. All of these "advantages," taken together, would cost far more than the AZT. Clearly the cost of the 076 regimen is beyond the reach of most of the resource-poor countries. Insistence on this standard would accomplish nothing other than to deny to resource-poor countries the possibility of developing therapies and preventions that they can afford. Moreover, it would preclude the participation of sponsors and investigators from industrialized countries in research and development programs designed to assist the resource-poor countries in developing affordable treatments and preventions.

Application of the "highest attainable and sustainable therapeutic method" standard is, in all relevant respects, a more suitable ethical standard. One of its chief advantages is that it tends to facilitate the efforts of resource-poor countries to develop needed therapies and preventions that are within their financial reach. Until the imbalances in the distribution of wealth among the nations of the world are corrected, this appears to be the best we can do.

ACKNOWLEDGMENTS

This work was supported in part by Grant PO1 MH/DA 56 826-01A1 from the National Institute of Mental Health and the National Institute on Drug Abuse.

NOTES AND REFERENCES

1. LEVINE, R.J. 1994. The impact of HIV infection on society's perception of clinical trials. Kennedy Inst. Ethics J. **4(2):** 93–98.
2. LEVINE, R.J. 1996. International codes and guidelines for research ethics: a critical appraisal. *In* The Ethics of Research Involving Human Subjects: Facing the 21st Century. H.Y. Vanderpool, Ed.: 235–259. University Publishing Group. Frederick, MD.
3. LEVINE, R.J. 1999. The need to revise the Declaration of Helsinki. N. Engl. J. Med. **341:** 531–534.
4. LEVINE, R.J. 1979. Clarifying the concepts of research ethics. Hastings Ctr. Rep. **9(3):** 21–26.
5. LEVINE, R.J. 1988. Ethics and Regulation of Clinical Research. Second edit. Yale University Press. New Haven, CT.
6. LURIE, P. & S.M. WOLFE. 1997. Unethical trials of interventions to reduce perinatal transmission of the human immunodeficiency virus in developing countries. N. Engl. J. Med. **337:** 853–856.
7. ANGELL, M. 1997. The ethics of clinical research in the third world. N. Engl. J. Med. **337:** 847–849.
8. LEVINE, R.J. 1998. The "best proven therapeutic method" standard in clinical trials in technologically developing countries. IRB: Rev. Hum. Subj. Res. **20(1):** 5–9.
9. This is necessarily an overly simplistic analysis of the justification of PEP. A thorough ethical analysis would entail taking into account all of the ethical standards embodied in (e.g.) the UNAIDS Guidance Document. Such an analysis is far beyond the scope of this article.

Achievable Standard of Care in Low-Resource Settings

C. LUO[a]

Department of Pediatrics and Child Health, University Teaching Hospital, RW1 Lusaka, Zambia

ABSTRACT: The gap between rich and resource-poor countries has continued to grow as reproductive care providers integrate interventions to limit mother-to-child transmission (MTCT) of HIV in a manner consistent with existing information. There are two major reasons for this difference: access to prophylactic antiretroviral therapy (ARV) for HIV-infected pregnant mothers and availability of alternative feeding for babies. In resource-poor settings, these options are beyond reach for the majority of the women. Infant and under-five mortality rates from other infections are high in these settings and breastfeeding remains the norm. Answering the question, What is an achievable standard of care in resource-poor settings? still remains a major challenge today. Dialogue has begun in most resource-poor settings to address the key elements in the package of interventions to reduce MTCT of HIV. These elements include the following: (1) overall prevention of HIV in mothers and fathers; (2) provision of good-quality voluntary testing and counseling (VCT) in antenatal clinics; (3) a comprehensive package of interventions during pregnancy, during labor, and after delivery, including screening for sexually transmitted diseases (STDs), family planning, and—where possible—ARVs; (4) provision of infant and maternal nutrition within the socioeconomic realities; (5) advocacy and program communication; and (6) other supportive measures, including community mobilization to address issues such as stigmatization of and violence against HIV-infected women. This paper discusses the challenges faced by most resource-poor settings in integrating some of these activities into reproductive care services.

INTRODUCTION

Although HIV/AIDS remains a problem globally, the epidemic is concentrated mainly in Africa and has the most devastating consequences in sub-Saharan Africa.[1] During 1998 it was estimated that 5.8 million persons were newly infected with HIV, and 590,000 of these new infections occurred in children.[1] Of the 3 million infants infected with HIV since the beginning of the pandemic, about 90% are in Africa, as a result of high HIV prevalence rates among pregnant women and the high fertility rates.[2] Nearly all the infections in children are acquired through mother-to-child transmission (MTCT) during pregnancy, labor, and breastfeeding. Trends in infant and under-five mortality rates indicate that previous gains realized with child survival strategies in southern Africa are being eroded by the AIDS epidemic.[3]

[a]Current address for correspondence: Chewe Luo, M.D., UNICEF, P.O. Box 20678, Gaborone, Botswana. Voice: (267) 352752/351909.

cluo@unicef.org

TABLE 1. HIV prevalence in antenatal clinics[a]

Country	City	Inhabitants (millions)	VCT centers	Sample (*n*)	HIV Prevalence	Year
Burkina Faso	Dobo Dioullasso	0.4	1	4000	9.2	1999
Cote D'Ivoire	Abidjan	2.5	1	2500	14.0	1995
Kenya	Nairobi	2.0	6	1807	15.0	1996
	Mombasa	0.5	2	200	12.5	1995
Tanzania	Dar-es-Salaam	3.0	4	3000	12.0	1994
Malawi	Blantyre	0.4	2	814	30.0	1997
Zambia	Lusaka	1.5	10	595	27.5	1994
Zimbabwe	Harare	1.5	0	1800	28.0	1996
South Africa	Soweto	3.0	1	15000	18.3	1997
	Durban	2.0	8	3351	27.0	1997
Thailand	Bangkok	8.0	20	40000	2.3	1996

[a]Adapted from Cartoux *et al.*[4]

The gap between rich and resource-poor countries has continued to grow in the implementation of interventions for MTCT of HIV consistent with existing information. There are two major reasons for this difference: access to prophylactic anti-retroviral therapy (ARV) for HIV-infected pregnant mothers and availability of alternative feeding for babies. In resource-poor settings these options are beyond reach for the majority of the women. Infant and under-five mortality rates from other infections are high in these settings and breastfeeding remains the norm. The answer to the question What is an achievable standard of care in resource-poor settings? still remains a major challenge today.

ANTENATAL PREVALENCE AND TRANSMISSION

MTCT of HIV in Africa is occurring as a direct consequence of failed preventive interventions among women. In most of southern Africa, antenatal prevalence rates are extremely high and continue to rise (TABLE 1). The number of cases in India and Southeast Asia also appear to be rising rapidly.

Before ARV drugs became the standard of care for pregnant women infected with HIV, the MTCT of HIV rates in rich countries where few women breastfeed were between 15 and 20% in Western Europe and between 20 and 25% in the United States.[5] With advances in care, the transmission rate in these Western countries is now under 8%. In Africa, however, where breastfeeding is the norm, various studies have indicated rates between 25 and 40%,[6] whereas among nonbreastfeeding women in Thailand and Brazil the rates are reported to be 18 and 13%.[7,8] Apart from increased risk among breastfeeding populations, various studies have shown that a number of factors play a role in MTCT of HIV (TABLE 2).

With the high rates of transmission, policy makers in high-HIV-prevalence, low-income countries are under extreme pressure to provide practical and affordable in-

TABLE 2. Risk factors associated with MTCT[a]

Strong evidence	Less evidence of effect
Maternal	
Viral load	Viral strain
HIV clinical status	Immune response
HIV immune status	Nutritional status
Labor and delivery	
Prematurity	Other diseases
Mode of delivery	Obstetric procedures
	Duration of rupture of membranes
Postpartum	
Breast-feeding	Duration of labor
	Washing the neonate

[a]Adapted from Newell.[9]

terventions for MTCT of HIV. They have a clear moral, ethical, and humanitarian obligation; but the enormous logistic and economic constraints make some of these interventions difficult to implement.

INTERVENTIONS FOR REDUCTION OF MTCT

Dialogue has begun in most resource-poor settings to address key issues in the implementation package of interventions to reduce MTCT of HIV. The key elements of the package include the following:

- overall prevention of HIV in mothers and fathers;

- provision of good-quality voluntary testing and counseling (VCT) in antenatal clinics;

- a comprehensive package of interventions during pregnancy, during labor and after delivery, including screening for sexually transmitted diseases (STDs), family planning, and—where possible—ARVs;

- provision for infant and maternal nutrition within the socioeconomic realities;

- advocacy and program communication; and

- other supportive measures including community mobilization to address issues such as stigmatization of and violence againstHIV-infected women.

Some of these elements are discussed in this paper.

PREVENTION OF HIV IN MOTHERS AND FATHERS

One of the many challenges facing resource-poor countries is finding ways to reduce the increasing incidence of new infections. In other words, how can the epidemic be slowed down? Some of the interventions that have been shown to be effective are general promotion and use of condoms[10] and syndromic treatment of STDs.[10] Establishing an effective intervention program requires political commitment, including resource mobilization.[11]

The issues in HIV/AIDS control go far beyond the health sector. Human rights, knowledge and attitude about sex, the general status of women, migration, poverty, and income levels are all major concerns in HIV/AIDS control. Clearly, the spread of HIV is a dynamic process requiring a multifactorial approach. There are some convincing signs that the epidemic is slowing down in some resource-poor countries. Uganda and Tanzania, now showing a downward trend in HIV prevalence, were among the first countries in sub-Saharan Africa to have an open attitude toward HIV and to promote HIV education. Awareness of HIV is now widespread in these countries, and there is a trend toward fewer sexual partners, increased use of condoms for casual sex, and control of STDs.[12]

Voluntary Counseling and Testing

The critical element in prevention of MTCT of HIV is the identification, through confidential counseling and testing, of women infected with HIV. Good-quality VCT involves staff who are trained in counseling skills; adequate staff time; laboratory capacity for testing including trained staff, laboratory facilities, and availability of HIV test kits; availability of a private room or space for pre- and post-counseling waiting; and facilities that are spouse- or partner-friendly. In the majority of resource-poor countries, these elements are lacking, and establishment of these systems will need evaluation before VCT implementation can be scaled up.

Good counseling has several positive benefits for the pregnant mothers and their spouses or partners:

- The couple can make informed decisions including whether to continue having children.

- For HIV-negative women, VCT provides an opportunity to reinforce educational efforts to help them remain negative.

- VCT also provides an opportunity for dialogue with woman's spouse or partner as well as her family.

- HIV-positive women can be referred to community groups involved in HIV/ AIDS advocacy and control activities.

- HIV-positive women can discuss the management options for the pregnancy, the expected pregnancy outcome, and other care issues.

A recent review of various studies indicated that acceptance rates for HIV testing are over 70% in resource-poor settings with the exception of one study in Blantyre in Malawi where the rate was found to be 53%.[4] Ideally, pre- and post-test counseling should be provided within the reproductive health package. This, however, re-

TABLE 3. Approaches to preventing MTCT of HIV[a]

Proven effective	Theoretically effective
Antiretroviral therapy (singly or combination)	Preventing new infection in childbearing women, especially when breastfeeding
Caesarean section delivery	Reducing number of sexual partners
Avoidance of breastfeeding	Reducing frequency of sexual intercourse during pregnancy
	Immuno-therapy
	Vitamin A
	Avoidance of scalp electrodes and fetal blood sampling
	Cleansing of the birth canal

[a]Adapted from Newell.[9]

quires a lot of time and the already overburdened staff might see the service as an obstacle for provision of other services. The challenge, therefore, remains to urgently evaluate what models of counseling are needed without causing staff burnout.

These models might include community-based pre- and post-test clubs, using groups such as church support groups. For this system to work, referral systems will need to be established between the health facility and the community groups. Pre-test group discussion in the antenatal clinics while the women are waiting is another possible model.

Algorithms adopted for VCT should consider the ultimate goal of ensuring that as many women as possible obtain their test results if a positive impact is to be achieved. Rapid tests are becoming increasingly cheaper and easy to perform and have the advantage that the results are available on the same day. A return rate of 100% was achieved in three ANC clinics in Lusaka, Zambia using pre-test discussion and the rapid test algorithm.[12] The disadvantage with same-day pre- and post-test counseling is that the woman might be inadequately prepared for the results and, if the spouse is not involved during testing, some of the women will not discuss the test results with them for fear of blame, violence, and possible divorce.

COMPREHENSIVE PACKAGE OF CARE BEFORE, DURING, AND AFTER DELIVERY FOR RESOURCE-POOR SETTINGS

Care interventions that have been shown to reduce MTCT of HIV include reducing maternal viral load with prophylactic antiretroviral therapy, reducing exposure during delivery by delivering women by elective cesarean section, and avoidance of breastfeeding. Other supportive interventions, though not known to reduce transmission, have been shown to improve pregnancy outcomes. These are listed in TABLE 3 as theoretically effective.[8]

Antiretroviral Therapy

Emerging data in studies both in the rich and resource-poor settings strongly indicate that ARVs are extremely effective in the prevention of MTCT. The administration of zidovudine (AZT) during pregnancy, labor, and after delivery to the baby for one week resulted in a 67% reduction in infection among infants of mothers enrolled in the AIDS Clinical Trial Group Protocol (076) in the United States.[14] This therapy, however, costs about U.S. $1000 per pregnancy.

Shorter regimens studied in Thailand and Africa have shown a 50% reduction in nonbreastfeeding women in Thailand, 37% at 3 months of age in Cote d'Ivoire, and 32% at 6 months in Cote d'Ivoire and Burkina Faso.[15–17] In both Cote d'Ivoire and Burkina Faso breastfeeding is the norm. The average cost of the AZT therapy in Thailand is U.S. $50 per pregnancy.

Although antiretroviral prophylactic therapy has become the standard of care in rich countries, very few pregnant mothers in resource-poor settings have access to these drugs except in a very few countries such as Botswana, Thailand, and Brazil. Most countries in resource-poor settings can only afford a few dollars per person per year on health.[18] The health sector is struggling to cope with the background burden of disease unrelated to HIV. Though access to antenatal care may be good, few pregnant women report early enough for other routine supportive interventions such as malaria treatment, de-worming, iron and folate supplementation, and multi-vitamin supplementation. Compared to antenatal care, fewer women will come back to deliver at a health facility.

The important question that still remains unanswered is, Who sets the standard of care in a world that has so many inequalities? Access to AZT prophylactic therapy during pregnancy in resource-poor settings is just one of the many inequalities.

The situation has become brighter with the new hope created by niverapine therapy. A recent study in Uganda using a single dose of niverapine during delivery and one dose to the baby within 72 hours demonstrated a 47% reduction in transmission at 3 months of age when compared to AZT given in a similar regime.[19] This treatment has been estimated to cost U.S. $4 per pregnancy. The reality, however, is that other than the expense, for these therapies to be integrated in the reproductive care package, systems will have to be strengthened during implementation for the impact on MTCT of HIV to be realized. For niverapine there is still the issue of drug resistance to be addressed when the drug is licensed for use. Proper control measures will have to be put in place so that the drug is not used singly in the treatment of AIDS patients. The other question is whether niverapine is the magic bullet to be given to all pregnant women without screening in low-resource settings where VCT may be too expensive. The consequences of not counseling the women will have to be weighed against the provision of blanket treatment.

Cesarean Section and Other Practices during Labor in March 1998

In March 1998, a European randomized trial was terminated because preliminary results indicated a reduction in transmission from 10.7% to 1.7% among infants born by elective cesarean section.[20] No deaths or major morbidity was reported. However, cesarean section as an intervention for the reduction of MTCT of HIV has to be weighed against the risk of the operation itself, the expertise available, the prevalence of HIV infection among pregnant women, and overall maternal mortality in the setting. In resource-poor countries with high HIV burden and high fertility rates, these results have to be interpreted with caution. Other practices to be discouraged during labor include artificial rupture of membranes, fetal sampling, instrumental deliveries, and episiotomies.[2]

Limiting Breastfeeding

In resource-poor countries breastfeeding is still the norm in the majority of the communities. The current WHO-UNAIDS-UNICEF guidelines recommend that HIV-positive pregnant women be counseled about feeding options so that they are able to make an informed choice. The pertinent question that arises from this statement is Do these women have a choice in low-resource settings? Formula feeding is not only expensive for the women, but also the health services will need to intensify education efforts about sterilization of water and equipment as well as preparation and storage of milk. If instructions are not followed, feeding with formula may lead to severe malnutrition and life-threatening infectious diseases. In addition, because breastfeeding is the norm in most resource-poor settings, women opting not to breastfeed run the risk of being ostracized and stigmatized. Community groups should be mobilized to support HIV-infected women opting to formula feed.

The debate at the moment is whether women in resource-poor settings should exclusively breastfeed for 6 months followed by complete cessation of breastfeeding to reduce HIV transmission through breastfeeding. This question requires further evaluation.

Vaginal Cleansing during Labor

Most HIV infections in children occur during the time of delivery, and free and cell-bound virus has been found in cervical and vaginal secretions. Theoretically, this mode of transmission could be aborted by cleansing the vagina with an antiseptic or virucidal agent such as chlorhexidine. The intervention using chlorhexidine to cleanse the vagina has potential for low-income countries, because it is cheap enough to be provided to all women without prior VCT.

The study in Malawi by Biggar *et al.,* however, did not show any benefit in reducing MTCT of HIV except in women who had prolonged rupture of membranes (over 4 hours).[21] Another study is planned for Zambia using higher concentrations. A preliminary evaluation of the highest concentration of chlorhexidine that is safe is under way in South Africa.

Supplementation with Micronutrients

In a study by Semba *et al.,* a clear association between maternal vitamin A deficiency and not only MTCT of HIV but also infant mortality was demonstrated.[22,23] Nevertheless, follow-up vitamin A and multivitamin supplementation trials have not shown a reduction in HIV transmission rate.[23–25] Despite these findings, vitamin supplementation is still beneficial in HIV-infected pregnant mothers because of other outcomes.[25] These include improved maternal CD4 counts, reduced morbidity and mortality of the infants, reduced low-birthweight rate (prematurity and intrauterine growth retardation), reduced fetal loss, and increased maternal hemoglobin.

These outcomes are important and should form the basis for promoting multivitamin supplementation in the minimum package of care for resource-poor countries.

CONCLUSION

The most effective ways of reducing mother-to-child transmission according to what is currently known is to reduce viral load through prophylatic ARV therapy and avoidance of breastfeeding. However, these approaches are beyond reach for the majority of HIV-infected women. It is projected that by 2010, if the spread of HIV has not been contained, AIDS will increase infant mortality by 25% and under-five mortality by 100% in the regions most affected by HIV.[26] It is urgent that avenues for ensuring the access of women to these interventions be explored in addition to the implementation of behavioral interventions to reduce the number of infections in women. The strengthening of already existing systems must be the focus in order for the impact to be realized.

UNAIDS is currently working in 10 countries in Africa to assess the feasibility of integrating activities aimed at reducing MTCT of HIV including ARVs in existing reproductive care services. The mother–child package in this initiative has a number of elements:

- provision of good-quality voluntary and confidential counseling and HIV testing for women and their partners including counseling on feeding options;

- integration of a minimal package of care including AZT and formula into antenatal, delivery, and child-care services;

- formation and strengthening of community support networks for mothers and children;

- advocacy and program communication through sensitization of policy makers, health managers, and community leaders to the scope of the problem and possible solutions;

- monitoring and evaluation of operational experiencs; and

- economic evaluation and assessment of impact.

UNAIDS is also working with pharmaceutical companies to try to make AZT/ARV affordable for pregnant mothers.

REFERENCES

1. UNAIDS/WHO. 1998. AIDS Epidemic Update. December. WHO. Geneva.
2. UNAIDS/WHO 1998. UNAIDS Technical Update. October. Mother to child transmission of HIV. WHO. Geneva.
3. TIMAEUS, I.M. 1998. Impact of the HIV epidemic on mortality in sub-Sahara Africa: evidence from national surveys and censuses. AIDS **12**(Suppl. 1): S15–S27.
4. CARTOUX, M., N. MEDA, P. VAN DE PERRE, *et al.* 1998. Acceptability of voluntary HIV testing by pregnant women in developing countries: an international survey. AIDS **12:** 2489–2493.
5. DAVIS, S.F., R.H, BYERS, M.L. LINDERGREN, *et al.* 1995. Prevalence and incidence of vertically acquired HIV infection in the United States. JAMA **274:** 952–955.

6. THE WORKING GROUP ON MOTHER TO CHILD TRANSMISSION OF HIV. 1995. Rates of mother to child transmission of HIV in Africa, America and Europe: results from 13 perinatal studies. J. Acquir. Immune Def. Syndr. Hum. Retro. **8(5):** 506–510.

7. PHOOLCHAROEN, W. 1998. HIV/AIDS prevention in Thailand: success and challenges. Science **280:** 1873–1874.

8. TESS, B.H., L.C. RODRIGUES, M. NEWELL, *et al.* 1998. Breast-feeding, genetic, obstetric and other risk factors associated with mother to child transmission of HIV in Sao Paulo State, Brazil. AIDS **12:** 513–520.

9. NEWELL, M. 1999. How can we prevent mother to child transmission of HIV infection? WHO Bull. **33(3):** 1–3.

10. THE WORLD BANK. 1997. Confronting AIDS: public priorities in a global epidemic. A World Bank Policy Research Report. World Bank. Washington, D.C.

11. GROSSKURTH, H., F. MOSHA, J. TODD, *et al.* 1995. Impact of sexually transmitted diseases on HIV infection in rural Tanzania: a randomized control trial. Lancet **346:** 530–536.

12. ASSIMIWE-OKIROR, G., A.A. OPIO, J. MUSINGUZI, *et al.* 1997. Change in sexual behavior and decline in HIV infection among pregnant women in urban Uganda. AIDS **11:** 1757–1763.

13. BHAT, G.J., S. MCKENNA, H. TERENUMA, *et al.* Same day testing and counseling improves overall acceptability among prenatal women in Zambia. XII World AIDS Conference. Geneva. June–July (Abstr. 33282).

14. CONNOR, E.M., R.S. SPERLING, R. GELBER, *et al.* 1994. Reduction of maternal infant transmission of human immuno-deficiency virus type 1 with zidovudine treatment. Pediatrics AIDS Clinical Trials Group Protocol 076 Study Group. N. Engl. J. Med. **331:** 1173–1180.

15. DABIS, F., P. MSELLATI, N. MEDA, *et al.* 1999. Six-month efficacy, tolerance and acceptability of a short regimen of oral zidovudine to reduce vertical transmission of HIV in breast fed children in Cote d'Ivoire and Burkina Faso. Lancet **353:** 786–792.

16. WITKOR, S.Z., E. EKPINE, K.M. SHARON, *et al.* 1999. Short course oral zidovudine for the prevention of mother to child transmission of HIV-1 in Abidjan, Cote d'Ivoire: a randomised trial. Lancet **353:** 781–785.

17. SHAFFER, N.R., R. CHUACHOOWONG, P.A. MOCK, *et al.* 1999. Short course zidovudine for perinatal HIV-1 transmission in Bangkok, Thailand: a randomised controlled trial. Lancet **353:** 773–780.

18. THE WORLD BANK. 1993. Investigating in Health. World Development Report. Oxford University Press. New York.

19. NATIONAL INSTITUTES OF HEALTH. 1999. Press release. July. NIH. Bethesda, MD.

20. EUROPEAN MODE OF DELIVERY COLLABORATION. 1999. Elective caesarian section versus vaginal delivery in preventing vertical HIV-1 transmission: a randomised clinical trial. Lancet **3538:** 1035–1039.

21. BIGGAR, R.J., P.G. MIOTTI, T.E. TAHA, *et al.* 1996. Perinatal intervention trial in Africa: effect of birth canal cleansing intervention to prevent HIV transmission. Lancet **347:** 647–1650.

22. SEMBA, R.D., P.G. MIOTTI, J.D. CHIPANGWI, *et al.* 1994. Maternal vitamin A deficiency and mother to child transmission of HIV-1. Lancet **343:** 1593–1597.

23. SEMBA, R.D., P.G. MIOTTI, J.D. CHIPANGWI, *et al.* 1995. Infant mortality and maternal vitamin A deficiency during human immunodeficiency virus infection. Clin. Infect. Dis. **21:** 996–972.

24. COUTSOUDIS, A. 1999. Late breaker. XIX IVACG Meeting. Durban, South Africa.

25. FAWZI, W.W., R.L. MBISE, E. HERTMARK, *et al.* 1999. A randomised trial of vitamin A supplements in relation to mortality among human immuno deficiency virus-infection and uninfected children in Tanzania. Paediatr. Infect. Dis. J. **18:** 127–133.

26. UNAIDS/AIDS. 1999. HIV in pregnancy.

Organizational Approaches to the HIV/AIDS Crisis

MARTHA F. ROGERS[a] AND P. LYNNE STOCKTON

Centers for Disease Control and Prevention, National Center for HIV, STD and TB Prevention, Division of HIV/AIDS Prevention, Atlanta, Georgia, USA

ABSTRACT: The Centers for Disease Control and Prevention (CDC) has played a major role in controlling the HIV/AIDS epidemic in the United States. After implementation of perinatal zidovudine therapy in 1994, the efforts of the CDC and others produced a dramatic decline in perinatal HIV transmission. However, in recent years, approximately 300 perinatally infected infants have been born annually in the United States. To further reduce this number, the CDC has identified four prevention goals: improve prenatal care, recommend HIV testing, ensure treatment for HIV-infected pregnant women, and ensure follow-up care. To address these goals, the CDC launched a prevention plan consisting of surveillance, research, outreach strategies, grant programs, evaluation efforts, and policy development. Globally, the CDC tailors this plan to meet the needs of developing countries. The CDC provides technical assistance to international organizations to help develop, implement, and evaluate global prevention programs. Specific international sites are targeted for new research and programs to reduce perinatal HIV transmission.

INTRODUCTION

The Centers for Disease Control and Prevention (CDC) has played a large role in controlling the HIV/AIDS epidemic in the United States. A combination of surveillance, research, outreach strategies, grant programs, evaluation efforts, and policy development has contributed to the overall success. Perinatal transmission is just one focus of the CDC's HIV prevention efforts, and in this area tremendous progress has been made. The CDC's efforts to maximally reduce perinatal transmission of HIV are by no means limited to the United States; however, this paper focuses on the CDC's domestic efforts. The implications can be, and have been, extrapolated globally despite major differences in circumstances and resources.

THE PEDIATRIC HIV/AIDS EPIDEMIC IN THE UNITED STATES

To date, marked reduction in pediatric AIDS cases has been one of the most important successes in the fight against AIDS. In fact, this prevention success has led the CDC to consider expanding its goals. If the chain of care from prenatal through follow-up can be strengthened so that every pregnant women receives HIV screening

---

[a]Address for correspondence: Martha F. Rogers, M.D., Centers for Disease Control and Prevention, 1600 Clifton Road, MS D21, Atlanta, GA 30333.

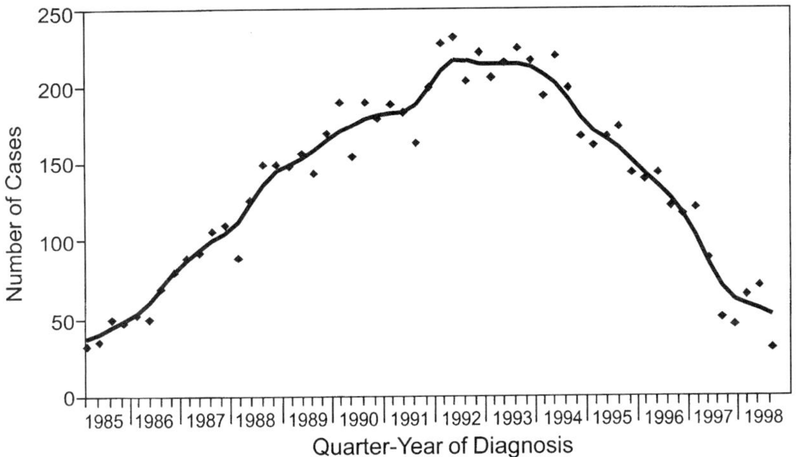

FIGURE 1. Perinatally acquired AIDS cases by quarter-year of diagnosis: 1985–1998, United States. Adjusted for reporting delays and redistribution of NIRs. Data reported through March 1999.

and treatment (if indicated), elimination of perinatal transmission of HIV will be possible.

The CDC estimates that more than 16,000 perinatally infected children have been born in the United States since the beginning of the HIV/AIDS epidemic.[1] In fact, perinatal transmission accounts for most pediatric HIV infections. The number of perinatally infected children grew rapidly from the 1980s to the early 1990s, peaked in 1992, and sharply declined thereafter. The decline followed the dramatic prevention breakthrough in 1994, when the results of the Pediatric AIDS Clinical Trials Group protocol number 076 showed that the antiretroviral drug zidovudine (ZDV or AZT) administered to HIV-infected pregnant women and their newborns reduces the risk for perinatal HIV transmission by two-thirds (FIG. 1).[1]

In response to this highly effective preventive measure, the U.S. Public Health Service (USPHS) in 1994 published guidelines for zidovudine use to reduce perinatal HIV transmission and in 1995 recommended universal counseling and voluntary HIV testing of all pregnant women and treatment for those found to be infected.[2,3] Rapid dissemination and widespread implementation of these guidelines produced a steep and sustained decline in the incidence of perinatal AIDS. Consequently, by 1997, the incidence of pediatric AIDS cases had dropped 67% below the peak incidence of 1992.[1]

Despite the dramatic decline, however, children are still being born with HIV infection. The CDC estimates that 300 HIV-infected babies are born each year in the United States. To respond to the challenge of ensuring healthy babies free of HIV infection, the CDC has identified several prevention needs and developed a plan to address them.

PREVENTION NEEDS

Improve Prenatal Care

A CDC study conducted between 1993 and 1996 identified lack of prenatal care as a critical obstacle to full implementation of USPHS guidelines. This Surveillance to Evaluate Prevention (STEP) project showed that HIV-infected pregnant women are less likely than uninfected pregnant women to receive prenatal care. Among the general U.S. population, prenatal care is late or absent in 4% of pregnant women; yet among HIV-infected women, prenatal care is absent in up to 15% of women tested before delivery.[4] African-American and Hispanic women and women who used illicit drugs during pregnancy are at highest risk for not receiving prenatal care. Reaching these women in particular is a critical first step in preventing perinatal transmission of HIV.

Encourage Testing for HIV

Another barrier to HIV prevention occurs when women receive prenatal care that does not include counseling or testing for HIV. An Institute of Medicine (IOM) study, published in 1999, found that many providers considered the counseling process onerous and that they felt they had neither the time nor the skills needed to counsel patients.[5] The CDC's Pregnancy Risk Assessment Monitoring System (PRAMS) confirmed that testing was not consistently being offered. This ongoing, state-based surveillance system collects information about maternal behaviors, attitudes, and experiences. Data collected from 1996 through 1997 from 14 participating states showed that 63.4% to 86.7% of women were counseled about HIV during pregnancy and 58% to 80.7% were actually tested. Frequency of offering testing varied by state of residence (legislation), provider type (public or private), and mothers' economic status (Medicaid recipient or not) and demographic characteristics (race/ethnicity, education).[6] Another CDC study showed that among women who were offered HIV testing, one of the major reasons for declining was not perceiving that the provider thought testing to be important.[7] Educating providers about the value of HIV testing of pregnant women will take us another step closer to universal prenatal screening.

Ensure Treatment for HIV-Infected Women

On the heels of the 1994 finding that perinatal zidovudine therapy reduces HIV transmission came the challenge of ensuring access to, availability of, and adherence to therapy. Data from the national HIV reporting system collected from 1993 to 1997 found that the percentage of pregnant women tested for HIV infection and subsequently receiving zidovudine increased sharply, from 7% to 91%.[1] The CDC STEP study showed that from 1993 through 1996, among women in whom HIV infection was diagnosed before delivery, the proportion offered prenatal zidovudine increased from 27% to 85%; intrapartum zidovudine, from 5% to 75%; and neonatal zidovudine, from 5% to 76%. Less than 5% of women refused treatment, and 6% discontinued treatment during pregnancy.[4] This marked increase in zidovudine use was temporally associated with an equally dramatic decline in perinatal AIDS cases.

These impressive results stress the importance of providing therapy for all HIV-infected women and their children.

Ensure Follow-up Care

Case management and follow-up care are critical for ensuring that women adhere to their therapy regimens. Women need to be educated about the importance of adhering to therapy and that timely treatment can prolong their own lives as well as improve the chances their babies will be born free of infection. They also need to be educated about how HIV can be transmitted through breastfeeding. Other basic education about HIV and risk assessment should be incorporated into routine prenatal care whenever possible. This educational approach will increase compliance with follow-up care for HIV-infected women, their infants, and family members. It can also help uninfected women reduce their risk for ever acquiring HIV, the ultimate goal in reducing perinatal transmission.

THE CDC'S HIV PREVENTION PLAN

The CDC's plan to further reduce perinatal transmission includes a number of components: surveillance, research, outreach, grant programs, evaluation, and policy development. The following paragraphs describe each of these components.

Surveillance

The CDC administers a national AIDS/HIV surveillance system, which gathers, analyzes, and disseminates AIDS and HIV case report data. These data are forwarded to the CDC from state and local health departments. The data include demographics, mode of exposure, laboratory data, AIDS-defining conditions, and zidovudine use by mothers and infants. Since 1985, many states have conducted HIV surveillance using the same methods as for AIDS surveillance. But enhanced surveillance is needed, including surveillance of perinatally exposed and infected children in all states in order to monitor effectiveness of perinatal prevention programs designed to maximally reduce perinatal transmission. Only after all states report on AIDS cases and HIV infections can the U.S. perinatal HIV epidemic be completely understood. Part of the CDC's supplemental funds for prevention of perinatal transmission of HIV will go toward enhancing pediatric surveillance in the 26 states with the greatest burden of pediatric HIV disease.

Research

Research has shown inadequate prenatal care to be a major reason that an unacceptably high incidence of perinatal HIV transmission persists in certain areas of the United States.[4] Therefore, if pediatric HIV infection is to be eliminated, innovative approaches must be developed to increase and improve prenatal care. In addition, research is needed to improve implementation of intrapartum interventions for those women who do not receive care until labor and delivery. The Perinatal AIDS Collaborative Transmission Studies (PACTS) infrastructure developed by the CDC over the past 12 years has laid the foundation for such a research and intervention effort, launched in the spring of 1999. In this project, called MIRIAD (Mother Infant Rapid Intervention at Delivery), the CDC will investigate (1) a 24-hour counseling and voluntary rapid HIV testing program, (2) the feasibility of obtaining informed consent during labor, and (3) the rapid implementation and assessment of antiretroviral therapy given at labor and delivery and to the neonate. Results will be coordinated with those from a new Bangkok Perinatal Study for late registrants and will lead to best-practice recommendations.

Outreach

The CDC provides consultation and technical assistance in planning, implementing, and evaluating prevention activities. These services are provided directly and indirectly through prevention partners. The CDC provides these partners with up-to-date scientific information; assistance with program design, implementation, and evaluation; and assistance with collaboration with other programs. These outreach efforts target women who may not be accessing prenatal care (e.g., women who are substance abusers, incarcerated, non-English speaking, uninsured, homeless, teen-aged, or unaware of or in denial about their risk for HIV infection and potential perinatal transmission). The goal is to increase the number of women who obtain prenatal care; who know their own and their infants' HIV status; and who receive appropriate prevention, treatment, and care services.

Grant Programs

In July 1999, the CDC announced a program for Prevention of Perinatal Transmission of HIV. This program has provided 16 jurisdictions with $6.3 million in funding to supplement current awards for HIV prevention in state and city health departments reporting the greatest prevalence of HIV (seroprevalence in 1994 $\geq 2/1000$ or ≥ 150 perinatally acquired cases by June 1998). The grant recipients will coordinate activities with relevant national, regional, state, and local HIV prevention programs. They will collect and review data, offer education, interventions, outreach, and linkages with service providers. In turn, the CDC will provide scientific information, consultation, and technical assistance for planning, implementing, and evaluating prevention activities. The CDC will share lessons learned through meetings of the grantees, workshops, conferences, newsletters, Internet sites, and communications with project officers.

Evaluation

The CDC will continue to assist in the design and implementation of program evaluation activities, monitoring the effects of interventions at the national and local levels. Specifically, the CDC's HIV/AIDS evaluation program workgroup will work directly with grant recipients to develop strategies for (1) evaluating processes and monitoring outcomes of interventions to determine whether objectives are being met and (2) evaluating the overall effectiveness of programs. Specific outcomes to be evaluated include the following:

- use of prenatal care,
- HIV testing rates,

- access and adherence to therapy to reduce perinatal HIV transmission,
- access and adherence to therapy for the mother's own health,
- use of HIV-related services during the perinatal period, and
- adherence by HIV-infected women to recommendations to avoid breastfeeding.

To improve future programs, the CDC also conducts overall national evaluations of the activities supported by its programs.

Policy Development

Complex sources of medical care, financing mechanisms, and organizations that influence care must be taken into account when instituting policies for reducing perinatal HIV transmission. Yet the fact that the U.S. healthcare system is itself undergoing dramatic changes in structure, funding, and service delivery presents both challenges and opportunities. In response to these challenges, the CDC is using scientific advances, recommendations from the Instituite of Medicine and from a broad representation of consultants to revise the USPHS recommendations for prevention of perinatal HIV transmission. Other CDC policy activities include encouraging and monitoring state laws and regulations and promoting Medicaid-managed care contract language that will encourage HIV prevention activities.

INTERNATIONAL INVOLVEMENT

The above-mentioned domestic efforts have global implications as well. Almost immediately after antiretroviral therapy was proven to effectively reduce perinatal transmission in the United States, the CDC immediately began researching ways to simplify the regimen and lower its cost to make treatment more affordable and practical for women in developing countries. Indeed, studies in Thailand and Côte d'Ivoire have shown a shorter regimen of zidovudine to be safe and effective in reducing perinatal transmission, offering a practical treatment alternative in developing countries.[8,9]

More opportunities for the CDC's international involvement have emerged since July 1999 when the Clinton administration announced a $100 million increase in U.S. support to address the global AIDS pandemic. This Leadership and Investment in Fighting an Epidemic (LIFE) initiative builds on the existing U.S. investment in HIV/AIDS programs in sub-Saharan African countries and India. It involves an unprecedented collaboration among the United States Agency for International Development, the Department of Health and Human Services, and the Department of Defense toward achieving the goals of the Joint United Nations Programme on AIDS (UNAIDS). One of these goals is to increase from 1% to 50% the proportion of HIV-infected women having access to perinatal transmission interventions.

The CDC's other international activities involve providing technical assistance to the United Nations Children's Fund, UNAIDS, and the World Health Organization to help develop, implement, and evaluate pilot perinatal prevention programs. The effects of breastfeeding also need to be evaluated, especially in countries where women have no alternative ways to nourish their newborns. New research is planned at international field sites to address breastfeeding issues.

CHALLENGES AHEAD

Although much success has been achieved, several challenges remain.

- increasing prenatal care,

- making HIV counseling and testing the standard of care among all prenatal care providers,

- evaluating rapid testing of women in labor,

- improving adherence to complex treatment regimens,

- monitoring the emergence of resistance to and potential toxicity of antiretroviral agents, and

- improving surveillance to target and evaluate interventions.

Through continued surveillance, research, education, outreach, programs, evaluations, and policies, the CDC is addressing each of these issues. Only by addressing each link in the chain of events leading to perinatal transmission of HIV infection can we extend our goal from reduction to elimination.

REFERENCES

1. LINDEGREN, M.L. 1999. Trends in perinatal transmission of HIV/AIDS in the United States. JAMA **282:** 531–538.
2. CENTERS FOR DISEASE CONTROL AND PREVENTION. 1994. Recommendations of the Public Health Service Task Force on use of zidovudine to reduce perinatal transmission of human immunodeficiency virus. Morbid. Mortal. Wkly. Rep. **43**(No. RR-11): 1–21.
3. CENTERS FOR DISEASE CONTROL AND PREVENTION. 1995. U.S. Public Health Service recommendations for human immunodeficiency virus counseling and voluntary testing for pregnant women. Morb. Mortal. Wkly. Rep. **44**(No. RR-7): 1–14.
4. CENTERS FOR DISEASE CONTROL AND PREVENTION. 1998. Success in implementing public health service guidelines to reduce perinatal transmission of HIV—Louisiana, Michigan, New Jersey, and South Carolina, 1993, 1995, and 1996. Morbid. Mortal. Wkly. Rep. **47:** 688–691.
5. INSTITUTE OF MEDICINE & NATIONAL RESEARCH COUNCIL. 1999. Reducing the Odds: Preventing Perinatal Transmission of HIV in the United States. National Academy Press. Washington, DC.
6. CENTERS FOR DISEASE CONTROL AND PREVENTION. 1999. Prenatal discussion of HIV testing and maternal HIV testing—14 states, 1996–1997. Morbid. Mortal. Wkly. Rep. **48:** 401–404.
7. FERNANDEZ, M.I. *et al.* 1998. Acceptance of HIV testing among women in prenatal care in Miami, New York City, and Connecticut. Conference Record of the 12th World AIDS Conference. Geneva. Abstract No. 43142. July 2.
8. SCHAFFER, N. *et al.* 1999. Short-course zidovudine for perinatal HIV-1 transmission in Bangkok, Thailand: a randomised controlled trial. Bangkok Collaborative Perinatal HIV Transmission Study Group. Lancet **353(9155):** 773–780.
9. WIKTOR, S.Z., *et al.* 1999. Short-course oral zidovudine for prevention of mother-to-child transmission of HIV-1 in Abidjan, Cote d'Ivoire: a randomised trial. Lancet **353(9155):** 781–785.

Future Directions for NIH-Supported Pediatric AIDS Research

NEAL NATHANSON[a] AND ROBERT W. EISINGER

Office of AIDS Research, National Institutes of Health, United States Department of Health and Human Services, Bethesda, Maryland 20892, USA

ABSTRACT: The Office of AIDS Research (OAR) at the National Institutes of Health (NIH) is responsible for the coordination of AIDS research. In June 1999, the OAR, in conjunction with the NIH Institutes and Centers, initiated a review of NIH-sponsored pediatric AIDS research. This article discusses a number of important priorities for future clinical research in NIH-sponsored pediatric AIDS in both developed and developing countries. These have the potential to significantly prevent perinatal transmission, reduce adolescent infections, and impact treatment of pediatric infections.

The Office of AIDS Research has the responsibility, in collaboration with the various Institutes and Centers, to formulate guidelines for AIDS research funded by the National Institutes of Health (NIH). In fiscal year 1999, the total NIH AIDS research budget was about $1.8 billion, of which about half was devoted to fundamental research in basic biomedical and behavioral subjects such as virology and immunology. The remainder of the AIDS budget was used to support more clinically oriented studies, including trials of therapeutics and preventive interventions. Of the clinical component, $184 million focused on studies of HIV infection and AIDS in pediatric populations, ages 0–21 years.

Periodically, the Office of AIDS Research, in conjunction with the NIH Institutes and Centers, reviews specific components of the AIDS research program to ascertain the state of knowledge and to determine future directions for research, after identifying scientific opportunities and gaps, as well as public health needs. We recently initiated such a review of the NIH-sponsored pediatric AIDS program, in collaboration with several Institutes, particularly the National Institute of Child Health and Human Development and the National Institute of Allergy and Infectious Diseases. Meeting in June 1999, about 50 representatives from academia, industry, and community constituency groups, working with NIH staff, reviewed existing pediatric AIDS research programs and developed a series of recommendations and priorities. In recognition of the international dimension of the epidemic, the Working Group included representatives from the United States and abroad. The report of this group is available on the NIH website.[1]

[a]Address for correspondence: Office of AIDS Research, Building 2, Room 4W02, 2 Center Drive, Bethesda, MD 20892-0234.

nathansn@od.nih.gov

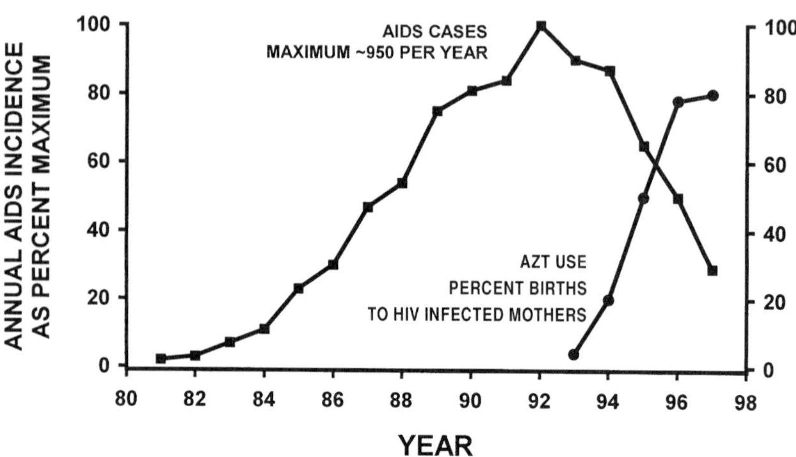

FIGURE 1. Pediatric AIDS, ages 0–13 years, United States, 1980–1997, and use of AZT for treatment of HIV-infected pregnant women. Data from the Centers for Disease Control and Prevention.

The comments presented here have been distilled from the discussions conducted during the review, but do not represent the formal recommendations of the review panel. Instead, we have attempted to focus on some of the issues that were considered during the review process. In particular, we will attempt to highlight what appear to be the most important priorities for future clinical research in NIH-sponsored pediatric AIDS. As an introduction, it is important to take cognizance of the current status of pediatric AIDS, both in developed and developing countries.

EPIDEMIOLOGIC CONSIDERATIONS

The incidence of pediatric AIDS in the United States is summarized in FIGURE 1, which shows that pediatric cases peaked in the early 1990s at about 1,000 cases per year, or about 2% of all new AIDS cases. The introduction of perinatal intervention in 1994, based on the use of an azidothymidine (AZT) regimen in the antepartum, intrapartum, and postpartum periods, together with formula feeding to avoid postnatal transmission, has led to a drastic reduction in perinatal AIDS to about 20% of its highest level, or about 200 new cases in 1997, the last year for which data are currently available.[2] Although it is unclear whether pediatric AIDS can be eliminated, it certainly can be held to minimal levels using regimens available to HIV-infected pregnant women in the United States.[3] Similar results have been observed in Europe.

The situation is totally different in the developing world, as reflected in the incidence of HIV/AIDS shown in FIGURE 2 for sub-Saharan Africa, the most heavily affected region of the world. Not only is the prevalence of HIV/AIDS much higher, but it is increasing each year (in contrast to developed countries, where the number of infected persons has stabilized for roughly the last 10 years). In addition, pediatric infections represent a much higher proportion of all infections, that is, >10% in sub-

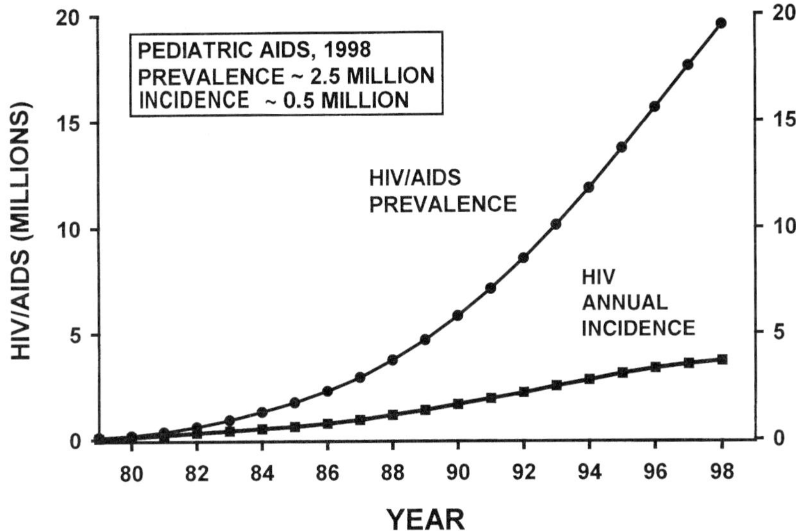

FIGURE 2. HIV incidence and prevalence of HIV/AIDS in sub-Saharan Africa, 1980–1998. Pediatric infections and cases represent more than 10% of the total. Based on data from UNAIDS, 1998.

Saharan Africa in contrast to <2% in the United States in 1998. For sub-Saharan Africa, it is estimated that there were ~500,000 new perinatal infections in 1998 alone and that there were 1–2 million children living with HIV/AIDS during the same year.

These drastic differences between the United States and sub-Saharan Africa in the patterns of pediatric AIDS indicate that the research priorities must be quite different for the developed and developing countries. In addition, disparities in medical care mandate a radically different strategy in the two settings.

PRIORITIES FOR NIH-SUPPORTED PEDIATRIC AIDS RESEARCH

The following remarks are focussed on issues involving pediatric AIDS, since a review of the broad AIDS research program at the NIH is beyond the scope of this discussion. It is important to note that the NIH brings a global vision to its AIDS research program, which has a substantial moiety dedicated to problems that are specific to developing countries.

By general consensus, the Working Group divided pediatric AIDS research into components in order to facilitate analysis and develop recommendations. First, this area of research was divided according to three age groups: perinatal (0–2 years), pediatric (2–13 years), and adolescent (13–21 years). The research then was further divided between treatment and prevention research, and into research relevant to the United States and research relevant to developing countries. This breakdown, into 12 separate rubrics, is shown in TABLE 1. At present, the program of pediatric AIDS research supported by NIH is a broad one, which involves both treatment and preven-

TABLE 1. NIH-supported pediatric AIDS research divided into rubrics, with suggested areas of highest priority for future expansion

	United States		Developing countries	
	Therapy	Prevention	Therapy	Prevention
Perinatal < 2 years	High			High
Pediatric 2–13 years	High			
Adolescent 13–21 years		High		High

tion, for different age groups, in the United States and abroad. The focus of this discussion is to identify the highest priorities for further expansion of research to address critical opportunities and challenges.

United States: Therapy

Although significant progress has been made in reducing perinatal transmission, there is a need to expand therapeutics research, particularly efforts focused on HIV-infected infants and young children. Further research should include studies of pharmacokinetics, pediatric drug formulations, the merits of early versus delayed treatment, the various combinations of multiple drugs, and the emergence of drug-resistant HIV strains. In addition, the potential toxicity of antiviral drugs must be studied further in infants and young children, who may be at increased risk for toxicity than adults, and it is important to conduct long-term studies to detect any possible effects of exposure to antiretrovirals. Animal studies also may be useful to study the effects of antiretroviral drugs administered ante or postpartum.

United States: Prevention

With the development of successful therapeutic regimens for the prevention of perinatal transmission, the focus now needs to shift to prevention of infection in adolescents. This involves a variety of approaches, beginning with the identification of and access to at-risk adolescents, followed by attempts to reduce risk behaviors by interventions at the level of the individual, the group, the community, and the society. For those at risk of infection through sexual transmission, efforts should be directed to delay the onset of sexual activity, to reduce the number of partners, and to emphasize safer sex, including the use of condoms. For those at risk of infection through injecting drugs, the emphasis should be on drug withdrawal programs combined with transmission prevention programs, such as those that may involve needle exchange, the single use of needles and syringes, and the use of bleach.

Developing Countries: Perinatal Prevention

In the developing world, the focus should be on expanding prevention efforts, since economic considerations make therapy inaccessible to most persons. Improved perinatal interventions must continue to be a high priority, with emphasis on the sim-

　　　　　

TABLE 2. Three successive studies of regimens designed to prevent perinatal transmission

Trial	Regimen[a]	Transmission	Percent efficacy	Cost[b]	Reference
PACTG 076 USA AZT	AP, IP, PP Placebo	8.3% 25.5%	67%	700	Connor *et al.*[4]
Petra SS Africa AZT/3TC	AP, IP, PP Placebo	8.6% 17.2%	50%	50	Saba *et al.*[5]
HIVNET 012 Uganda Nevaripine	IP, PP [AZT]	13.1% 25.1%	>48%	4	Jackson *et al.*[6]

[a]ABBREVIATIONS: AP, antepartum; IP, intrapartum; PP, post partum; SS, sub-Saharan. Uganda trial: no placebo control was used, and the AZT arm is taken as representing the minimum rate if a placebo control had been included.
[b]Cost estimates in US dollars after R. Knox, *Boston Globe*, July 15, 1999.

plicity and low cost of these regimens. TABLE 2 illustrates three successive studies of regimens to interrupt perinatal transmission. The first study, PACTG 076, provided the most effective prevention, and it is now estimated that, when combined with ancillary measures, such as cesarean section, it may be possible to reduce transmission to ~2%, which would approximate 90% efficacy.[4] However, this optimal regimen is too expensive and impractical for developing countries with limited availability of medical care. The PETRA (perinatal transmission) study indicated that considerable efficacy could be obtained with a restricted regimen and that the combination of intra- and short-term postpartum intervention was quite effective.[5] The HIVNET 012 study further extends this approach and shows that nevirapine, substituted for AZT and 3TC, is efficacious and can further simplify the regimen and reduce costs.[6]

These perinatal trials stand as models of the potential contribution of research to practical interventions for developing countries. Further work is needed to explore regimens designed to prevent postpartum transmission by breastfeeding in countries where it is practiced. Vaccines, passive immunization with high-titer antibodies, or continued drug treatment of mother and infant are examples of potential interventions deserving further study.

Developing Countries: Prevention of Adolescent Transmission

In developing countries most transmission among adults is through heterosexual contact, particularly in the 13- to 21-year-old age group. In this instance, prevention involves behavioral alteration, implemented at the level of the individual, the group, and the community. Recent experience in several developing countries, such as Uganda and Thailand, indicate that risk behaviors can be modified, and HIV transmission can be substantially reduced. These precedents justify additional investments in research designed to identify culturally and ethnically specific programs that reduce heterosexual transmission and also investments in programs to translate research studies into widely applied programs for public health prevention.

COMMENTS

In conclusion, it should be re-emphasized that this preliminary and brief report is based on discussions conducted in June 1999 by an external review of the NIH-supported pediatric AIDS research programs. It does not represent the final consensus report, scheduled to be released in the fall of 1999. Nevertheless, it may be concluded that there are a number of important priorities for future investment in NIH-sponsored pediatric AIDS research. Future studies have the potential to significantly contribute to prevention of perinatal transmission, reduction in adolescent infection rates, and treatment of pediatric infections, not only in the United States, but also in developing nations where the epidemic continues to spread at an alarming rate.

REFERENCES

1. WORKING GROUP TO REVIEW THE NIH PERINATAL, PEDIATRIC, AND ADOLESCENT HIV RESEARCH PRIORITIES. 1999. Report of the Working Group to Review the NIH Perinatal, Pediatric, and Adolescent HIV Research Priorities. Office of AIDS Research, National Institue of Allergy and Infectious Diseases, and the National Institute of Child Health and Human Development. http://www.nih.gov/od/oar/public/pubs/pedreport.pdf
2. LINDEGREN, M.L. *et al.* 1999. Trends in perinatal transmission of HIV/AIDS in the United States. JAMA **282:** 531–538.
3. MOFENSON, L.M. 1999. Can perinatal HIV infection be eliminated in the United States? JAMA **282:** 577–579.
4. CONNOR, E.M. *et al.* 1994. Reduction of maternal–infant transmission of human immunodeficiency virus type 1 with zidovudine treatment. Pediatric AIDS Clinical Trials Group Protocol 076 Study Group. N. Engl. J. Med. **331(18):** 1173–1180.
5. SABA, J. *et al.* 1999. A multicentre, randomized, double-blind, placebo-controlled clinical trial to evaluate efficacy, tolerance and effectiveness of three drug regimens using zidovudine plus lamivudine for the prevention of mother-to-child transmission of HIV-1. The PETRA Study. Presentation at the Sixth Conference on Retroviruses and Opportunistic Infections. Abstract No. 57. Chicago, IL, Jan. 31–Feb. 4.
6. JACKSON, B. *et al.* 1999. A Phase IIB randomized, controlled trial to evaluate the safety, tolerance, and HIV vertical transmission rates associated with short course nevirapine (NVP) vs. short course zidovudine (ZDV) in HIV infected pregnant women and their infants in Uganda. Executive Summary. Press Release, National Institute of Allergy and Infectious Diseases, July 21, 1999.

Evaluating the Safety of Interventions for Prevention of Perinatal Transmission of HIV

THOMAS R. FLEMING[a]

Department of Biostatistics, University of Washington, Seattle, Washington 98195, USA

ABSTRACT: Efficient approaches are needed for obtaining reliable insights into the safety, in developing and developed country settings, of interventions for prevention of mother-to-child transmission (MCT) of HIV. A randomized trial designed with an appropriate sample size and adequate duration of follow-up provides a powerful tool for obtaining causal evidence regarding the safety and efficacy of MTC prevention interventions. Such trials are ideal for detecting adverse effects (AEs) that occur in the short or moderate term and with moderate to high frequency. Passive and active surveillance procedures, where practical, can provide valuable insights regarding long-term or rare AEs. Ideally, surveillance procedures should be carefully planned sufficiently early to allow prospective definition and uniform collection of important classes of AEs, enhancing the sensitivity and specificity of these surveillance data.

INTRODUCTION

In clinical research targeting the prevention of mother-to-child transmission (MCT) of human immunodeficiency virus (HIV), the primary goals include identification of convenient and affordable interventions that could be widely accessible to at-risk populations and a reliable assessment of the safety as well as efficacy of these interventions. An important challenge, then, is identifying efficient and informative approaches that provide reliable and timely insights into the causal influence of these interventions on measures of benefit and risk.

Given these goals, the focus of this manuscript is on the significant challenges relating to evaluating the safety of promising interventions to prevent MCT. Potentially useful approaches for studying adverse effects are discussed, motivated by experiences from the setting of evaluating the safety of childhood vaccines. The usefulness of these approaches in assessing risk in the context of benefit is illustrated from the settings of the childhood acellular pertussis vaccine, treatment of moderate to severe asthma, and treatment of Wilms' Tumor in children.

The challenges in implementing these approaches for studying adverse effects in the MCT setting are explored. In this setting, we consider the influence of magnitude of benefit on the level of sensitivity required in evaluating risk. Recommendations for a scientifically and ethically responsible approach to safety assessment in MCT trials are discussed.

[a]Address for correspondence: Thomas R. Fleming, Ph.D., University of Washington, Department of Biostatistics, Box 357232, 1705 N.E. Pacific Street, HSB Room F-600, Seattle, WA 98195-7232.

APPROACHES TO STUDYING ADVERSE EFFECTS

The setting of childhood vaccines provides important motivation for several informative approaches for studying adverse effects (AEs), as well as experience regarding their usefulness and limitations. These approaches include passive and active surveillance systems as well as randomized clinical trials.

Adequately Sized "Pre-Marketing" Randomized Clinical Trials

The randomized clinical trial provides an ideal approach to assessing the causal influence of an intervention on the risk of AEs that occur in the short or moderate term and with moderate to high frequency. Randomization of assignment to experimental and control regimens eliminates the systematic occurrence of imbalances between interventions in baseline characteristics of study participants. Although randomly occurring imbalances can arise, these are highly likely to induce only small levels of confounding in those clinical trials having moderate to large sample sizes. Elimination of confounding allows one to conclude that the intervention is causally inducing any differences in safety risks, rather than being uncertain about whether these differences could be attributable to factors that led to the choice to use or not use the intervention, an uncertainty that is routinely present in most observational databases.

Although randomization is a powerful tool for enabling assessments of the causal role of interventions in inducing safety risks, some limitations of the randomized trial must be recognized:

Inability to detect rare or low-frequency events

Suppose an experimental intervention induces a threefold increase in the rate of a given serious AE, relative to the control. If that AE occurs on the control regimen with moderate frequency (i.e., in 10 per 1000 participants), this threefold increase would correspond to having an increase in the rate in the experimental intervention to 30 per 1000 participants. Assuming the goal is to have a 90% chance to detect this threefold increase using a statistical procedure having a 2.5% chance of arriving at a false positive conclusion, then the trial would be required to have $2n = 2000$ to 5000 participants, where we denote the sample size on each regimen of the trial by n (hence $2n$ being the sample size in a two-armed trial). The following table provides some motivation for why vaccine trials in children have typically had large sample sizes. Specifically, sample sizes ranging from 2000 to 50,000 would be required to detect threefold increases when rates of AEs in the control regimen range from 10/1000 to 1/1000 (TABLE 1).

Inability to detect long-term adverse effects

Randomized trials of childhood vaccines typically follow participants for safety risks occurring in the first 30–90 days post vaccination. Thus, latent or long-term effects would likely go undetected.

Effect of incomplete follow-up on loss of integrity of the randomization

Although randomization provides a balance in baseline characteristics between the intervention groups, in turn enabling an unbiased assessment of the influence of

TABLE 1. Rationale for large sample size for vaccine trials in children

Frequency	Increase in rate	$2n$
Low–moderate	1/1000 to 3/1000	20,000–50,000
Moderate	10/1000 to 30/1000	2,000–5,000
High	100/1000 to 300/1000	200–500

an intervention on safety risks, the assurance of this unbiasedness will be lost if uniform follow-up of study participants is not achieved. Providing safety monitoring only in those in whom follow-up is most readily achievable can lead to very misleading conclusions about the true safety risks and the relative safety risks of the interventions. Those participants with missing follow-up information can readily have experienced very different risks of adverse effects than those who are followed. Even if the two interventions have the same fraction of participants in whom safety information is missing, bias can still arise in the assessment of relative safety risks if the cause of the missing information differs between these two groups.

The problem of bias arising from incomplete follow-up is especially serious when one is attempting to detect an increase in a relatively low-frequency event having clinical significance that is very important but not so extreme as to ensure capture through passive surveillance, such as high fever, or even meningitis or sepsis. Uniform follow-up of clinical trial participants should be required at least to ensure detection of short-term safety risks. In addition, it is strongly encouraged that uniform follow-up be extended to achieve uniform capture of significant adverse events that would occur over a moderate period of follow-up.

These limitations of randomized clinical trials in detecting rare or long-term adverse events provide motivation for additional approaches to monitoring safety risks through use of passive and active surveillance systems.

"Post Marketing" Passive Surveillance Systems

Surveillance systems provide approaches for detecting previously unrecognized AEs or increases in the rate of known AEs, as well as an opportunity to identify characteristics of individuals associated with high rates of reactions. In 1988, in order to ensure passive surveillance of AEs associated with the administration of licensed vaccines in the United States, the Department of Health and Human Services established the Vaccine Adverse Event Reporting System (VAERS). The VAERS is a single system for collection and analysis of reports on all serious AEs, implemented by the Center of Disease Control and the Food and Drug Administration.[1]

Because health care providers are required to report serious AEs to the VAERS, this passive surveillance system has some desirable properties. These include timeliness of information, uniformity of reporting procedures, and the national coverage by the system.

Important limitations of this passive surveillance system must also be recognized. To estimate the rate of occurrence of any AE,[2] one needs reliable estimates of both the numerator (i.e., the number of participants experiencing the given AE) and the denominator (i.e., the number of participants receiving the intervention). Because passive surveillance involves voluntary submission of AEs, there is substantial underreporting. The variable accuracy and completeness of submitted information further weakens the reliability of estimates of the numerator. Meanwhile, the passive surveillance system does not provide any information on the denominator. Other limitations of passive surveillance also exist. These include the lack of a valid comparator group to obtain direct evidence regarding the casual role of the intervention in the occurrence of the AEs, as well as frequent lack of adequate information regarding the role of dose and schedule and the role of concomitant medications.

Passive surveillance systems are best suited to identifying previously undetected AEs when (a) the occurrence of the AE would be extraordinarily unusual in the absence of the intervention, (b) the intervention induces a very large increase in the rate of the occurrence of the AE, or (c) there is a clear temporal relationship between administration of the intervention and appearance of the AE.

Recognizing the limitations of a passive surveillance system, its role would usually be in "signal detection" or "hypothesis generation." Confirmatory information would frequently be sought through evidence provided by active surveillance.

"Post Marketing" Active Surveillance Systems

Active surveillance systems can provide important evidence regarding an intervention's effect on rare AEs, (i.e., AEs occurring at a rate of 0.01 to 0.1 per 1000 individuals in the absence of the intervention). Active surveillance is often based on use of large prospective cohorts or large linked databases. For childhood vaccines, for example, the linking of automated databases from health maintenance organizations has provided a database of over 500,000 children having active follow-up over an extended period of time.

Advantages of active surveillance systems include: (a) providing safety information on a large, well-defined population over an extended period; (b) having more complete information on both numerators (i.e., the number of participants experiencing an AE) and denominators (i.e., the number receiving the intervention); (c) achieving a reduction in reporting bias, since the record is made before the AE occurs; and (d) speed and low cost.

An active surveillance system has its disadvantages as well. These include: (a) lack of a randomized comparator group; (b) lack of adequate confounder information (e.g., maternal smoking history when exploring the relationship of an intervention with occurrence of SIDS); (c) concerns regarding outcome specificity (e.g., is a report of seizures truly an event?); and (d) concerns regarding outcome sensitivity (e.g., would occurrences of fever or attention deficit disorder be reliably captured?).

An effective strategy for safety monitoring that will be sensitive to detecting and estimating the frequency of rare as well as frequent AEs, and of long-term as well as immediate events, should involve the conduct of randomized clinical trials having high-quality follow-up of participants, and implementation of systems to perform both passive and active surveillance.

ILLUSTRATIONS: ASSESSING RISK IN THE CONTEXT OF LEVEL OF BENEFIT

In this section, the usefulness of previously discussed approaches for monitoring safety risks in infants and children are illustrated in several clinical settings. Attention is also drawn to how the expected magnitude of benefit influences the level of sensitivity required in evaluating risk.

Acellular Pertussis Vaccine in Infants: Balancing Important Benefits to a Small Minority versus Rare but Significant Risks

The efficacy of acellular pertussis vaccines was established in three randomized clinical trials involving over 100,000 infants in the 1990s in Italy and Sweden.[3–5] In the two trials having a control vaccine without a pertussis component, the acellular pertussis vaccines reduced the risk of pertussis over a one- to two-year interval approximately from 5% to 1%. This translates into prevention of approximately 40 cases of pertussis per 1000 infants receiving the vaccine.

It was important to ensure that safety risks associated with the acellular pertussis vaccines did not substantially offset this magnitude of benefit derived from reducing the risk of pertussis. Although it was straightforward to establish that minor short-term injection site reactions, drowsiness, anorexia, or pain occurred at the expected rate of approximately 10%, it was a significant challenge to assess impact on rare but severe AEs. Through sample sizes that exceeded $n = 25,000$ infants on each acellular pertussis vaccine regimen and on the control regimen, the randomized clinical trials were adequately powered to detect a tripling in any events that would be expected to occur on the control regimen at a rate of the 0.5–1.0 per 1000 infants. Thus, these trials were able to rule out such increases in the rate of convulsions/seizures, high fever, hypotonic/hyporesponsive episodes, and invasive bacterial infections such as meningitis and sepsis.

Even with such large randomized clinical trials, post marketing surveillance would be necessary to determine whether the acellular pertussis vaccines increase the rate of certain severe neurological and allergic reactions. This would be particularly important given historical concerns about the possible adverse effects of whole-cell pertussis vaccines on the risk of encephalitis, anaphylaxis, and SIDS. Because these events occur at a rate of approximately 0.1 per 1000 infants, detecting a three-fold increase would require monitoring of 200,000 vaccine recipients in post marketing surveillance. Such surveillance is currently under way.

Treatment of Moderate to Severe Asthma: Balancing Moderate Benefits to a Large Majority versus Rare but Significant Risks

As in the pertussis setting, in the management of patients with moderate to severe asthma, a treatment-induced increase in mortality would be unacceptable. This is true even if that asthma therapy provides widespread improvement in quality of life. As a result, when the possibility of such an increase in mortality has been suggested by prior clinical evidence, regulatory authorities have required a randomized clinical trial be conducted in moderate to severe asthma patients to reliably rule out the mortality increase. With a background rate of 1.3 asthma-related deaths per 1000 person years, detecting a tripling (i.e., an increase of 2–3 deaths per 1000 person years) requires a randomized trial with $2n = 20,000$ participants to be followed for one year. Such a trial is time- and resource-intensive. However, the risk of bias inherent with the alternative use of active or passive surveillance would make detection of such an important yet small increase in mortality difficult to conclusively investigate by post-marketing surveillance approaches.

When assessing benefit against risk for an experimental intervention, the magnitude of the clinical benefit has considerable influence on the level of risk that would be acceptable. Although the prevention of a case of pertussis or the improvement in asthma-related quality of life is important, neither clinical benefit is close in magnitude to the importance of the prevention of HIV infection and its subsequent morbidity and mortality. On the other hand, a consideration of benefit to risk in the setting of Wilms' Tumor, where effective interventions against this fatal disease can enable children to experience a full and healthy life, would present greater similarities to the benefit-to-risk issues arising in the setting of prevention of perinatal transmission of HIV.

Treatment of Wilms' Tumor in Children with Stage II–III Disease: Balancing Frequent Profound Benefits versus Frequent Significant Risks

Over 20 to 30 years of research, as regimens in Wilms' tumor have evolved from radiation plus single-agent chemotherapy to radiation plus triple-agent chemotherapy, mortality in children with stage II or III disease has been reduced from 70% to 10%. With the prevention of 60 deaths per 100 treated children, substantial safety risks could be tolerated. The most frequent are acute hematologic toxicities that are very serious, although usually manageable.

The enormous advances that were achieved through mortality reductions in the early generation clinical trials in Wilms' tumor resulted in a clear judgment that benefit-to-risk profiles were favorable even though these treatment regimens induced substantial AEs. However, the benefit-to-risk issues have been complex in more recent clinical trials in this disease setting.

These complex issues are illustrated by an important third-generation clinical trial involving the randomization of $2n = 560$ children, with stage II or III disease, either to the standard two-agent chemotherapy regimen (using dactinomycin plus vincristine) or to that regimen with the addition of adriamycin.[6] In these children, only a small improvement in four-year survival was provided by the addition of adriamycin, with this benefit predominantly appearing in the stage III setting. Fortunately, in this randomized trial in which children were randomized between October 1979 and August 1986, long-term assessments are still ongoing in order to identify long-term safety risks. Over 15 to 20 years of follow-up, congestive heart failure has been identified in approximately 1% of children receiving adriamycin (personal communication, Norman Breslow and Bin Nan). This contributed to the abandonment of this agent in the primary treatment regimen for children with low-stage Wilms' tumor.

Interestingly, in the same trial, in the small group of children with a presenting diagnosis of clear cell sarcoma of the kidney, the addition of adriamycin to the two-agent chemotherapy regimen led to a very substantial reduction in six-year mortality, approximately from 70% to 33%.[7] Thus, for these children who are treated with adriamycin, even if a small percentage would experience significant long-term adverse effects, the prevention of 30–40 deaths per 100 children would lead to the judgment that the addition of adriamycin improves the benefit-to-risk profile.

The clinical trials in this area illustrate the importance of assessing long-term safety risks, and illustrate that interventions providing significant reductions in morbidity or mortality may have favorable benefit-to-risk safety profiles even though substantial safety risks exist.

ASSESSING RISK IN THE CONTEXT OF BENEFIT IN MCT TRIALS

In clinical trials targeting prevention of MCT of HIV, effective interventions can provide profoundly important benefits to infants and children. As in the setting of Wilms' tumor, in early generation trials, these benefits can be so significant that benefit-to-risk profiles may be very favorable even when safety risks are substantial, whereas in later generation trials when net gains in efficacy become more modest, these benefit-to-risk issues become much more complex. We will explore these issues in the MCT setting by considering both recent results from the HIVNET 012 single-dose nevarapine trial as well as the proposals for subsequent trials.

In the HIVNET 012 clinical trial,[8] an experimental short-course nevarapine (NVP) regimen involving a single oral dose to the mother at the initiation of labor and a single oral dose to the infant after delivery was compared to a short-course zidovudine (ZDV) regimen. At 14–16 weeks of age, the HIV transmission rates on NVP versus ZDV were 13% versus 25%. Although transmission rates were not reported at 6 months, for illustrative purposes one might project these to be 16% versus 26%.

Consider two strategies for implementation of the NVP regimen. In strategy #1, assume NVP is offered to any HIV-infected mother and her infant (i.e., to all M+/I pairs). By this strategy, the morbidity/mortality of HIV disease would be prevented in 100 infants for each 1000 M+/I pairs treated. In settings in which prevalence of HIV is high in pregnant women and adequate counseling/testing infrastructure is not yet in place, a more effective, affordable, and convenient approach (strategy #2) might be to provide the NVP regimen to all mothers and infants (i.e., to all M/I pairs). With strategy #2, if 30% of pregnant women are HIV infected, the morbidity/mortality of HIV disease would be prevented in 30 infants for each 1000 M/I pairs treated.

In the setting of strategies #1 and #2, minimum requirements for safety monitoring would be detection of an intervention-induced increase in serious, nonreversible AEs occurring at a rate of 20–30 per 1000 mother/infant pairs. An increase in the AE rate from 1 per 1000 to 31 per 1000 mother/infant pairs would require following $2n$ = 750 mother/infant pairs. Interestingly, this coincides with the sample size of the HIVNET 012 trial. These analyses suggest that sample sizes from carefully conducted clinical trials having long-term safety monitoring could satisfy minimum requirements for safety monitoring when the experimental regimen provides very large effects on clinical endpoints of profound importance. As observed earlier, requirements for safety monitoring become more complex in later generation trials. For illustration, we will consider second-generation trials, first in the developing country setting and then in the developed country setting.

In developing countries, where breastfeeding provides continued risk between birth and six months, a second-generation trial might address whether the addition of an intervention to reduce transmission due to breastfeeding (e.g., continued dosing with NVP through six months) could further reduce the HIV transmission rate at

TABLE 2. Sample sizes ($2n$) required to detect a 0.5% increase in serious adverse effects occurring in mother/infant pairs

Rate of adverse effects		Example of adverse effect
Control vs. Experimental	$2n$	
0.1/1000 vs. 5.1/1000	4,300	Mitochondrial dysfunction
1/1000 vs. 6/1000	5,800	Stevens-Johnson syndrome
10/1000 vs. 15/1000	20,700	Renal–bone toxicity
50/1000 vs. 55/1000	88,500	Non-HIV-related deaths
(0.1/1000 vs. 1/1000	28,500	Mitochondrial dysfunction)

six months. If very successful, this trial of $2n = 4000$ mother/infant pairs could establish that the additional intervention further reduces the HIV transmission rates at 6 months from 16% to 12%. With strategy #1, involving treatment of all M+/I pairs with the single-dose NPV regimen plus this additional intervention, the use of the additional intervention would lead to the prevention of the morbidity/mortality of HIV disease in 40 additional infants for each 1000 M+/I pairs treated. With strategy #2 involving treatment of all M/I pairs, the use of the additional intervention would prevent the morbidity/mortality of HIV disease in 12 additional infants for each 1000 M/I pairs treated, if we continue to assume the prevalence of HIV infection is 30% among pregnant women. (It is immediately apparent that implementation of strategy #1 would be preferred over strategy #2 unless the intervention added to reduce transmission during breastfeeding does not substantially compromise the safety, convenience, and affordability of the single-dose NVP regimen).

In developed countries, a second-generation trial might address whether the addition of the single-dose NVP regimen to standard antiretroviral therapy (ART) would further reduce transmission rates. Such a study, the #316 trial in the AIDS Clinical Trials Group, is currently under way. If transmission rates at six months are reduced from 5% on ART to 3.75% on ART + NVP, then the addition of a single-dose NVP regimen would prevent the morbidity/mortality of HIV disease in 12 additional infants for each 1000 M/I pairs treated. Interestingly, this is identical to the benefit achieved in the second-generation trial in the developing country setting through the implementation in all M/I pairs of the intervention to prevent breastfeeding transmission (i.e., through strategy #2).

In these second-generation trials in the developing or developed country settings, it is apparent that minimum requirements for safety monitoring would be detection of an increase of approximately 5 per 1000 mother/infant pairs in the rate of serious, nonreversible AEs due to the additional intervention.

In TABLE 2, sample sizes, $2n$, are provided for detecting a 0.5% increase in the rate of AEs that occur at various baseline rates in the control "standard of care" setting. An increase in the AE rate from 0.1 to 5.1 per 1000 M/I pairs, corresponding to possible increases in the risk of mitochondrial dysfunction with use of ZDV[9] or from 1 to 6 per 1000 M/I pairs (corresponding to increases in the risk of Stevens-Johnson syndrome that could occur with exposure to extended high doses of NVP) could be detected in properly sized randomized clinical trials having procedures adequate to provide long-term safety monitoring. On the other hand, when baseline rates are higher, such as the 5% non-HIV death rate in developing countries, increases in the rate of AEs would need to be greater than 0.5% to be detectable by randomized trials. Active surveillance systems also would not be well suited to detect an increase of only 0.5% from a 5% rate on the control "standard-of-care" regimen, due to difficulties in discerning signal from bias.

For completeness, the last line in TABLE 2 addresses the setting in which a 10-fold increase, rather than a 50-fold increase, is observed when the baseline rate is very low (i.e., 0.1/1000). In such a setting, passive or active surveillance might provide the preferred approach for detection.

STUDYING ADVERSE EVENTS IN MCT CLINICAL TRIALS: CHALLENGES AND RECOMMENDATIONS

In first-generation MCT trials, if substantial reductions are achieved in the rate of HIV transmission, long-term monitoring of the cohorts from the original randomized trials could provide adequate safety data. Although supportive safety data from large-scale surveillance studies would be informative, such data probably would not be necessary in order to establish that the intervention has a favorable benefit-to-risk profile. This in particular would be true when evaluating short-course interventions, such as the single-dose NVP regimen, which can be expected to have very favorable safety profiles. However, in future generation clinical trials, when evaluating more intensive interventions intended to improve on the existing standard of care, the incremental benefit will tend to be of smaller magnitude, whereas the probability of important increases in safety risks could be much greater. This would lead to the need for greater sensitivity in safety monitoring to obtain precise and unbiased estimates of incremental increases in risk.

Other challenges must also be faced in monitoring the safety of interventions in the setting of MCT of HIV. It is of significant public health importance to achieve broad implementation of safe and effective interventions to reduce transmission of HIV, particularly in developing countries where the need is by far the greatest. Because results of safety evaluations might not be reliably extrapolated from one setting to another, it is important to ensure that adequate monitoring of safety occurs in these developing countries. Considerable challenges result due to the high background rate of health risks in such settings. In the evaluation of safety, detecting a signal in the presence of substantial noise can be quite difficult.

Randomized trials, if designed with appropriate sample sizes and adequate duration of follow-up, provide a powerful tool for obtaining causal evidence regarding the safety and well as efficacy of interventions to prevent transmission of HIV. Such trials are ideal for detecting AEs that occur in the short or moderate term and with moderate to high frequency. In many settings, achieving uniform follow-up for two to five years post-randomization, rather than for simply 30–90 days post completion of the study interventions, will provide important additional insights into those benefits and risks that are not immediately apparent, such as effects on survival or on occurrence of neurological complications.

The most significant adverse influence on the reliability of safety assessments from randomized trials is bias resulting from missing information. Providing safety monitoring only in those in whom follow-up is most readily achievable can lead to very misleading conclusions about the true safety risks and the relative safety risks of the interventions. By ensuring high-quality follow-up of all randomized participants (or at least in all randomized participants within selected clinical sites judged most capable of providing high-quality follow-up), one can obtain the most informative source of safety information, particularly in the setting of developing countries where the infrastructure required for active and passive surveillance is often quite limited.

Procedures for passive and active surveillance, where practical, can provide valuable insights regarding long-term or rare AEs. Ideally, these procedures should be carefully planned sufficiently early to allow for prospective rather than retrospective data capture. This would also allow guidance to be provided prospectively regarding the definition of certain AEs, such as mitochondrial dysfunction, where problems relating to sensitivity and specificity must be minimized for results to be interpretable.

Considerable excitement has been generated by recent results from clinical trials evaluating convenient and affordable interventions that have been established to be effective in substantially reducing the risk of MCT of HIV. In turn, several challenges must be addressed. Efforts are required to achieve broad access, in those settings of greatest need, to interventions established to have a favorable benefit-to-risk profile. Further research is needed to identify interventions providing even greater reductions in the risk of MCT of HIV while maintaining safety, convenience, and affordability. Finally, the procedures must be planned prospectively to ensure that safety can be reliably evaluated in a timely manner in both developed and developing country settings.

ACKNOWLEDGMENT

We thank Arthur Ammann for enlightening discussion. We also thank Norman Breslow, Bin Nan, and Tracy Bergemann for helpful information relating to the research in Wilms' tumor. This research was supported by the National Institutes of Health Grant RO1 AI-29168.

REFERENCES

1. CHEN, R.T., S.C. RASTOGI, J.R. MULLEN, et al. 1994. The vaccine adverse event reporting system (VAERS). Vaccine 12: 542–550.
2. MITCHELL, A.A. 1990. Adverse drug effects and drug epidemiology. In Pediatric Pharmacology: Therapeutic Principles in Practice. W.B. Saunders. Baltimore, MD.
3. GRECO, D., S. SALMASO, P. MASTRANTONIO, et al. 1996. A controlled trial of two acellular vaccines and one whole-cell vaccine against pertussis. N. Engl. J. Med. 334: 341–348.
4. GUSTAFSSON, L., H.O. HALLANDER, P. OLIN, et al. 1996. Controlled trial of a two-component acellular, a five-component acellular and a whole-cell pertussis vaccine. N. Engl. J. Med. 334: 349–355.
5. OLIN, P., F. RASMUSSEN, L. GUSTAFSSON, et al., for the Ad Hoc Group for the Study of Pertussis Vaccines. 1996. Randomized controlled trial of two-component, three-com-

ponent, and five-component acellular pertussis vaccines compared with whole-cell pertussis vaccine. Lancet **350:** 1569–1577.

6. D'ANGIO, G.J., N. BRESLOW, B. BECKWITH, *et al.* 1989. Results of the Third National Wilms' Tumor Study. Cancer **64:** 349–360.

7. GREEN, D.M., N.E. BRESLOW, J.B. BECKWITH, *et al.* 1994. Treatment of children with clear-cell sarcoma of the kidney: a report from the National Wilms' Tumor Study Group. J. Clin. Oncol. **12:** 2132–2137.

8. GUAY, L.A., P. MUSOKE, T. FLEMING, *et al.* 1999. Intrapartum and neonatal single-dose nevirapine compared with zidovudine for prevention of mother-to-child transmission of HIV-1 in Kampala, Uganda: HIVNET 012 randomized trial. Lancet **354:** 795–802.

9. BLANCHE, S., M. TARDIEU, P. RUSTIN, *et al.* 1999. Persistent mitochondrial dysfunction and perinatal exposure to antiretroviral nucleoside analogues. Lancet **354 (9184):** 1084–1089.

Lack of Evidence of Mitochondrial Dysfunction in the Offspring of HIV-Infected Women

Retrospective Review of Perinatal Exposure to Antiretroviral Drugs in the Perinatal AIDS Collaborative Transmission Study

MARC BULTERYS,[a,g] STEVEN NESHEIM,[b] ELAINE J. ABRAMS,[c] PAUL PALUMBO,[d] JOHN FARLEY,[e] MARGARET LAMPE,[a] MARY GLENN FOWLER,[a] AND THE PERINATAL SAFETY REVIEW WORKING GROUP[f]

[a]Epidemiology Branch, Division of HIV/AIDS Prevention, National Center for HIV/STD/TB Prevention, Centers for Disease Control and Prevention, Atlanta, Georgia 30333, USA

[b]Department of Pediatrics, Emory University, Atlanta, Georgia 30303, USA

[c]Harlem Hospital and Columbia University, New York, New York 10037, USA

[d]Department of Pediatrics, University of Medicine and Dentistry of New Jersey, Newark, New Jersey 07103, USA

[e]Department of Pediatrics, University of Maryland, Baltimore, Maryland 21201, USA

ABSTRACT: A recent report suggesting mitochondrial dysfunction among eight HIV-exposed but uninfected children exposed perinatally to nucleoside reverse transcriptase inhibitors (NRTIs) prompted a review within the Perinatal AIDS Collaborative Transmission Study (PACTS). A standardized retrospective review was conducted of 118 deaths at <5 years. Deaths were classified as unrelated to mitochondrial dysfunction (Class 1), unlikely related (Class 2), possibly related (Class 3), or likely related or proven (Class 4). Among 35 deaths recorded in HIV-uninfected or indeterminate children, none were classified in either Class 2, 3, or 4. We also reviewed signs or symptoms consistent with possible mitochondrial dysfunction among 1,954 living uninfected children. Only one child was in Class 3 and two siblings were in Class 2; none had perinatal antiretroviral drug exposure. We found no evidence indicating that uninfected infants exposed to perinatal NRTIs died of mitochondrial disorders or that living exposed children had symptoms of mitochondrial dysfunction.

[f]See Appendix for list of members of the Perinatal Safety Review Working Group.

[g]Corresponding author: Marc Bulterys, MD, PhD, Mother-Child Transmission & Pediatric and Adolescent Studies Section, Epidemiology Branch, Division of HIV/AIDS Prevention, Centers for Disease Control and Prevention, 1600 Clifton Road, Mailstop E-45, Atlanta, GA 30333, USA. Voice: 404-639-4980; fax: 404-639-6127.

zbe2@cdc.gov

BACKGROUND

Administration of antiretroviral drugs during pregnancy is recommended for HIV-infected women for their own health, and zidovudine (ZDV) is recommended for both HIV-infected mothers and their newborn infants for prevention of perinatal HIV transmission.[1,2] Follow-up through the first 5 years of life of children who participated in the Pediatric AIDS Clinical Trials Group (PACTG) protocol 076 has revealed no differences in growth, immune function, or cognitive development between those who were exposed to ZDV and those who received a placebo, and no cancers were detected in this group or in a longitudinal observational cohort.[3,4]

Nucleoside reverse transcriptase inhibitors (NRTIs), however, have well-described toxicity to mitochondrial function in animal models,[5] and NRTIs have been associated with mitochondrial dysfunction in patients receiving long-term treatment.[6] A recent report[7] by clinical investigators in France suggested mitochondrial dysfunction among 8 HIV-uninfected infants who were exposed to NRTIs in the perinatal period, including two neurologically related deaths among infants perinatally exposed to ZDV/3TC combination therapy. This concerning French report prompted an extensive review of data from major perinatal HIV cohorts in the United States to determine if any similar cases had occurred in the US. To carry out this comprehensive review, the U.S. Perinatal Safety Review Working Group was constituted in February 1999 and included representative investigators from each of the major US perinatal cohorts, and Centers for Disease Control and Prevention (CDC) and National Institutes of Health (NIH) staff, with consultation from mitochondrial experts.[8]

The Perinatal Safety Review Working Group reviewed all deaths in children <5 years of age in five large HIV-exposed perinatal studies, including the CDC population-based pediatric HIV surveillance project, the Pediatric Spectrum of Disease project, the Women and Infants Transmission Study, and the PACTG cohort.[8] As part of this review, a detailed retrospective review was also conducted in the Perinatal AIDS Collaborative Transmission Study (PACTS) for all children who died and were born to HIV-infected women between 1986 and 1998. In addition, we reviewed signs or symptoms consistent with possible mitochondrial dysfunction among 1,954 living HIV-exposed but uninfected children enrolled in PACTS.

METHODS

Description of Cohort

PACTS is a prospective cohort study of HIV-infected women and their children, funded by the CDC and carried out in seven hospitals in four U.S. cities (Atlanta, Baltimore, Newark, and New York).[9] The study enrolled HIV-infected women during pregnancy, at delivery, or within 60 days following delivery. Data collection began in 1985 in New York City, 1987 in Baltimore and Newark, and 1990 in Atlanta. Enrollment of new mother-infant pairs ended on September 30, 1998. HIV-infected children continue to be followed, whereas follow-up for HIV-uninfected children varied between 24 and 36 months after birth among PACTS sites. A minimum of twice-yearly study visits included monitoring of anthropometric indices, certain laboratory parameters, HIV-related conditions, medications and immunizations received, and reasons for any hospitalization in the interim period.

Definition of HIV Infection Status

For this analysis, a child was classified as HIV-infected if (1) at least two blood specimens drawn on different dates tested positive for HIV by DNA polymerase chain reaction (PCR), coculture, or p24 antigen assay; (2) at least one specimen tested positive for anti-HIV antibody in a child over 18 months of age; (3) the child had AIDS; or (4) the child died from an HIV-related cause.[9] A child was classified as HIV-uninfected if (1) at least two specimens drawn on different dates (at least one after 6 weeks of age) tested negative for HIV by PCR or coculture; (2) at least two specimens drawn on different dates after 6 months of age or at least one specimen drawn after 18 months of age tested negative for anti-HIV antibody by enzyme immunoassay (EIA); or (3) at least one specimen drawn after 6 months of age tested negative for anti-HIV antibody by EIA and at least one specimen tested negative for HIV by PCR or coculture. Children who failed to meet the criteria for infection or absence of infection were considered indeterminate.

Antiretroviral Exposure Categories

Perinatal antiretroviral drug exposure was classified in six categories. Data were abstracted from prenatal, delivery, and pediatric medical records. Exposure was categorized as "none" if there was no antiretroviral use during pregnancy and the first 6 weeks of life in the infant. Any use of ZDV as monotherapy during pregnancy or in the first 6 weeks of life was categorized as "ZDV" exposure. Any combination of drugs that included ZDV and 3TC to either mother or infant was categorized as "ZDV+3TC" exposure. Other antiretroviral drug combinations were categorized as "other" exposure. Those mother-infant pairs with no recorded information about perinatal antiretroviral prophylaxis (the "unknown" category) were subdivided into two time periods before and after March 1, 1994. The majority of infants born prior to March 1994 with "unknown" exposure likely had no exposure, as antiretroviral treatment of HIV-infected pregnant women was uncommon in the US prior to the announcement of the results of the PACTG 076 trial.[9–11]

Death Data Review

Records of all children in the PACTS who died under the age of 60 months and were born before December 31, 1998 were reviewed. Death records were obtained, as were records of autopsies, if performed. Computerized hospitalization ICD-9 codes and outpatient study clinic records were reviewed, and local pediatric investigators were questioned if there were ambiguities.

The Working Group met weekly by conference call beginning in March 1999 to review data on all cohort children who died before 5 years of age.[8,12] All deceased children were then classified by consensus as having illness that was considered (1) *unrelated* to mitochondrial dysfunction (class 1); (2) *possibly, but unlikely related*: limited signs, symptoms, and/or laboratory data that are consistent with mitochondrial dysfunction, but mitochondrial disease unlikely (class 2); (3) *consistent* with mitochondrial disease: signs, symptoms, and/or laboratory data in which a mitochondrial disorder might reasonably be included in the differential diagnosis (class 3); or (4) *likely related or proven* due to mitochondrial dysfunction: signs, symptoms, and/or laboratory data suggestive of mitochondrial dysfunction, or proven due to mitochondrial dysfunction (class 4).[8] Sudden infant death syndrome (SIDS) was a separate category. If the information available was insufficient to allow classification, investigators made contact with pediatricians involved in the child's care, and new available data were reviewed.

Living HIV-Uninfected Children Data Review

The majority of HIV-exposed but uninfected children in PACTS were followed 24–36 months after birth. Prior to 1991, these children were followed indefinitely since birth. Study visits for HIV-exposed children were scheduled at 1 month, 2 months, 4 months, 6 months, and every 3–6 months thereafter. An extensive database search and manual review included (1) all ICD-9 hospitalization codes beyond 3 months of age (with a specific focus on neurologic findings and other signs and symptoms possibly related to mitochondrial dysfunction) and (2) recorded study visit data on possible "HIV-related" conditions (i.e., failure to thrive, weight loss >10%, developmental delay, progressive motor deficits, impaired brain growth, hepatitis or abnormal liver function, cardiomyopathy, nephropathy, neutropenia, and thrombocytopenia). Serial laboratory data were also reviewed for evidence of severe anemia (i.e., hemoglobin <7 g/dl).

For children with at least one recorded sign or symptom consistent with mitochondrial dysfunction on at least two occasions (except for "failure to thrive" if a likely infectious cause was identified), standardized queries were sent to pediatric investigators at each of the participating sites. Queries were also sent for children with evidence of severe anemia (i.e., hemoglobin <7 g/dl) at any time point during the first 3 years of life. Further clinical information was then reviewed by the Perinatal Safety Review Working Group. The common definitions that were used in the death data review to categorize perinatal exposure to antiretroviral drugs and to classify possible mitochondrial dysfunction[8,12] were also used in the PACTS living children review. Heightened vigilance of pediatric clinic directors for possible mitochondrial disease manifestations also resulted in at least two referrals for a more intensive workup and examination by a pediatric neurologist.

RESULTS

Between 1985 and 1998, a total of 2,665 mother–infant pairs were enrolled in PACTS. Of these, 352 (13.2%) were classified as HIV-infected, 353 (13.2%) remained with indeterminate HIV status, and 1960 (73.5%) were classified as HIV-uninfected.

Review of Deaths in PACTS

A standardized format is used to present data from the death review in PACTS (TABLES 1–5), similar to the death reviews in other cohorts participating in the U.S. Perinatal Safety Review Working Group (see related papers in this issue). TABLE 1

TABLE 1. Number of HIV-exposed children and cumulative incidence of death (%) recorded by 5 years of age and stratified by infant HIV infection status; PACTS cohort

Number of children and deaths examined (%)							
Uninfected		Indeterminate		Infected		All	
Total	Deaths	Total	Deaths	Total	Deaths	Total	Deaths
1960	6 (0.31%)	353	29 (8.2%)	352	83 (24%)	2665	118 (4.4%)

TABLE 2. History of perinatal antiretroviral drug exposure among 2,665 HIV-exposed children; PACTS cohort

Number of children (%) in designated perinatal drug exposure category						
None	Unknown born before Mar 1, 1994	Unknown born after Mar 1, 1994	ZDV alone	ZDV+3TC	Other	All
1376 (52%)	73 (3%)	42 (2%)	958 (36%)	164 (6%)	52 (2%)	2665

presents the number and cumulative incidence of death recorded by 5 years of age and stratified by infant HIV status. A total of 118 deaths were reviewed for a cumulative incidence of 44.3 deaths/1,000 live births in the entire cohort. It is evident from TABLE 1 that mortality was much higher in the HIV-infected and indeterminate groups than in the uninfected children. Among the 118 deaths, 5% were in HIV-uninfected children, 70% in infected children, and 25% in HIV-indeterminate children.

TABLE 2 shows that approximately half the children born in PACTS were not exposed to perinatal antiretroviral drugs. Of the remainder, the most common perinatal exposure was to ZDV monotherapy (36%). A relatively small proportion of infants (6%) was exposed to ZDV plus 3TC *in utero*, and none of these received the combination therapy during the first 6 weeks of life.

TABLES 3–5 present a summary of our findings of the death data review in PACTS. Among children who were HIV-uninfected or indeterminate, 6 and 29 deaths were recorded, respectively (TABLES 3 and 4). None of these deaths was classified by the Working Group in either class 2, 3, or 4. Five indeterminate and 1 HIV-uninfected child died of SIDS (cumulative incidence of SIDS = 2.6 per 1,000 live births). Among deceased HIV-infected children, 14 children were classified in class 2 and 14 children in class 3 (TABLE 5). The high proportion of deaths in HIV-infected children that were classified as class 3 probably reflects the similarity of symptoms and signs of HIV/AIDS to those of mitochondrial dysfunction. Cardiomyopathy and encephalopathy were particularly common among these children. Perinatal ZDV or other antiretroviral use did not increase the risk of being classified in class 2 or 3.

Review of Living HIV-Uninfected Children in PACTS

The total duration of active follow-up of HIV-uninfected children between 0 and 5 years of age was 2,716 child-years, and only 35% of the child-year follow-up was in individuals with perinatal exposure to NRTIs (TABLE 6). Of the 1,954 living unin-

TABLE 3. Classification of deaths by perinatal antiretroviral drug exposure: HIV-uninfected infants in the PACTS cohort

| | Number of deaths in designated antiretroviral exposure category | | | | | | |
	None	Unknown, born before March 1, 1994	Unknown, born after March 1, 1994	ZDV alone	ZDV+3TC	Other	All
Class 1	4	0	0	1	0	0	5
Class 2	0	0	0	0	0	0	0
Class 3	0	0	0	0	0	0	0
Class 4	0	0	0	0	0	0	0
SIDS	1	0	0	0	0	0	1
Total	5	0	0	1	0	0	6

TABLE 4. Classification of deaths by perinatal antiretroviral drug exposure: HIV-indeterminate infants in the PACTS cohort

| | Number of deaths in designated antiretroviral exposure category | | | | | | |
	None	Unknown, born before March 1, 1994	Unknown, born after March 1, 1994	ZDV alone	ZDV+3TC	Other	All
Class 1	13	0	0	9	1	1	24
Class 2	0	0	0	0	0	0	0
Class 3	0	0	0	0	0	0	0
Class 4	0	0	0	0	0	0	0
SIDS	3	0	0	2	0	0	5
Total	16	0	0	11	1	1	29

TABLE 5. Classification of deaths by perinatal antiretroviral drug exposure: HIV-infected infants in the PACTS cohort

| | Number of deaths in designated antiretroviral exposure category | | | | | | |
	None	Unknown, born before March 1, 1994	Unknown, born after March 1, 1994	ZDV alone	ZDV+3TC	Other	All
Class 1	38	4	0	12	0	0	54
Class 2	10	0	0	4	0	0	14
Class 3	12	0	0	2	0	0	14
Class 4	0	0	0	0	0	0	0
SIDS	0	0	0	0	0	0	0
Uncertain	1	0	0	0	0	0	1
Total	61	4	0	18	0	0	83

TABLE 6. Duration of active follow-up (in child-years) by perinatal antiretroviral drug exposure: HIV-uninfected children, 0–5 years of age, in the PACTS cohort

	None	ZDV alone	ZDV+3TC	Other	Unknown	Total
Number of children	1003	739	116	35	67	1960
Child-years of follow-up						
0–6 months of age	295.2	252.8	36.9	14.1	16.4	615.4
7–12 months of age	275.3	207.9	14.2	8.1	11.2	516.7
13–18 months of age	254.4	173.7	7.3	5.9	10.4	451.7
19–24 months of age	221.3	118.8	0.7	2.6	8.9	352.3
25–36 months of age	353.5	104.4	0.0	2.2	14.0	474.1
37–48 months of age	192.6	33.5	0.0	0.0	5.7	231.8
49–60 months of age	63.6	8.4	0.0	0.0	1.7	73.7
Total	1655.9	899.4	59.1	32.9	68.2	2715.5

fected children followed in the PACTS cohort, standardized queries were sent to pediatric clinic directors for 33 (1.7%) children with symptoms or signs consistent with possible mitochondrial dysfunction. After a comprehensive review of all clinical data, two (0.1%) of these children were classified in class 2 (both had transient signs or symptoms lasting less than 12 months) and one child (0.05%) in class 3. The latter child was born in 1991, had persistent epilepsy and developmental delay (documented from 22 until at least 46 months of age), and had no perinatal antiretroviral drug exposure. The two living children with transient signs or symptoms (class 2) were siblings born 1 year apart, and neither of them had documented perinatal antiretroviral drug exposure. Further investigations are still ongoing for 2 children, whereas all remaining children have been classified in class 1.

DISCUSSION

In this systematic review of the PACTS database, which included over 2,600 children of HIV-infected mothers and 118 recorded deaths, we found no evidence suggesting that uninfected infants exposed to NRTIs in the perinatal period died of illnesses that resembled mitochondrial disorders. This same conclusion was reached by the Perinatal Safety Review Working Group after careful review of deaths in all five U.S. studies.[8] More specifically, no cases similar to the two infants with progressive neurologic disorders reported by Blanche *et al.*[7] were uncovered.

The PACTS consortium has also undertaken a careful review of symptoms and diagnoses among living uninfected children in the cohort. Preliminary findings indicate no cases of living HIV-uninfected children with symptoms we could definitively attribute to mitochondrial dysfunction. However, the sensitivity of our case findings among living children may be suboptimal, and currently we cannot rule out the possibility that some PACTS children exposed to perinatal NRTIs might have developed transient mitochondria-related dysfunction. Continued observation and follow-up is underway.

The benefits of antiretroviral drugs administered to HIV-infected women during pregnancy and of ZDV administered to the neonate during the first 6 weeks of life for the prevention of perinatal HIV transmission are high given ZDV's proven effectiveness and safety profile to date and the fatal nature of HIV infection.[1,13] The French cases of possible mitochondrial dysfunction associated with NRTI exposure are of great concern, but similar cases have not been noted in U.S. multicenter perinatal cohorts to date despite an exhaustive review. Therefore, current USPHS recommendations for the reduction of perinatal HIV transmission remain unchanged, and women should likewise be provided the best antiretroviral drug regimen for care of their own health during pregnancy in consultation with their health care provider.[1] Offering of antiretroviral therapy, whether primarily to treat maternal HIV infection or to reduce perinatal transmission, should be accompanied by a discussion of the known and unknown short- and long-term benefits and potential risks of such therapy. Within this context, the need for long-term follow-up and monitoring for late toxicities for both mother and infant should be stressed.[14]

ACKNOWLEDGMENTS

The authors gratefully acknowledge other members of the Perinatal AIDS Collaborative Transmission Study: *Emory University, Atlanta*: Vickie Grimes, Francis Lee, Michael Lindsay, Andre Nahmias, Mary Sawyer; *New York City Perinatal HIV Transmission Collaborative Study*: Mahrukh Bamji, Susan Champion, Mary Ann Chiasson, Joanna Dobrosycki, Louise Kuhn, Genevieve Lambert, Ellie Schoenbaum, Mayris Webber, Jeremy Weedon; *University of Maryland, Baltimore*: Sue Hines, Peter Vink; *University of Medicine and Dentistry of New Jersey, Newark*: Arlene Bardeguez, Thomas Denny, James Oleske; and *Centers for Disease Control and Prevention, Atlanta*: Joanne Ethier-Ives, Marcia Kalish, Sherry Orloff, Richard Respess, Martha Rogers, R.J. Simonds, Jeffrey Wiener.

REFERENCES

1. CENTERS FOR DISEASE CONTROL AND PREVENTION. 1998. Public Health Service Task Force recommendations for the use of antiretroviral drugs in pregnant women infected with HIV-1 for maternal health and for reducing perinatal HIV-1 transmission in the United States. Morbid. Mortal. Wkly. Rep. **47(RR-2):** 1–30.
2. CENTERS FOR DISEASE CONTROL AND PREVENTION. 1998. Guidelines for the use of antiretroviral agents in HIV-infected adults and adolescents. Morbid. Mortal. Wkly. Rep. **47(RR-5):** 39–82.
3. CULNANE, M., M.G. FOWLER, S.S. LEE, *et al.* 1999. Lack of long-term effects of in utero exposure to zidovudine among uninfected children born to HIV-infected women. JAMA **281:** 151–157.
4. HANSON, I.C., T.A. ANTONELLI, R.S. SPERLING, *et al.* 1999. Lack of tumors in infants with perinatal HIV-1 exposure and fetal/neonatal exposure to zidovudine. J. AIDS Hum. Retrovir. **20:** 463–467.
5. LEWIS, W. & M.C. DALAKAS. 1995. Mitochondrial toxicity of antiviral drugs. Nature Med. **1:** 417–422.
6. BRINKMAN, K., H.J. TER HOFSTEDE, D.M. BURGER, *et al.* 1998. Adverse effects of reverse transcriptase inhibitors: mitochondrial toxicity as common pathway. AIDS **12:** 1735–1744.

7. BLANCHE, S., M. TARDIEU, P. RUSTIN, *et al.* 1999. Persistent mitochondrial dysfunction and perinatal exposure to antiretroviral nucleoside analogues. Lancet **354:** 1084–1089.
8. PERINATAL SAFETY REVIEW WORKING GROUP. 2000. Nucleoside exposure in the offspring of HIV-infected women receiving antiretroviral drugs: Absence of clear evidence for mitochondrial disease in children who died before five years of age in five United States cohorts. Submitted to Lancet.
9. SIMONDS, R.J., R. STEKETEE, N. NESHEIM, *et al.* 1998. Impact of zidovudine use on risk and risk factors for perinatal transmission of HIV. AIDS **12:** 301–308.
10. LANSKY, A., J.L. JONES, P.C. WAN, *et al.* 1998. Trends in zidovudine prescription for pregnant women infected with HIV. J. AIDS Hum. Retrovir. **18:** 289–292.
11. LINDEGREN, M.L., R.H. BYERS, JR., P. THOMAS, *et al.* 1999. Trends in perinatal transmission of HIV/AIDS in the United States. JAMA **282:** 531–538.
12. SMITH, M. FOR THE PERINATAL SAFETY REVIEW WORKING GROUP. 1999. Presented at the Second Conference on Global Strategies for the Prevention of HIV Transmission from Mothers to Infants in Montreal, Canada, September 1–6.
13. BULTERYS, M. & M.G. FOWLER. 2000. Prevention of HIV infection in children. Pediatr. Clin. N. Am. **47:** 241–260.
14. WORKSHOP ON DETECTION OF POTENTIAL TOXICITIES FOLLOWING PERINATAL EXPOSURE TO ANTIRETROVIRALS. 1999. Report from the Workshop on Detection of Potential Toxicities following Perinatal Exposure to Antiretrovirals. Office of AIDS Research, National Institutes of Health. Bethesda, Maryland, January 19–20.

Appendix

MEMBERS OF PERINATAL SAFETY REVIEW WORKING GROUP

MARC BULTERYS, M.D., Ph.D., Epidemiology Branch, Division of HIV/AIDS Prevention, Centers for Disease Control and Prevention, *Atlanta, Georgia.*

SANDRA K. BURCHETT, M.D., Children's Hospital/Harvard Medical School, *Boston, Massachusetts.*

MARY CULNANE, M.S., CRNP, Pediatric Medicine Branch, Division of AIDS, National Institute of Allergy and Infectious Diseases, National Institutes of Health, *Bethesda, Maryland.*

BETHANN CUNNINGHAM-SCHRADER, M.S., Frontier Science and Technology Research Foundation, Inc., *Amherst, New York.*

KENNETH DOMINGUEZ, M.D., M.P.H., Epidemiology Branch, Division of HIV/AIDS Prevention, Centers for Disease Control and Prevention, *Atlanta, Georgia.*

LISA DUNKLE, M.D., Bristol-Myers Squibb Pharmaceutical Research Institute, *Wallingford, Connecticut.*

LINDA DRAPER, Frontier Science and Technology Research Foundation, Inc., Amherst, New York.

MARY GLENN FOWLER, M.D., M.P.H., Epidemiology Branch, Division of HIV/AIDS Prevention, Centers for Disease Control and Prevention, *Atlanta, Georgia.*

CELINE HANSON, M.D., Department of Pediatrics, Baylor College of Medicine, *Houston, Texas.*

ELOI KPAMEGAN, Ph.D., Clinical Trials and Surveys Corp., *Baltimore, Maryland.*

MARY LOU LINDEGREN, M.D., Surveillance Branch, Division of HIV/AIDS Prevention, Surveillance and Epidemiology, Centers for Disease Control and Prevention, *Atlanta, Georgia.*

LOUISE MARTIN-CARPENTER, M.S.; Glaxo Wellcome Research and Development, *Research Triangle Park, North Carolina.*

KENNETH MCINTOSH, M.D., Children's Hospital, Harvard Medical School, *Boston, Massachusetts* (Chair).

JAMES MCNAMARA, M.D., Pediatric Medicine Branch, Division of AIDS, National Institute of Allergy and Infectious Diseases, National Institutes of Health, *Bethesda, Maryland.*

GEORGE MCSHERRY, M.D., Department of Pediatrics, University of Medicine and Dentistry of New Jersey Medical School, *Newark, New Jersey.*

WENDY G. MITCHELL, M.D., Keck School of Medicine, University of Southern California School of Medicine and Childrens Hospital Los Angeles, *Los Angeles, California.*

LYNNE M. MOFENSON, M.D., Pediatric, Adolescent and Maternal AIDS Branch, National Institute of Child Health and Human Development, National Institutes of Health, *Bethesda, Maryland.*

JAMES M. OLESKE, M.D., M.P.H., Department of Pediatrics, UMD/New Jersey Medical School, *Newark, New Jersey.*

PHILLIP RHODES, Ph.D., Statistics and Data Management Branch, Division of HIV/AIDS Prevention, Centers for Disease Control and Prevention, *Atlanta, Georgia.*

DAVID E. SHAPIRO, Ph.D., Center for Biostatistics in AIDS Research, Harvard School of Public Health, Boston, Massachusetts.

MARY E. SMITH, M.D., Pediatric Medicine Branch, Division of AIDS, National Institute of Allergy and Infectious Diseases, National Institutes of Health, *Bethesda, Maryland.*

BARBARA STYRT, M.D., MPH, Division of Antiviral Drug Products, CDER, Food and Drug Administration, Rockville, Maryland.

Drug Safety during Pregnancy and in Infants

Lack of Mortality Related to Mitochondrial Dysfunction among Perinatally HIV-Exposed Children in Pediatric HIV Surveillance

MARY LOU LINDEGREN,[a] PHILIP RHODES, LAURA GORDON, PATRICIA FLEMING, STATE AND LOCAL HEALTH DEPARTMENT HIV/AIDS SURVEILLANCE PROGRAMS, AND THE PERINATAL SAFETY REVIEW WORKING GROUP

Division of HIV/AIDS Prevention-Surveillance and Epidemiology, National Center for HIV/STD/TB Prevention, Centers for Disease Control and Prevention, Atlanta, Georgia 30333, USA

ABSTRACT: The objectives were to assess whether any deaths reported among perinatally exposed, uninfected, or indeterminate children were consistent with mitochondrial dysfunction. and to characterize perinatal exposure to antiretrovirals among children born in the last five years and reported to perinatal HIV surveillance. Population-based HIV/AIDS surveillance data on perinatally exposed children born in 1993 through 1998 from 32 states with HIV reporting and from a special HIV surveillance project in Los Angeles County and in 22 hospitals in New York City were used. The classifications of exposure and deaths were consistent with the investigation of deaths across all US cohorts. Deaths were ascertained from recent matches with death registries in each state. Causes of death were ascertained from death certificates, autopsy records when available, and medical records. None of the 98 deaths (1.1%) among 9067 perinatally exposed uninfected or indeterminate children born from 1993 through 1998 and reported through pediatric HIV surveillance died of conditions that were consistent with mitochondrial dysfunction. This included 679 children exposed to zidovudine (ZDV) and 3TC, 277 exposed to other antiretroviral combinations, 4512 exposed to ZDV alone, 927 with no antiretroviral exposure, and 2672 with unknown exposure—1128 of whom were born before March 1994 and were unlikely to have been exposed to ZDV. No deaths attributable to mitochondrial dysfunction were found through this evaluation of population-based HIV surveillance data. Long-term follow-up of antiretroviral-exposed children has been recommended by the Public Health Service. This evaluation highlights the contribution of population-based surveillance to the evaluation of potential toxicities associated with maternal antiretroviral use.

BACKGROUND

The findings of the PACTG 076 trial in 1994 demonstrating that zidovudine (ZDV) therapy given to HIV-infected women and their newborn reduced perinatal transmis-

[a]Address for correspondence: Mary Lou Lindegren, M.D., Reporting and Analysis Section, Surveillance Branch, Division of HIV/AIDS Prevention-Surveillance and Epidemiology, Centers for Disease Control and Prevention, Mailstop E-47, 1600 Clifton Road, Atlanta, GA 30333.

sion from 25% to 8% was a major prevention breakthrough in the HIV epidemic.[1,2] Rapid implementation of the Public Health Service (PHS) guidelines for the use of ZDV to reduce perinatal HIV transmission and universal, routine HIV counseling and voluntary testing of pregnant women have resulted in a dramatic decrease in perinatal HIV transmission in the United States in the last 5 years.[3–5] Shorter courses of ZDV used in Thailand and West Africa and, more recently, a single dose of Nevirapine at labor and a single dose to the infant after birth have also been effective.[6–8]

Theoretical concerns regarding the potential for carcinogenicity and mitochondrial toxicity of ZDV have led the PHS since 1994 to recommend the long-term follow-up of children exposed to ZDV and other antiretrovirals *in utero*.[9,10] Many HIV-infected pregnant women are now receiving combination antiretroviral therapy for treatment of their own infection, but the long-term safety of using these drugs in pregnancy is not known.[10,11] However, after 4 years of follow-up in PACTG protocol 076, no differences in immunologic, neurocognitive, and growth parameters between infants exposed to ZDV and those not exposed were detected.[12] Data from the Women and Infants Transmission Study Observational Cohort and Pediatric AIDS Clinical Trials Group 076/219 show no tumors in populations of perinatally HIV-exposed, antiretrovirus-exposed children followed up to 7 years of age.[13]

Nucleoside-analogue reverse transcriptase inhibitors (NRTIs) are known to inhibit DNA polymerase gamma and can cause mitochondrial depletion.[14] Among HIV-infected persons who have been treated chronically with NRTIs, these mitochondrial toxicities have included myopathy and more severe, sometimes fatal cases involving pancreatitis, liver failure, and lactic acidosis.[14–17] In most cases, these toxicities were reversed with drug discontinuation, but in some cases toxicity persisted after drug discontinuation.[14]

In 1999, French researchers reported the deaths of two uninfected infants born to HIV-infected mothers who had received ZDV and 3TC during pregnancy but who died of severe progressive neurologic symptoms at about 1 year of age and who had mitochondrial dysfunction.[18] Six additional living children with mitochondrial dysfunction were subsequently described. Three of these were asymptomatic but had transient or persistent biochemical abnormalities. All had been exposed to NRTIs *in utero* and for varying times during the newborn period (4 to ZDV alone and 2 to ZDV and 3TC). The frequency of mitochondrial dysfunction reported by the French was much higher than expected in the general population.[18] As a result, a group of U.S. investigators, including staff from the Centers for Disease Control and Prevention (CDC), the National Institutes of Health (NIH), immediately began systematically reviewing deaths among perinatally exposed children who died at or before 5 years of age who were followed in five NIH and CDC databases.[19–21] This paper describes the results from one of the databases, the perinatal HIV/AIDS surveillance database, which assesses outcome in HIV perinatally exposed uninfected and indeterminate children born in 1993 through 1998.

METHODS

All states currently conduct AIDS surveillance, and 33 of the states also conduct confidential HIV surveillance (FIG. 1).[22] Thirty-one collect information on all HIV-

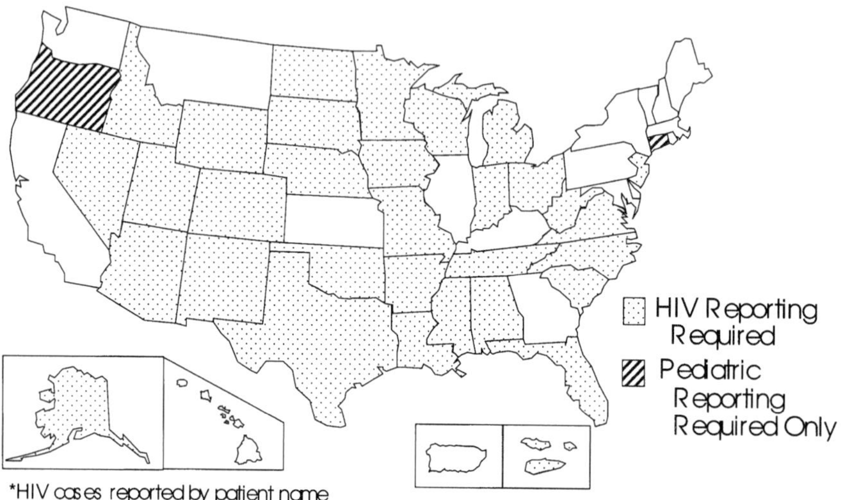

FIGURE 1. States with confidential HIV case surveillance, United States, June 1999.

infected persons, and two states collect information solely on children. Special HIV surveillance projects are located in Los Angeles County and in 22 hospitals in New York City.

These HIV-reporting areas monitor children born to HIV-infected mothers and follow-up to determine HIV infection and AIDS status. Data collected on children born to HIV-infected mothers include demographics, opportunistic illnesses, HIV diagnostic and immunologic tests, timing of maternal HIV testing, maternal anti-retroviral ZDV use during pregnancy, week started, use in labor/delivery, other anti-retrovirals received during pregnancy, neonatal ZDV use, child's antiretroviral treatment, PCP prophylaxis as well as birth history including receipt of prenatal care, prematurity, birth defects, birth weight, and type of delivery.

Ascertainment of data on mother-infant pairs can come from multiple sources and is actively collected. These include maternal HIV clinic, prenatal record, labor/delivery record, and newborn and pediatric records. Ascertainment of mother-infant pairs occurs through active case finding at pediatric sites and obstetric hospitals; HIV-infected women reported when pregnant; use of laboratory reporting of HIV tests; and matching the HIV/AIDS registry to the birth registry to identify births to HIV-infected women after their first positive test. The use of these methods provides very complete data on mother-infant pairs in most of these areas.[23]

Assessment of infant infection status is conducted by active follow-up of perinatally exposed children every 6 months until the child is determined to be uninfected, or if determined to be infected, follow-up continues until AIDS and death. The vital status of all cases is ascertained from active follow-up of cases, death certificate reviews, and matching to the death registry. Ascertainment of death is very complete as population-based surveillance data are matched to death registries routinely and were matched again for this study if not done recently. Information on causes of death was obtained from death certificates, autopsy reports, when performed, coroner's records, and information on death and other clinical conditions from medical record review.

Definitions of HIV Infection, Absence of HIV Infection, and Indeterminate Status

A child of any age was considered HIV-infected if the result of a detectable quantity was positive on two separate specimens, excluding cord blood, using any of the following HIV virologic tests: culture, detection of HIV nucleic acid-DNA or RNA, or p24 antigen ($\geq$1 mo of age), including neutralization assay.[24] Children with one positive virologic test were also considered to be infected with HIV if there were no subsequent negative HIV virologic or negative HIV antibody tests.[24] A child was also considered HIV-infected if the result for HIV antibody was positive on a screening test (e.g., repeatedly reactive enzyme immunoassay) followed by a positive confirmatory test for HIV antibody (e.g., Western blot or IFA) at 18 months of age or greater.[24] If laboratory data were unavailable, children were considered HIV-infected if they met the criteria included in the 1987 pediatric AIDS case definition.[24]

A child was considered not infected with HIV if at least one negative HIV antibody test was obtained at $\geq$6 mos of age or at least two negative HIV virologic tests (culture, detection of HIV nucleic acid-DNA or RNA) were obtained from separate specimens, both of which were performed at $\geq$1 month of age and one of which was performed at $\geq$ 4 months of age, or if one HIV virologic test performed at $\geq$4 months of age was negative *and* there were no positive HIV virologic tests and no AIDS-defining condition.[24] A child was also considered not infected with HIV if he/she had one positive HIV virologic test with at least two subsequent negative virologic tests, at least one of which was performed at $\geq$4 months of age or a negative HIV antibody test at $\geq$6 months of age.[24] A child who did not meet the criteria for HIV infection or "not infected with HIV" was classified as having indeterminate status.[24]

Antiretroviral Exposure Categories

Exposure to antiretrovirals was classified into six categories according to either receipt of antiretrovirals during pregnancy and in the first 6 weeks of life, as follows: none, ZDV monotherapy, ZDV and 3TC, other antiretroviral drug exposure, and those with unknown drug exposure born before March 1994 and those with unknown exposure born after March 1994. PACTG 076 results were announced in February 1994; therefore, we described those with unknown antiretroviral drug exposure born before March 1994, as they were less likely to have received antiretrovirals compared to those born after March 1994.

Classification of Deaths

The group of U.S. investigators (the Perinatal Safety Review Working Group) met weekly by conference call beginning in March 1999 and reviewed data on all the deaths among children who died before 5 years of age. Deaths were classified according to the likelihood that they were related to mitochondrial dysfunction.[19–21] These "mitochondrial" causes of death consisted of: neurologic, including seizures, encephalopathy, myopathy, progressive weakness, developmental delay, opthamaloplegia, blindness, deafness, ataxia, degenerative diseases of ganglia, hearing loss,

TABLE 1. Classification of deaths

Class 1: No evidence of mitochondrial disease
Class 2: Limited signs, symptoms, and /or laboratory data that are consistent with mitochondrial dysfunction but mitochondrial disease unlikely
Class 3: Signs, symptoms, and/or laboratory data where a mitochondrial disorder might reasonably be included in the differential diagnosis
Class 4: Signs, symptoms, and/or laboratory data suggestive of mitochondrial dysfunction or proven due to mitochondrial dysfunction
Class 5 or Sudden Infant Death Syndrome: No other known cause of death, no mitochondrial symptoms or signs during life, and when an autopsy was available, pathologic findings consistent with SIDS.

NOTE: Class 1: Child who died within 28 days of birth of prematurity or birth-related abnormalities or older children with clear explanations for death (e.g., trauma, bacterial meningitis, or complications of cardiac surgery).

Class 2: Child with one transient, nonprogressive, or clinically mild "mitochondrial" symptom.

Class 3: Child with a progressive or clinically severe "mitochondrial" symptom or two or more nonprogressive or clinically mild "mitochondrial" symptoms.

retinitis pigmentosa; cardiomyopathy, liver failure, pancytopenia, metabolic and lactic acidosis. Each death was reviewed by the perinatal safety review working group and classified according to the following (TABLE 1). Class 1 deaths were children who had no signs or symptoms consistent with mitochondrial dysfunction, including those who died within 28 days of birth of prematurity or birth-related abnormalities and older children with clear explanations for death (e.g. trauma, bacterial meningitis, or complications of cardiac surgery). Class 2 deaths were children with one transient, nonprogressive, or clinically mild "mitochondrial" symptom that was consistent with mitochondrial dysfunction but mitochondrial disease was unlikely. Class 3 deaths occurred among children with progressive or clinically severe "mitochondrial" symptoms or two or more nonprogressive or clinically mild "mitochondrial" symptoms where a mitochondrial disorder might reasonably be included in the differential diagnosis. Class 4 deaths were children with signs or symptoms suggestive of mitochondrial dysfunction or proven due to mitochondrial dysfunction. Class 5 consisted of children who died of Sudden Infant Death Syndrome (SIDS) with no other known cause of death, no "mitochondrial" symptoms or signs during life, and, when autopsy was available, pathologic findings consistent with SIDS.

Statistical Methods

In HIV surveillance, follow-up of exposed children is conducted for ascertainment of HIV infection status and vital status. In addition, the HIV surveillance registry is matched to the death registry and was matched again for this project, if not done recently. For calculation of person-years of follow-up for death ascertainment, if the patient died during the study period, the date of death was used as the last follow-up. If the patient was not dead or not lost to follow-up we calculated the time from birth to December 1998. If the patient was known to be lost to follow-up, we ordered all dates for each patient and chose the most recent date (i.e., date of last medical evaluation or

TABLE 2. Pediatric HIV surveillance: uninfected and indeterminate cases of children born from 1993 through 1998,[a] antiretroviral exposure characteristics

ARV exposure category	HIV status		
	Uninfected (*n*, %)	Indeterminate (*n*, %)	Total (*n*, %)
None	584 (11)	343 (10)	927 (10)
ZDV Only	2,871 (52)	1,641 (46)	4,512 (50)
ZDV + 3TC	223 (4)	456 (13)	679 (7)
Other ARV	95 (2)	182 (5)	277 (3)
Unknown[b]	1,744[b] (32)	928[c] (26)	2,672 (29)
Total	5,517 (100)	3,550 (100)	9,067 (100)

[a]Reported through March 1999.
[b]Of 1,744 uninfected children, 860 (49%) were born before March 1994.
[c]Of 928 indeterminates cases, 268 children (29%) were born before March 1994.

TABLE 3. Pediatric HIV surveillance: uninfected and indeterminate children born 1993–1998,[a] antiretroviral (ARV) exposure and vital status characteristics

ARV exposure	Uninfected		Indeterminate		Total	
	Deaths (*n*, %)	Live births	Deaths (*n*, %)	Live births	Death (*n*, %)	Live births
None	1 (0.2)	584	36 (10.5)	343	37 (4.0)	927
ZDV only	6 (0.2)	2871	30 (1.8)	1,641	36 (0.8)	4,512
ZDV + 3TC	0 (0.0)	223	3 (0.7)	456	3 (0.4)	679
Other	0 (0.0)	95	2 (1.1)	182	2 (0.7)	277
Unknown	2 (0.1)	1,744[a]	18 (1.9)	928[b]	20 (0.7)	2,672
Total	9 (0.2)	5,517	89 (2.5)	3550	98 (1.1)	9,067

[a]Of 1,744 uninfected children, 860 (49%) were born before March 1994.
[b]Of 928 indeterminates cases, 268 children(29%) were born before March 1994.

most recent laboratory test). The person-time for each patient was then added together to get the total person-years that each patient contributed to the study.

RESULTS

Through March 1999, 11,636 children born to HIV-infected mothers in 1993 through 1998 had been reported through HIV surveillance and special surveillance projects. Of these, 5,517 (47%) were uninfected, 3,550 (31%) were of indeterminate infection status, and 2,569 (22%) were HIV-infected. Overall, there were 98 (1.1%)

TABLE 4. Pediatric HIV surveillance: uninfected children born 1993 through 1998; classification of deaths by antiretroviral (ARV) exposure

Classification	Deaths (*n*) in designated antiretroviral exposure group					
	None	ZDV Only	ZDV + 3TC	Other ARV	Unknown	Total
Total deaths (*n*)	1	6	0	0	2	9
Class 1	1	6	—	—	1	8
Class 2	—	—	—	—	—	0
Class 3	—	—	—	—	—	0
Class 4	—	—	—	—	—	0
Class 5-SIDS	—	—	—	—	1	1
Total exposed	584	2,871	223	95	1,744	5,517

deaths among 9,067 HIV-exposed children born from 1993 through 1998 who were either HIV uninfected (9 deaths [0.2%] among 5,517 uninfected) or of indeterminate infection status (89 deaths [2.5%] among 3550 indeterminate cases).

Exposure Classification

Among the 5,517 uninfected children, 11% had no antiretroviral drug (ARV) exposure, 52% had ZDV exposure only, 4% had ZDV and 3TC, 2% had other ARV exposure, and exposure was unknown in 32%, 49% of whom were born before March 1994 when the results of the ACTG 076 trial became available, and thus it was unlikely that their mothers received ZDV for prevention of perinatal transmission (TABLE 2). Among 3,550 children of indeterminate status, 10% had no ARV exposure, 46% had ZDV only, 13% had ZDV and 3TC, 5% had other ARV, and exposure was unknown in 26% (29% of whom were born before March 1994). Overall, these population-based surveillance data included over 4,512 uninfected or indeterminate children with ZDV and 679 with ZDV and 3TC exposure (TABLE 3).

Uninfected Children

Death by Classification and Antiretroviral (ARV) Exposure

Of the nine deaths occurring in the 5,517 uninfected children born since 1993, eight were considered Class 1 (no evidence of mitochondrial disease) and one was Class 5 (SIDS) (TABLE 4). There were no deaths considered possible or suggestive of mitochondrial disease. Among the eight Class 1 deaths, six children received ZDV exposure only, one had no ARV exposure, and one had unknown ARV exposure. The SIDS death occurred in a child with unknown ARV exposure.

From birth years 1993 to 1998, there was a dramatic increase in ZDV use among the 5,517 uninfected children, mostly ZDV monotherapy (FIG. 2). Starting in 1997 and especially in 1998, increasing proportions of children were prenatally exposed to ZDV and 3TC as well as to other ARV combinations. Thus, many of the children exposed to ZDV and 3TC were born in more recent years.

TABLE 5. Follow-up (in person-years) of pediatric surveillance by antiretroviral exposure of HIV-uninfected children born 1993 through 1998

| | Antiretroviral exposure group | | | | | |
	None	ZDV Only	ZDV + 3TC	Other ARV	Unknown	Total
Live births	584	2,871	223	95	1,744	5,517
Class 3 or 4 deaths	0	0	0	0	0	0
	Duration of follow-up (person years)					
0–12 mo	580	2,829	205	89	1,734	5,437
12–24 mo	534	2,411	78	63	1,683	4,769
24–36 mo	451	1,667	6	33	1,566	3,723
36–48 mo	377	816	—	15	1,369	2,577
48–60 mo	197	97	—	4	650	948
Total	2,139	7,820	289	204	7,002	17,454

Uninfected Person-Years

Follow-up in person-years for all 5,517 uninfected children born since 1993, by ARV exposure status, was very complete through the first and into the second year of life (TABLE 5). Among the group with ZDV exposure only, there were 2,411 person -years of follow-up through 24 months of age and 7,820 person-years of follow-up through 60 months of age. Among those with ZDV and 3TC exposure, there were 205 person-years of follow-up by 12 months of age and 78 person-years at 24

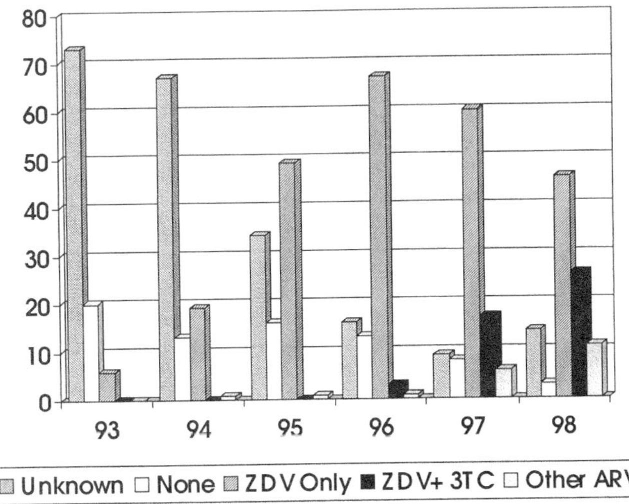

FIGURE 2. Antiretroviral exposure among uninfected children by birth year, pediatric HIV surveillance.

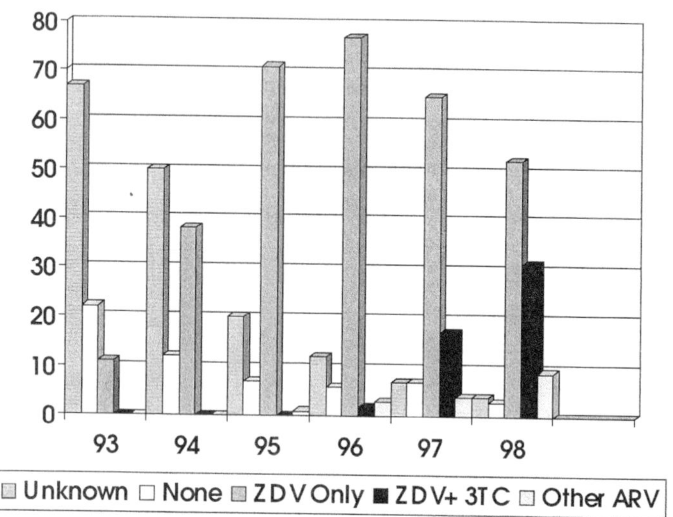

FIGURE 3. Antiretroviral exposure among indeterminate children by birth year, pediatric HIV surveillance.

months of age due to the recent birth of most of these children. Overall, there have been 17,454 person-years of follow-up of these HIV-uninfected children with no Class 3 or 4 deaths suggestive of mitochondrial dysfunction.

Indeterminate Deaths by Classification and Exposure

Of the 89 deaths among the 3,550 HIV indeterminate children born since 1993, 70 were considered Class 1 (no evidence of mitochondrial disease), 17 were SIDS, and two were Class 2 (mitochondrial disease unlikely) (TABLE 6). There were likewise no deaths considered possible or suggestive of mitochondrial disease (Class 3). Overall, the higher death rates that occurred among indeterminate cases were largely due to deaths among children who died in the first month of life before their infection status could be determined.

Among the 70 Class 1 deaths, 27 had no ARV exposure, 23 had ZDV only exposure, 3 had ZDV and 3TC exposure, 1 had other ARV exposure, and 16 had unknown ARV exposure. The Class 2 deaths occurred among one child with no ARV exposure and one child with ZDV exposure. The 17 SIDS deaths occurred among 8 children with no ARV exposure, 6 with ZDV exposure only, none with ZDV and 3TC, 1 with other ARV exposure, and 2 with unknown exposure.

ARV exposure category by year of birth among the 3,550 indeterminate cases in children born to HIV-infected mothers since 1993, similar to that seen in uninfected children, demonstrates a dramatic increase in ZDV, mostly monotherapy (FIG. 3). Starting in 1997 and especially in 1998, increasing proportions of children were exposed to ZDV and 3TC as well as to other ARV combinations. For both uninfected and indeterminate children, many children who had ZDV and 3TC exposures were born in more recent years.

TABLE 6. Pediatric HIV surveillance: indeterminate children born 1993 through 1998; classification of deaths by antiretroviral (ARV) exposure

Classification	Deaths (*n*) in designated antiretroviral exposure group					
	None	ZDV Only	ZDV + 3TC	Other ARV	Unknown	Total
Total deaths	36	30	3	2	18	89
Class 1	27	23	3	1	16	70
Class 2	1	1	—	—	—	2
Class 3	—	—	—	—	—	0
Class 4	—	—	—	—	—	0
Class 5-SIDS	8	6	—	1	2	17
Total	343	1,641	456	182	928	3,550

TABLE 7. Follow-up (in person-years) of pediatric surveillance by antiretroviral exposure of HIV-indeterminate children born 1993 through 1998

	Antiretroviral exposure group					
	None	ZDV Only	ZDV + 3TC	Other ARV	Unknown	Total
Live births	343	1,641	456	182	928	3,550
Class 3 or 4 deaths	0	0	0	0	0	0
Duration of follow-up (person years)						
0–12 mo	292	1,303	289	113	786	2,783
12–24 mo	203	735	52	28	618	1,636
24–36 mo	131	321	3	7	531	993
36–48 mo	82	118	1	4	421	626
48–60 mo	28	9	—	—	146	183
Total	736	2,486	345	152	2,502	6,221

Indeterminate Person-Years

Follow-up in person-years for the 3,550 indeterminate children born since 1993, by ARV exposure status, demonstrates an earlier fall-off in this group as 33% were born in 1998 and 24% in 1997 (TABLE 7). In addSition, there was a higher loss to follow-up in the indeterminate group, which may also contribute to less overall person-time. Among the group with ZDV exposure alone, there were 2,486 person-years of follow-up, and among ZDV and 3TC exposure, 345 person-years of follow-up. Overall, there have been 6,221 person-years of follow-up of these HIV indeterminate children in addition to the 17,454 person-years among uninfected children, and there have been no deaths categorized as Class 3 or 4 (possibly or suggestive of mitochondrial dysfunction).

DISCUSSION

None of the 98 observed deaths among 9,067 HIV-uninfected and indeterminate children could definitively be attributable to mitochondrial dysfunction. The database for this search included 4,512 with exposure to ZDV alone, 679 children exposed to ZDV and 3TC, 277 exposed to other ARV combinations, 926 with no ARV exposure, and 2,672 with unknown ARV exposure, most of whom were born before March 1994 and likely did not receive ARV. None of the five large databases at CDC and NIH evaluated by the Perinatal Safety Review Working Group (Perinatal AIDS Collaborative Transmission Study-PACTS, Pediatric AIDS Clinical trials-PACTG, Women and Infants Transmission Study, WITS, Pediatric Spectrum of Disease-PSD, and Pediatric HIV surveillance) found children who died of illnesses consistent with mitochondrial dysfunction as described by Blanche *et al.*[19–21]

Several other studies have also evaluated potential mitochondrial toxicities. New York State did not report any deaths among their cohort consistent with mitochondrial diseases.[25] There was no increased risk of neurologic symptoms in children exposed to ZDV and 3TC in the PETRA trial compared to children who received placebo.[26] Continued evaluation is ongoing to determine any evidence of mitochondrial dysfunction among the living children in several of the studies (PACTS, WITS, and PACTG).[19–21] Through population-based surveillance, HIV-uninfected children born in 1997 and 1998 who are still living are being evaluated for evidence of mitochondrial dysfunction in two states.

Several limitations of these data must be addressed. Ascertainment of perinatally exposed children may not be complete. However, data evaluated in 14 HIV reporting states showed that a median of 90% of estimated children born to an HIV-infected mother in 1995 were ascertained through HIV reporting.[5] Perinatal HIV exposure and infection reporting does not occur in all states. Recommendations for expansion to all states have been published by the CDC and the American Academy of Pediatrics.[24,27] Population-based surveillance for perinatal HIV exposure and infection enables timely monitoring of the extent and trends in the perinatal HIV epidemic among women and perinatally exposed children; assessing resources needed for prevention and care of both exposed and infected children; and targeting and evaluating implementation and effectiveness of perinatal prevention programs such as the use of ZDV and other antiretroviral therapies in pregnancy and the impact on perinatal transmission. Completeness of death ascertainment has been high among persons reported with HIV and AIDS.[24] In addition, death rates among HIV-exposed and uninfected children (11/1,000) less than 5 years of age were comparable to national rates of under 5 mortality (8.8/1,000 overall; 7.4/1,000 for white and 17.2/1,000 for blacks):[28] therefore, underascertainment of death is unlikely to be a large problem.

In the U.S., approximately 6,000 to 7,000 infants are born to HIV-infected women each year.[29,30] With the success of ZDV prophylaxis in the U.S., the elimination of perinatal HIV infection may be possible. Increasing numbers of children are also being exposed to combination therapies *in utero*. Over the next 10 years, 60,000 children will likely be exposed to multiple ARV *in utero*.[31] Population-based HIV/AIDS surveillance may help evaluate any potential significant toxicities from ARV use. Population-based surveillance provides a representative means of monitoring in all populations and communities, which will complement evaluations from facility-based observational cohorts and clinical trials. In addition to evaluating deaths, population-based perinatal HIV exposure and infection surveillance may be used to evaluate other potential toxicities such as birth defects and cancer by matching HIV perinatal antiretroviral registries to birth defects and cancer registries, as recommended by the Workshop on Detection of Potential Toxicities following Perinatal Exposure to Antiretrovirals.[31]

Safety of many ARV drugs during pregnancy is not known, and therefore, continued vigilance in examining deaths and in the long-term follow-up of ARV-exposed children, as recommended by the PHS, is critical. The report by Blanche raised concern about potential mitochondrial toxicity from NRTIs, but in the U.S. an association has not been established.[10,32] Data from the U.S. cohorts suggest that these effects, if related to perinatal ARV, are rare. Furthermore, new studies of rates of mitochondrial dysfunction in the general population may be higher than previously thought.[33] The data from France, however, emphasize the continued importance of the PHS recommendations for long-term follow-up of infants with *in utero* exposures to antiretroviral drugs.[10] Innovative surveillance strategies may play an important role in evaluating potential toxicities.[31]

REFERENCES

1. CONNOR, E.M., R.S. SPERLING, R. GELBER *et al.* 1994. Reduction of maternal-infant transmission of human immunodeficiency virus type 1 with zidovudine treatment. N. Engl. J. Med. **331:** 1173–1180.
2. SPERLING, R.S., D.E. SHAPIRO, R.W. COOMBS *et al.* 1996. Maternal viral load, zidovudine treatment, and the risk of transmission of human immunodeficiency virus type 1 from mother to infant. N Engl J Med. **335:** 1621–1629.
3. CENTERS FOR DISEASE CONTROL AND PREVENTION. 1994. Recommendations of the US Public Health Service Task Force on the use of zidovudine to reduce perinatal transmission of human immunodeficiency virus. Morb. Mortal. Wkly. Rep. **43**(RR-11): 1–20.
4. CENTERS FOR DISEASE CONTROL AND PREVENTION. 1995. US Public Health Service recommendations for human immunodeficiency virus counseling and voluntary testing for pregnant women. Morb. Mortal. Wkly. Rep. **44**(RR-7): 1–15.
5. LINDEGREN, M.L., R.H. BYERS, P. THOMAS *et al.* 1999. Trends in perinatal transmission of HIV/AIDS in the United States. JAMA **282:** 531–538.
6. GUAY, L.A., P. MUSOKE, T. FLEMING *et al.* 1999. Intrapartum and neonatal single-dose Nevirapine compared with zidovudine for prevention of mother-to-child transmission of HIV-1 in Kampala, Uganda: HIVNET012 randomized trial. Lancet **354:** 795–802.
7. SHAFFER, N., R. CHUACHOOWONG, P.A. MOCK *et al.* 1999. Short-course zidovudine for perinatal HIV-1 transmission in Bangkok, Thailand: a randomized controlled trial. Lancet **353:** 773–780.
8. WIKTOR, S.Z., E. EKPINI, J.M. KARON *et al.* 1999. Short course oral zidovudine for prevention of mother-to-child transmission of HIV-1 in Abidjan, Cote d'Ivoire: a randomized trial. Lancet **353:** 78–85.
9. CENTERS FOR DISEASE CONTROL AND PREVENTION. 1998. Public Health Service Task Force recommendations for the use of antiretroviral drugs in pregnant women infected with HIV-1 for maternal health and for reducing perinatal HIV-1 transmission in the United States. Morb. Mortal. Wkly. Rep. **47** (RR-2): 1–30.
10. CENTERS FOR DISEASE CONTROL AND PREVENTION 1998. U.S. Public Health Service Task Force Recommendations for the use of antiretroviral drugs in pregnant women infected with HIV-1 for maternal health and for reducing perinatal HIV-1 transmission in the United States. (http://www.hivatis.org/guidelines/perinatal/PerinatalFeb2500.pdf).

11. CENTERS FOR DISEASE CONTROL AND PREVENTION. 1998. Guidelines for the use of anti-retroviral agents in HIV-infected adults and adolescents. Morb. Mortal. Wkly. Rep. **47**(RR-5): 39–82.
12. CULNANE, M., M.G. FOWLER, S.S. LEE *et al.* 1999. Lack of long-term effects of *in utero* exposure to zidovudine among uninfected children born to HIV-infected women. JAMA **281:** 151–157.
13. HANSON, I.C., T.A. ANTONELLI, R.S. SPERLING *et al.* 1999. Lack of tumors in infants with perinatal HIV type 1 exposure and fetal/neonatal exposure to zidovudine. J. Acquir. Immune Defic. Syndr. Hum. Retrovir. **20:** 463–467.
14. BRINKMAN, K., J.M. HADEWYCN, D.M. BURGER *et al.* 1998. Adverse effects of reverse transcriptase inhibitors: mitochondrial toxicity as common pathway. AIDS **12:** 1735–1744.
15. ARNAUDO, E., M. DALAKA, S. SHANSKE *et al.* 1991. Depletion of muscle mitochondrial DNA in AIDS patients with zidovudine induced myopathy. Lancet **337:** 508–510.
16. CHURCH, J., W. MITCHELL & I. GONZALEZ-GOMEZ *et al.* 2000. Near-fatal metabolic acidosis, liver failure, and mitochondrial DNA depletion in HIV-infected children treated with combination antiretroviral therapy [abstr.]. Presented at the 7th Conference on Retroviruses and Opportunistic Infections. San Francisco, January 2000.
17. DALAKAS, M.C., I. ILLA, G.H. PEZESHPOUR *et al.* 1990. Mitochondrial myopathy caused by long-term zidovudine therapy. N. Engl. J. Med. **322:** 1098–1105.
18. BLANCHE, S., M. TARDIEU, P. RUSTIN *et al.* 1999. Persistent mitochondrial dysfunction and perinatal exposure to antiretroviral nucleoside analogues. Lancet **354:** 1084–1089.
19. MCINTOSH, K. 2000. Mitochondrial toxicity of perinatally adminstered zidovudine (abstr. S14). In Program and abstracts of the 7th Conference on Retroviruses and Opportunistic Infections. January–February, 2000. San Francisco, California.
20. PERINATAL SAFETY REVIEW WORKING GROUP. 2000. Nucleoside exposure in the offspring of HIV-infected women receiving antiretroviral drugs: absence of clear evidence for mitochondrial disease in children who died before five years of age in five United States cohorts. Submitted to Lancet.
21. SMITH, M. for the Perinatal Safety Review Working Group. 1999. Presented at the Second Conference on Global Strategies for the Prevention of HIV Transmission from Mothers to Infants. Montreal, Canada. September 1–6.
22. CENTERS FOR DISEASE CONTROL AND PREVENTION. 1998. HIV/AIDS Surveillance Rep. **10**(No.1): 1–40.
23. CENTERS FOR DISEASE CONTROL AND PREVENTION. 1998. Success in implementing PHS guidelines to reduce perinatal transmission of HIV-1993, 1995, and 1996. Morb. Mortal. Wkly. Rep. **47:** 688–691.
24. CENTERS FOR DISEASE CONTROL AND PREVENTION. 1999. CDC Guidelines for National Human Immunodeficiency Virus Case Surveillance, including monitoring of human Immunodeficiency virus infection and acquired immunodeficiency syndrome. Morb. Mortal. Wkly. Rep. **48** (RR-13): 1–31.
25. BIRKHEAD, G., N. WADE, STOFGER-ISSER *et al.* 2000. Review of deaths among a cohort of New York State infants exposed in the perinatal period to HIV and antiretroviral drugs [abstr.]. Presented at the 7th Cconference on Retroviruses and Opportunistic Infections. San Francisco, January 2000.
26. LANGE, J., R. STELLATO, K. BRINKMAN *et al.* 1999. Review of neurological adverse events in relation to mitochondrial dysfunction in the prevention of mother to child transmission of HIV: Petra Study [abstr. 250]. Presented at the Global Strategies for the Prevention of HIV Transmission from Mothers to Infants, September 1999. Montreal.
27. AMERICAN ACADEMY OF PEDIATRICS, Committee on Pediatric AIDS. 1998. Surveillance of pediatric HIV infection. Pediatrics **101:** 315–319.
28. ANDERSON, R.N. 1996. United States abridged life tables, 1996. National vital statistics reports; vol 47, no 13. Hyattsville, Maryland. National Center for Health Statistics. 1998.
29. BYERS, R.H., M.B. CALDWELL, S. DAVIS *et al.* 1998. Projection of AIDS and HIV incidence among children born infected with HIV. Stat. Med. **17:** 169–181.
30. DAVIS, S.F., R.J. BYERS, M.L. LINDEGREN *et al.* 1995. Prevalence and incidence of vertically acquired HIV infection in the United States. JAMA **274:** 952–955.

31. REPORT FROM THE WORKSHOP ON DETECTION OF POTENTIAL TOXICITIES FOLLOWING PERINATAL EXPOSURE TO ANTIRETROVIRALS. 1999. Office of AIDS Research, National Institutes of Health. Bethesda.
32. MORRIS, A.M. & A. CARR. 1999. HIV nucleoside analogues: new adverse effects on mitochondria? Lancet **354:** 1046–1047.
33. UUSIMAA, J., A.M. REMES, H. RANTALA *et al.* 2000. Childhood encephalopathies and myopathies: a prospective study in a defined population to assess the frequency of mitochondrial disorders. Pediatrics **105:** 598–603.

Appendix

MEMBERS OF PERINATAL SAFETY REVIEW WORKING GROUP

MARC BULTERYS, M.D., Ph.D.; Epidemiology Branch, Division of HIV/AIDS Prevention, Centers for Disease Control and Prevention, *Atlanta, GA.*

SANDRA K. BURCHETT, M.D.; Children's Hospital/Harvard Medical School, *Boston, MA.*

MARY CULNANE, M.S., C.R.N.P.; Pediatric Medicine Branch, Division of AIDS, National Institute of Allergy and Infectious Diseases, National Institutes of Health, *Bethesda, MD.*

BETHANN CUNNINGHAM-SCHRADER, M.S.; Frontier Science and Technology Research Foundation, Inc., *Amherst, NY.*

KEN DOMINGUEZ, M.D., M.P.H.; Epidemiology Branch, Division of HIV/AIDS Prevention, Centers for Disease Control and Prevention, *Atlanta, GA.*

LISA DUNKLE, M.D.; Bristol-Myers Squibb Pharmaceutical Research Institute, *Wallingford, CT.*

LINDA DRAPER; Frontier Science and Technology Research Foundation, Inc., *Amherst, NY.*

MARY GLENN FOWLER, M.D., M.P.H.; Epidemiology Branch, Division of HIV/AIDS Prevention, Centers for Disease Control and Prevention, *Atlanta, GA.*

CELINE HANSON, M.D.; Department of Pediatrics, Baylor College of Medicine, *Houston, TX.*

ELOI KPAMEGAN, Ph.D.; Clinical Trials and Surveys Corp., *Baltimore, MD.*

MARY LOU LINDEGREN, M.D.; Surveillance Branch, Division of HIV/AIDS Prevention, Surveillance and Epidemiology, Centers for Disease Control and Prevention, *Atlanta, GA.*

LOUISE MARTIN-CARPENTER, M.S.; Glaxo Wellcome Research and Development, *Research Triangle Park, NC.*

KENNETH MCINTOSH, M.D.; Children's Hospital, Harvard Medical School, *Boston, MA.*

JAMES MCNAMARA, M.D.; Pediatric Medicine Branch, Division of AIDS, National Institute of Allergy and Infectious Diseases, National Institutes of Health, *Bethesda, MD.*

GEORGE MCSHERRY, M.D.; Dept. of Pediatrics, University of Medicine and Dentistry of New Jersey Medical School, *Newark, NJ.*

WENDY G. MITCHELL, M.D.; Keck School of Medicine, University of Southern California School of Medicine and Childrens Hospital Los Angeles, *Los Angeles, CA.*

LYNNE M. MOFENSON, M.D.; Pediatric, Adolescent and Maternal AIDS Branch, National Institute of Child Health and Human Development, National Institutes of Health, *Bethesda, MD.*

JAMES M. OLESKE, M.D., M.P.H.; Department of Pediatrics, UMD/New Jersey Medical School, *Newark, NJ.*

PHILLIP RHODES, Ph.D.; Statistics and Data Management Branch, Division of HIV/AIDS Prevention, Centers for Disease Control and Prevention, *Atlanta, GA.*

DAVID E. SHAPIRO, Ph.D.; Center for Biostatistics in AIDS Research, Harvard School of Public Health, *Boston, MA.*

MARY E. SMITH, M.D.; Pediatric Medicine Branch, Division of AIDS, National Institute of Allergy and Infectious Diseases, National Institutes of Health, *Bethesda, MD.*

BARBARA STYRT, M.D., M.P.H.; Division of Antiviral Drug Products, CDER, Food and Drug Administration, *Rockville, MD.*

Lack of Definitive Severe Mitochondrial Signs and Symptoms among Deceased HIV-Uninfected and HIV-Indeterminate Children ≤ 5 Years of Age, Pediatric Spectrum of HIV Disease Project (PSD), USA

K. DOMINGUEZ,[a,k] J. BERTOLLI,[a] M. FOWLER,[a] V. PETERS,[b] I. ORTIZ,[c] S. MELVILLE,[d] T. RAKUSAN,[e] T. FREDERICK,[f] H. HSU,[g] P. D'ALMADA,[a] Y. MALDONADO,[h] C. WILFERT,[i] THE PSD CONSORTIUM, AND THE PERINATAL SAFETY REVIEW WORKING GROUP [j]

[a]*Epidemiology Branch, Division of HIV/AIDS Prevention, National Center for HIV/STD/TB Prevention, Centers for Disease Control and Prevention, Atlanta, Georgia 30333, USA*

[b]*Office of AIDS Surveillance, New York City Department of Health, New York, New York 10012, USA*

[c]*AIDS Surveillance Program, Puerto Rico Department of Health, Rio Piedras, Puerto Rico 00921, USA*

[d]*HIV/AIDS Division, Texas Department of Health, Austin, Texas 78756, USA*

[e]*Children's National Medical Center, Washington, D.C. 20010, USA*

[f]*Pediatric AIDS Surveillance Study, Los Angeles County Department of Health Services, Los Angeles, California 90012, USA*

[g]*Pediatric AIDS Surveillance Project, State Laboratories Institute, Jamaica Plain, Massachusetts 02130, USA*

[h]*Department of Pediatrics, Stanford University School of Medicine, Stanford, California 94305-5119, USA*

[i]*Pediatric Infectious Diseases, Duke University Medical Center, Durham, North Carolina 27710, USA*

ABSTRACT: **Background: In response to recent reports of mitochondrial dysfunction in HIV-uninfected infants exposed to antiretroviral (ARV) prophylaxis, the Perinatal Safety Review Working Group reviewed deaths in five large HIV-exposed perinatal cohorts in the United States to determine if similar cases of severe mitochondrial toxicity could be detected. We describe the results of this review for the PSD cohort.**

[j]See Appendix for list of members of Perinatal Safety Review Working Group.

[k]Address for correspondence: Kenneth L. Dominguez, MD, MPH, Mother-Child Transmission, Pediatric and Adolescent Studies Section, Epidemiology Branch, Division of HIV/AIDS Prevention, Centers for Disease Control and Prevention, 1600 Clifton Road, Mailstop E-45, Atlanta, GA 30333, USA. Voice: 404-639-6129; fax: 404-639-6127.

kld0@cdc.gov

Methods: Hospitalization, clinic and death records for deceased HIV-uninfected and HIV-indeterminate children who were less than 5 years of age were reviewed. Standard definitions were used to classify HIV infection status and the likelihood that signs and symptoms were related to mitochondrial dysfunction. Children were classified as having signs and symptoms that were considered (1) unrelated, (2) unlikely, (3) consistent with, or (4) likely related to mitochondrial disease. SIDS deaths were put into a separate category.

Results: 8,465 of 13,125 HIV-exposed children were either HIV-uninfected or HIV-indeterminate. Among the 84 deaths in the subgroup of 8,465 children, 9 were considered in Class 2 (unlikely), 4 were considered in Class 3 (consistent with), and none were considered in Class 4 (likely). 97% of those children who received ARV prophylaxis received zidovudine alone. None of the HIV-uninfected deaths were classified in 2, 3, or 4; and only one of these was exposed to ARV prophylaxis. Among the 3 HIV-indeterminate children who were classified in 3 (consistent with), 2 had no or unknown ARV exposure before 1994 when use of ZDV prophylaxis became the standard of care. Both HIV-uninfected and HIV-indeterminate children with ARV exposure or unknown exposure had lower mortality rates than children without ARV exposure.

Conclusion: Monoprophylaxis with ZDV was not associated with higher death rates in the cohort of 8,465 children or with any findings likely consistent with mitochondrial dysfunction among the 85 deaths. Ongoing monitoring of drug safety in large multi-site prospective cohort studies of HIV-exposed children is essential in the era of highly active antiretroviral therapy.

BACKGROUND

In the United States, the use of perinatal monoprophylaxis with zidovudine (ZDV) for the reduction of vertical transmission has shown no significant side effects within the first 5 years of life with widespread use since 1994.[1] However, in 1999, French investigators reported two HIV-exposed but uninfected infants who developed severe neurologic disease leading to death with evidence of mitochondrial dysfunction and who had been perinatally exposed to combination prophylaxis with ZDV and lamivudine in a clinical trial.[2] The French investigators later reported on six living HIV-uninfected children, four of whom were exposed to ZDV alone and two of whom were exposed to combination ZDV/3TC. These six children were also noted to have mitochondrial abnormalities on assays done on muscle biopsy.[2] Three of the six children were clinically asymptomatic at the time of last followup, but they had transient or persistent biochemical abnormalities.[2] Based on the two initial French cases, the Centers for Disease Control and Prevention (CDC) and the National Institutes of Health (NIH) rapidly began to look for any evidence of similar cases of deaths that may have occurred among HIV-exposed children in their major pediatric cohorts.

A Perinatal Safety Review Working Group (PSRWG) was formed to review and classify signs and symptoms that might be related to mitochondrial disease among HIV-exposed children in these cohorts. Their system of classification was described previously.[3] The review was limited to HIV-uninfected and HIV-indeterminate children. Cohorts from NIH and CDC were reviewed over a 6-month period, including the CDC's Pediatric Spectrum of HIV Disease (PSD) project.

PSD is a prospective, multi-site, medical record review study of HIV-exposed live-born children which started in 1988 and currently continues enrollment.[4] Pediatric charts of enrollees are reviewed every 6 months. The study is population-based in Los

TABLE 1. U.S. Drug Safety Working Group classification system for signs, symptoms, and laboratories

Class	Definition
1: Unrelated	No evidence of mitochondrial disease
2: Unlikely	Limited signs and symptoms, and/or laboratory data that are consistent with mitochondrial dysfunction, but mitochondrial disease unlikely.
3: Consistent with	Signs, symptoms, and/or laboratory data where a mitochondrial disorder might reasonably be included in the differential diagnosis.
4: Likely	Signs, symptoms and/or laboratory data suggestive of mitochondrial dysfunction, or proven due to mitochondrial dysfunction
SIDS	Sudden Infant Death Syndrome
Uncertain	Insufficient clinical/ and/or death information to assign to any class.

Angeles County, Massachusetts, and Washington, DC. In Puerto Rico, New York City, Texas, San Francisco, and North Carolina, it is hospital based and therefore does not capture all pediatric HIV-exposed children in those areas. Data from all eight sites were included in this review. As of September 1997, enrollment and follow-up of children were discontinued at the North Carolina and San Francisco sites.

METHODS

Criteria for Inclusion in PSD Review

Because there is a lag time of about 6 months in receiving and cleaning data, December 31, 1998 was chosen as the end-point date for analyzing the database to insure completeness of the data. We focused our study on deceased HIV-uninfected and deceased HIV-indeterminate children who were 5 years of age or less and enrolled in the study through 1998. In PSD, HIV-infected children were not included in the study review because of the difficulty in distinguishing those signs and symptoms related to HIV infection from those compatible with mitochondrial disease. The definitions for HIV-infection, HIV-uninfection, and HIV-indeterminate status for this study have been described elsewhere[3] and are consistent with the revised CDC HIV surveillance classification system.[5]

Signs and Symptoms

We collected information on signs and symptoms from hospitalization ICD-9 codes, outpatient clinic records, and death records. PSD data collection forms allow up to six hospitalizations and four ICD-9 codes per hospitalization to be entered for each 6- month period. As part of this routine data collection, PSD collects information on the following signs and symptoms not in the AIDS case definition which were of interest to this special study: (1) evidence of progressive neurologic disease, including (a) failure to progress or to achieve new milestones, (b) progressive motor deficits, and (c) impaired brain growth (acquired microcephaly or advancing brain atrophy on CT or NMR scan); (2) hepatitis; (3) cardiomyopathy; and (4) nephropathy. These symptoms were classified as in TABLE 1. The classification system was previously described.[3] In general, the higher the score between 1 and 4, the more likely the signs and symptoms were related to mitochondrial disease. Both a greater number of symptoms from different symptom categories (i.e., hepatic versus cardiac versus neurologic, etc.) and more progressive symptoms were associated with a higher classification score. Because the etiology of sudden infant death syndrome (SIDS) is by definition not determined, SIDS-related deaths were categorized in a separate category. For a death to be categorized as a SIDS-related death, no other known causes of death could be listed. If an HIV-exposed child was lost to follow-up after birth, that child was considered "uncertain."

Death Information

Death information in PSD is routinely abstracted from four main sources, including hospital record, death certificate, autopsy summary, and physician contact, as well as other sources. Four of six PSD sites conduct cross-matches of the PSD database with local vital statistics databases containing death certificate information to insure completeness of death information. Death information from all these sources and ICD-9 codes from all fields on the death certificates were included in this analysis. In addition, most deaths reported as SIDS deaths in the medical record or classified as such by the PSRWG were confirmed with autopsy reports from medical examiners.

Antiretroviral Exposure

Information on antiretroviral (ARV) exposure is also routinely collected on both infants and mothers. Although the overall study question for this analysis involved infant exposure during the first 6 weeks of life, PSD, for most of its history, had collected information in 6-month intervals without start or stop dates for medications. After April, 1998, PSD started collecting start and stop dates of ARV therapy or prophylaxis use. Therefore, for most children in this analysis, infant exposure to perinatal ARV was defined as exposure during the first 6 months of life. Because PSD is a pediatric medical record review study, information on maternal ARV exposure during the prenatal period is variable. Such information can only be abstracted from pediatric charts if it is noted in the pediatric chart or if copies of the mother's labor and delivery record were placed in the infant's chart. For this analysis, perinatal antiretroviral exposure was classified as ZDV alone, ZDV + 3TC, other combinations, unknown before March 1, 1994 or unknown on or after March 1, 1994. Before March 1, 1994, ZDV was not recommended by the U.S. Public Health Service as the standard of care to prevent perinatal transmission. By differentiating between unknown ARV exposures before and after this date, we can determine whether the majority of "unknowns" are likely to be due to missing information or are most likely children who did not receive ARV for prophylaxis purposes, because it was not a standard of care at the time.

TABLE 2. Number of live-born children and number and proportion (%) who died by HIV infection status

HIV-uninfected		HIV-indeterminate	
No. live-born	No. deaths (%)	No. live-born	No. deaths (%)
5,737	9 (0.16%)	2,728	75 (2.7%)

TABLE 3. Racial/ethnic classification of PSD cohort

Race/ethnicity	HIV-uninfected	HIV-indeterminate	Total
Black	3,086	1,694	4,780 (56%)
Non-black	2,592	9,84	3,580 (43%)
Other	59	50	109 (1%)
Total	5,737	2,728	8,465

TABLE 4. PSD person-years of follow-up by antiretroviral exposure and HIV infection status[a]

HIV infection status	Type of antiretroviral exposure					
	None	ZDV only	ZDV/3TC	Other	Unknown	Total
HIV-uninfected	507.8	s1,798.6	5.3	20.3	5,552.8	7,884.8
HIV-indeterminates	31.8	392.9	5.2	6.6	647.4	1,083.9
Total	539.6	2,191.5	10.5	26.9	6,200.2	8,968.7

[a]Includes children with a potential for ≥ 2 years of follow-up time based on time of enrollment and our December 31, 1998 endpoint for analysis and excludes children who: (1) died before they were enrolled or (2) were otherwise retroactively enrolled (e.g., among living children, those whose enrollment occurred more than 12 months after the date of last medical visit).

Follow-up of HIV-Exposed Children

In PSD, HIV-infected children are followed indefinitely as long as they stay in the catchment area of the hospital where they are followed. The majority of HIV-uninfected children in the cohort were also followed indefinitely; however, in 1998, the PSD protocol was changed so that children were no longer followed once they were determined to be HIV-uninfected. HIV-indeterminate children are followed as long as they continue to be HIV-indeterminate. HIV-infected children are followed indefinitely. We calculated follow-up rates for the children in our study in terms of person-years of follow-up by antiretroviral exposure and HIV status. Our follow-up calculations included only those children with a potential for 2 years of follow-up time based on time of enrollment and our December 31, 1998 end-point date for analysis, and excluded children who (1) died before they were enrolled, or (2) were otherwise retroactively enrolled (e.g., among living children whose enrollment occurred more than 12 months after the date of the last medical visit).

RESULTS

A total of 13,125 HIV-exposed children were enrolled in PSD between 1988 and 1998, of which 43.7% were HIV-uninfected, 35.6% were HIV-infected, and 20.8% were HIV-indeterminate. There were 877 deaths for a death rate of 66.8 deaths/1,000

TABLE 5. PSD Months of follow-up by percentile and HIV infection status

HIV infection status	No. of children[a]	No. months of follow-up by percentile		
		25%	50%	75%
Uninfected	5,681	14	19	30
Indeterminate	2,601	2	5	10
Uninfected + indeterminate	8,282	6	16	25

[a]One hundred eighty-three children were not included in the calculation because they died on the first day of life or had inaccurate or missing dates of follow-up.

TABLE 6. Perinatal antiretroviral drug exposure

HIV status	Number of children (%) by perinatal drug exposure category						
	None	ZDV alone	ZDV + 3TC	Other	Unknown born before 3/94	Unknown born after 2/94	Total
HIV-indeterminate	92	1,250	36	43	720	587	2,728
	(3)	(46)	(1)	(2)	(26)	(22)	(100)
HIV- uninfected	201	1,871	15	17	3102	531	5,737
	(4)	(33)	(0)	(0)	(54)	(9)	(100)
Total	293	3,121	51	60	3,822	1,118	8,465
	(3)	(37)	(1)	(1)	(45)	(13)	(100)

live births for the entire cohort. Among the 877 deaths, 1.0% were HIV-uninfected, 90.4% were HIV-infected, and 8.6% were HIV-indeterminate. Analysis was restricted to the subcohort of 8,465 children, of whom 5,737 were HIV-uninfected and 2,728 were HIV-indeterminate (TABLE 2). In this subcohort, nine deaths occurred among the HIV-uninfected children and 75 deaths among the HIV-indeterminate children. In addition, 56% of the subcohort was black, non-Hispanic (TABLE 3). A total of 7,884.8 person-years of follow-up were accrued from among HIV-uninfected children, and 1,083.9 persons-years of follow-up from among the HIV-indeterminate children (TABLE 4). The median follow-up time for live-born children in the PSD cohort was as follows: 19 months (HIV-uninfected), 5 months (HIV-indeterminate), and 16 months (HIV-uninfected and HIV-indeterminate combined) (TABLE 5).

ARV exposure among the 8,465 live-born children is characterized in TABLE 6. Among HIV-uninfected and HIV-indeterminate children combined, 39% of children received some perinatal ARV prophylaxis, that is, 37% received ZDV alone, 1% received ZDV and 3TC, and 1% received some other ARV. Within each HIV status group, the proportions receiving different ARV were similar, except that higher proportions of HIV-indeterminate children received ZDV alone (46% of HIV-indeterminate versus 33% of HIV-uninfected children) and had unknown ARV status on or after March 1, 1994 (22% of HIV- indeterminate versus 9% of HIV-uninfected children). By contrast, higher proportions of HIV-uninfected children had unknown ARV exposure status before March 1, 1994 (54% of HIV-uninfected versus 26.4% of HIV-indeterminate children). Seventy-seven percent of 4,490 children with unknown antiretroviral exposure were in the "Unknown before 3/94" category. The proportions of children whose maternal perinatal ARV exposure status was noted in the pediatric medical record were 54% (4,573) for ZDV alone, 27% (2,245) for ZDV and 3TC, and 42% (3,545) for ARVs other than ZDV or 3TC.

TABLE 7. Classification of deaths by perinatal antiretroviral drug exposure: HIV-uninfected infants

Mitochondrial disease class	Number of deaths in designated antiretroviral exposure group						
	None	ZDV alone	ZDV+3TC	Other	Unknown born before 3/94	Unknown born after 2/94	Total
Class 1 (unrelated)	3	1	-	-	5	-	9
Class 2 (unlikely)	-	-	-	-		-	-
Class 3 (consistent with)	-	-	-	-	-	-	-
Class 4 (likely)	-	-	-	-	-	-	-
SIDS	-	-	-	-	-	-	-
Unknown	-	-	-	-	-	-	-
Total	3	1	-	-	5	-	9

TABLE 8. Classification of deaths by perinatal antiretroviral drug exposure: HIV-indeterminate infants

Mitochondrial disease class	Number of deaths in designated antiretroviral exposure group						
	None	ZDV alone	ZDV+3TC	Other	Unknown born before 3/94	Unknown born after 2/94	Total
Class 1 (unrelated)	3	13	1	-	27	6	50
Class 2 (unlikely)	1	2	-	-	6	-	9
Class 3 (consistent with)	2	1	-	-	1	-	4
Class 4 (likely)	-	-	-	-	-	-	-
SIDS	1	1	-	-	5	-	7
Unknown	2	2	-	-	1	-	5
Total	9	18	1	-	0	6	75

TABLE 9. Mortality rates by exposure category (deaths/1,000 live-born children)

HIV Status	Antiretroviral exposure status						
	None	ZDV alone	ZDV+3TC	Other	Unknown born before 3/94	Unknown born after 2/94	Total
Indeterminate	97.8	15.2	27.8	...	55.6	10.2	27.5
Uninfected	14.9	0.5	...	...	1.6	...	1.6
Total	40.9	6.4	19.6	...	11.8	5.4	9.9

ARV exposure and classification of symptoms of the nine HIV-uninfected deceased children is shown in TABLE 7. All of the children were Class 1 (unrelated), and only one had ARV exposure. This child was exposed to ZDV alone. Five of the children were born before March 1, 1994 and had unknown ARV exposure status.

ARV exposure and classification of symptoms of the 75 HIV-indeterminate deceased children are shown in TABLE 8. Nineteen or 25% of children had ARV exposure, of which 18 were exposed to ZDV alone and one to ZDV + 3TC. Of 46 children with unknown ARV exposure status, 87% were born before March 1, 1994. The following proportions of deceased children were categorized into one of six classifications: 67% (Class 1: unrelated), 12% (Class 2: unlikely), 5% (Class 3: consistent with), 0% (Class 4: likely), 9% (SIDS), and 7% (unknown).

Description of HIV-Indeterminate Deaths in Class 3 (consistent with)

CASE 1. This child was born in 1991 and died at 5 months of age of pneumonia, unspecified septicemia, and unspecified respiratory disease. Hepatitis and cardiomyopathy had been noted on clinic visits. It is unknown whether the mother received antiretrovirals during pregnancy; however, the child had no exposure to antiretrovirals after birth, and birth had occurred prior to the 1994 recommendations on the use of ZDV for the prevention of perinatal HIV transmission.[6]

CASE 2. This child was born in 1984 and died at 5 months of age of cardiac arrest, at which time pneumothorax and pneumopericarditis were present. The child also had failure-to-thrive and hepatitis. Neither mother nor child could have had exposure to antiretrovirals based on the child's year of birth.

CASE 3. This child was born in 1993 and died at 3 months of age of unknown cause. Hospitalization and clinic information note a history of acidosis, lack of expected normal physiologic development, and failure to thrive. Neither mother nor child had exposure to antiretrovirals at the time of birth.

Mortality

The death rate (deaths/1,000 live-born HIV-exposed children) was 9.9 for the combined cohort of HIV-indeterminate and HIV-uninfected children, 1.6 for HIV-uninfected children, and 27.5 for HIV-indeterminate children (TABLE 9). The highest death rates in both HIV-uninfected and HIV-indeterminate children were among those who had no exposure to antiretrovirals with rates of 14.9 and 97.8, respectively. The death rates among those HIV-indeterminate and HIV-uninfected children who received ARVs or in whom ARV exposure was unknown had much lower death rates than did those who had no ARV exposure.

Seven deaths were classified as SIDS among the 8,465 live-born HIV-uninfected and HIV-indeterminate children. This corresponds to a rate of 0.83 SIDS deaths/ 1,000 live-born HIV-exposed children.

DISCUSSION

The PSD project brings a number of inherent strengths to this analysis. It provides good ascertainment of the signs and symptoms of interest to this study. It routinely collects information on progressive neurologic disorders, cardiomyopathy, failure to thrive, and nephropathy. It also insures completeness of death information by cross-checking with death databases. In addition, PSD has a large number of enrolled children, with a large group of children with no ARV exposure for comparison.

PSD's large sample size of 8,465 children is adequate for detecting severe mitochondrial signs and symptoms with a prevalance as rare as 1/5,000 children. The probability of detecting a single case of severe mitochondrial dysfunction is 82%, assuming a prevalence of 1/5,000. This probability increases to 100% at prevalences as high as 1/1,000 or 1/100. Considering that French investigators found a prevalence of deaths associated with mitochondrial signs and symptoms of 1/100 after exposure to combination AZT/3TC, and assuming that the probability of detecting such an event with exposure to monoprophylaxis with AZT might be somewhere between 1/100 and 1/5,000, it is reassuring that no such event was definitively diagnosed in our cohort.

Some constraints of the PSD project are the limited information available on maternal prenatal exposure to ARVs and the longer follow-up of HIV-infected children than of HIV-uninfected and HIV-indeterminate children, particularly in the last year of the study. Another constraint is that most children exposed to ARVs were exposed to AZT alone. Only a small number of children were exposed to combination perinatal ARV prophylaxis, thereby limiting the ability to assess the potential risk of exposure to combined ARV prophylaxis.

The overall mortality rate (deaths/1,000 live-born children) of 9.9 in our combined cohort of HIV-uninfected and HIV-indeterminate children was similar to the under-5-year mortality rate in the US in 1996 of 8.8 and to that between whites (7.4) and blacks (17.2).[7] As would be expected, HIV-indeterminate children had a much higher overall mortality rate than did HIV-uninfected children (27.5 versus 1.6) because some of the HIV-indeterminate children were undoubtedly HIV-infected, with clinical findings consistent with HIV infection but lacking laboratory confirmation at the time of death. The fact that both HIV-indeterminate and HIV-uninfected infants who received ZDV or ZDV/3TC had lower death rates than did those infants who received no ARVs may indicate, in part, that ZDV or ZDV/3TC exposure was protective against conditions that could lead to death, including opportunistic infections among indeterminate children who were truly HIV infected and that exposure to ZDV or ZDV/3TC therapy might be a marker for better access to health care and better living conditions that might result in lower mortality rates.

The SIDS rate (SIDS deaths/1,000 live-born children) of 0.83 for the PSD cohort is within the documented range of SIDS rates in the US. SIDS rates for black non-hispanic, white non-hispanic, and hispanic children were, respectively, 2.3, 1.2, and 1.0 in 1988 and 1.6, 0.7, and 0.5 in 1996 (Personal communication: Schoendorf, National Center for Health Statistics, linked Birth Death records, 1996).

CONCLUSION

This retrospective analysis indicates that monoprophylaxis with ZDV was not associated with higher death rates or any definitively diagnosed mitochondrial symptoms in a cohort of HIV-uninfected or HIV-indeterminate HIV-exposed children. Assuming a prevalence of severe mitochondrial disorders of 1/5,000 or higher, the sample size of 8,465 children should be considered adequate to detect a single such event. Among both HIV-uninfected and HIV-indeterminate HIV-exposed children, those with ZDV exposure had lower death rates than did those with no ARV exposure. The vast majority of children who received prophylaxis were given ZDV alone.

The effect of combination therapy could not be fully studied in the deceased cohort because of the small number of children and mothers using combination therapy. No deceased children had signs and symptoms definitively attributed to mitochondrial disease. There was no evidence suggesting mitochondrial dysfunction among deceased HIV-uninfected children in either the ARV-exposed or ARV-unexposed group. Among the three deceased HIV-indeterminate children with signs and symptoms possibly related to mitochondrial disease, two had no documented ARV exposure or were born before 1994 when ZDV prophylaxis was not the standard of care. In addition, the SIDS deaths in our cohort were unlikely related to mitochondrial dysfunction, as they were consistent with national SIDS rates and were not preceded by clinical illness consistent with mitochondrial dysfunction.

This analysis underscores the importance of maintaining large multi-site prospective cohort studies of HIV-exposed and HIV-infected children in the era of highly active antiretroviral therapy (HAART) therapy. As the number of newly HIV-infected children and pediatric AIDS clinical trials decrease, the role of large multi-site epidemiologic cohort studies in monitoring emerging issues such as drug safety and drug resistance increases in importance.

ACKNOWLEDGMENTS

The authors acknowledge the dedicated staff of the Pediatric Spectrum of Disease Project, the United States Perinatal Safety Working Group, and particularly the leadership of Dr. Ken McIntosh of Boston's Children's Hospital in helping to review the cases used in this paper. The authors also acknowledge the assistance of Dr. Philip Rhodes of the CDC in calculating person-years of follow-up, that of Dr. Bob Byers and Dr. John Karon in calculating the probability of detecting a mitochondrial event in the PSD sample size, and that of Petra Walton of the CDC in the preparation of this manuscript.

REFERENCES

1. CONNOR, E.M., R.S. SPERLING, R. GELBER *et al.* 1994. Reduction of maternal-infant transmission of human immunodeficiency virus type 1 with zidovudine treatment. N. Engl. J. Med. **331:** 1173–1180.
2. BLANCHE, S., M. TARDIEU, P. RUSTIN *et al.* 1999. Persistent mitochondrial dysfunction and perinatal exposure to antiretroviral nucleoside analogues. Lancet **354:** 1084–1089.
3. PERINATAL SAFETY REVIEW WORKING GROUP. 2000. Absence of clear evidence for mitochondrial disease in children who died before five years of age in five United States cohorts. J. Acquir. Immunodef. Syndr. In press.
4. CALDWELL, M.B., L. MASCOLA, W. SMITH *et al.* 1992. Biologic, foster, and adoptive parents: caregivers of children exposed perinatally to human immunodeficiency virus in the United States. The Pediatric Spectrum of Disease Clinical Consortium. Pediatrics **90(4):** 603–607.
5. CENTERS FOR DISEASE CONTROL AND PREVENTION. 1999. CDC Guidelines for national human immunodeficiency virus case surveillance, including monitoring for human immunodeficiency virus infection and acquired immunodeficiency syndrome. M.M.W.R. **48:** 29–31.
6. CENTERS FOR DISEASE CONTROL AND PREVENTION. 1994. Recommendations for the use of zidovuding to reduce perinatal transmission of human immunodeficiency virus. M.M.W.R. **43:** 1–20.
7. ANDERSON, R.N. 1998. United States abriged life tables, 1996. Natl. Vital Stat. Rep. 47(13). National Center for Health Statistics. Hyattsville, MD.

Appendix

LIST OF MEMBERS OF PERINATAL SAFETY REVIEW WORKING GROUP

MARC BULTERYS, M.D., Ph.D.; Epidemiology Branch, Division of HIV/AIDS Prevention, Centers for Disease Control and Prevention, *Atlanta, Georgia.*

SANDRA K. BURCHETT, M.D.; Children's Hospital/Harvard Medical School, *Boston, Massachusetts.*

MARY CULNANE, M.S., C.R.N.P.; Pediatric Medicine Branch, Division of AIDS, National Institute of Allergy and Infectious Diseases, National Institutes of Health, *Bethesda, Maryland.*

BETHANN CUNNINGHAM-SCHRADER, M.S.; Frontier Science and Technology Research Foundation, Inc., *Amherst, New York.*

KENNETH DOMINGUEZ, M.D., M.P.H.; Epidemiology Branch, Division of HIV/AIDS Prevention, Centers for Disease Control and Prevention, *Atlanta, Georgia.*

LISA DUNKLE, M.D.; Bristol-Myers Squibb Pharmaceutical Research Institute, *Wallingford, Connecticut.*

LINDA DRAPER; Frontier Science and Technology Research Foundation, Inc., *Amherst, New York.*

MARY GLENN FOWLER, M.D., M.P.H.; Epidemiology Branch, Division of HIV/AIDS Prevention, Centers for Disease Control and Prevention, *Atlanta, Georgia.*

CELINE HANSON, M.D.; Department of Pediatrics, Baylor College of Medicine, *Houston, Texas.*

ELOI KPAMEGAN, Ph.D.; Clinical Trials and Surveys Corp., *Baltimore, Maryland.*

MARY LOU LINDEGREN, M.D.; Surveillance Branch, Division of HIV/AIDS Prevention, Surveillance and Epidemiology, Centers for Disease Control and Prevention, *Atlanta, Georgia.*

LOUISE MARTIN-CARPENTER, M.S.; Glaxo Wellcome Research and Development, *Research Triangle Park, North Carolina.*

KENNETH MCINTOSH, M.D.; Children's Hospital, Harvard Medical School, *Boston, Massachusetts.*

JAMES MCNAMARA, M.D.; Pediatric Medicine Branch, Division of AIDS, National Institute of Allergy and Infectious Diseases, National Institutes of Health, *Bethesda, Maryland.*

GEORGE MCSHERRY, M.D.; Dept. of Pediatrics, University of Medicine and Dentistry of New Jersey Medical School, *Newark, New Jersey.*

WENDY G. MITCHELL, M.D.; Keck School of Medicine, University of Southern California School of Medicine and Childrens Hospital Los Angeles, *Los Angeles, California.*

LYNNE M. MOFENSON, M.D.; Pediatric, Adolescent and Maternal AIDS Branch, National Institute of Child Health and Human Development, National Institutes of Health, *Bethesda, Maryland.*

JAMES M. OLESKE, M.D., MPH; Department of Pediatrics, UMD/New Jersey Medical School, *Newark, New Jersey.*

PHILLIP RHODES, Ph.D.; Statistics and Data Management Branch, Division of HIV/AIDS Prevention, Centers for Disease Control and Prevention, *Atlanta, Georgia.*

DAVID E. SHAPIRO, Ph.D.; Center for Biostatistics in AIDS Research, Harvard School of Public Health, *Boston, Massachusetts.*

MARY E. SMITH, M.D.; Pediatric Medicine Branch, Division of AIDS, National Institute of Allergy and Infectious Diseases, National Institutes of Health, *Bethesda, Maryland* .

BARBARA STYRT, M.D., M.P.H.; Division of Antiviral Drug Products, CDER, Food and Drug Administration, *Rockville, Maryland.*

A Comparision of Genetic Mitochondrial Disease and Nucleoside Analogue Toxicity

Does Fetal Nucleoside Toxicity Underlie Reports of Mitochondrial Disease in Infants Born to Women Treated for HIV Infection?

RICHARD H. HAAS[a]

Departments of Neurosciences and Pediatrics, University of California, San Diego, La Jolla, California 92093-0935

ABSTRACT: Recent reports of mitochondrial disease in infants whose mothers were treated in pregnancy with nucleoside analogues are of concern. Chronic nucleoside analogue treatment of adults has long been known to cause mitochondrial DNA depletion with the risk of multisystem disease. Combination nucleoside analogue treatment regimens may have the greatest risk of toxicity. This paper briefly presents the underlying biochemical etiologies and phenotypes of some common genetic mitochondrial diseases in order to provide a comparison with reports of infant toxicity. A standardized method for the diagnosis and evaluation of mitochondrial disease is discussed. A hypothesis, with predictions of the effects of antenatal nucleoside analogue treatment on the fetus, is presented and future directions for research on this problem are suggested.

INTRODUCTION

Reports of mitochondrial disease resulting from nucleoside analogue treatment highlight the fact that mitochondrial disease may be acquired, in this case as an unintended consequence of antiretroviral therapy. One of the earliest examples of drug-induced mitochondrial disease with a devastating consequence was the report in 1983 of irreversible Parkinson's disease in young people exposed to the toxin 1-methyl-4-phenyl-1,2,3,6-tetrahydropyridine (MPTP).[1] The mechanism is thought to be the result of inhibition of complex I (NADH-coenzyme Q oxidoreductase) of the electron transport chain.[2] More recently, zidovudine (AZT)-induced mitochondrial myopathy was noted in patients chronically treated 6 months or longer.[3] There is evidence that the mechanism is mitochondrial DNA (mtDNA) depletion.[4] The spectrum of AZT mitochondrial toxicity includes hepatopathy, cardiotoxicity, and lactic acidosis following long-term treatment. Other nucleoside analogues produce similar toxic effects with extension to include bone marrow failure, peripheral neuropathy, and pancreatitis.[5] The most florid example of nucleoside toxicity resulted from the use of the reverse trancriptase inhibitor fluoro-iodoarauracil (FIAU) for the treatment of hepatitis B infection.[6] Toxic effects included severe lactic acidosis, encephalopathy, myopathy, and cardiomyopathy with lipid storage, pancreatitis, and peripheral neuropathy. Fatal acute liver toxicity occurred in 5 of 15 patients treated for 8–12 weeks with FIAU. The mechanism of toxicity is by potent inhibition of mitochondrial DNA polymerase γ, leading to mtDNA depletion in human cells[7,8] and a woodchuck animal model.[9]

In February 1999 the French AIDS study group, ANRS, reported the deaths of 2 non-HIV–infected infants born to mothers treated with two nucleoside analogue reverse transcriptase inhibitors (AZT and thiacytidine [3TC]) from the thirty-second week of gestation to 6 weeks postpartum. There were 445 mother/infant pairs treated in this study. In a recent report,[10] an additional six infants with features of mitochondrial disease were found in the French perinatal cohort of 1,754 nucleoside analogue-treated HIV sero-positive mothers.[10]

This paper presents an overview of mitochondrial metabolism and the role of mitochondrial DNA in human disease. Examples of the spectrum of genetic mitochondrial disease phenotypes, an approach to the diagnosis of mitochondrial disease, discussion of the French report, and a personal case of an infant with a mitochondrial disease phenotype following prenatal and postnatal AZT treatment are presented. A hypothesis with a prediction of the timing and effects of prenatal exposure to nucleoside analogues and future research directions are discussed.

MAJOR MITOCHONDRIAL FUNCTIONS

Mitochondria play an integral role in cellular metabolism. In addition to making ATP, the cellular energy currency, mitochondria also play a crucial role in intermediary metabolism. The terminal metabolism of carbohydrates and amino acids occurs in the mitochondria where interconversion of fats, carbohydrates, and amino acids occurs. The beta oxidation pathway for fats is contained within the mitochondria.

FIGURE 1 provides an overview of important oxidative metabolic pathways. Carbohydrate carbon skeletons enter oxidative metabolism through the citric acid cycle via pyruvate and the important regulatory enzyme, pyruvate dehydrogenase (PDH). The products of fat metabolism provide an energy source that enters the electron transport chain at complex I (NADH), at coenzyme Q (ETFred), and via the citric acid cycle (acetyl CoA). Uridine, important for cellular pyrimidine production, is linked to the electron transport chain through the activity of the Q-linked enzyme dihydroorotate coenzyme Q oxidoreductase (DHO-QO) (FIG. 1). As a consequence of electron transport, most of the cell's free radicals are produced in mitochondria where reactive oxygen species can damage proteins and DNA. Another cellular destructive activity linked to mitochondria is programmed cell death. The release of mitochondrial cytochrome *c* is an irreversible apoptotic event.[11]

Mitochondrial DNA encodes and the mitochondrial ribosomal system manufacturers several important proteins in the electron transport chain. The contribution of nuclear and mtDNA genes to the coding of polypeptides of the electron transport chain is detailed in TABLE 1. The mtDNA gene contribution is critical, encoding a number of important subunits. For this reason, mtDNA mutations and damage can have serious cellular consequences. Lastly, mitochondrial DNA is replicated within mitochondria utilizing the mitochondrial polymerase. It is this activity that gives rise to the toxicity of nucleoside analogues.

OXIDATIVE PHOSPHORYLATION LINKED PATHWAYS

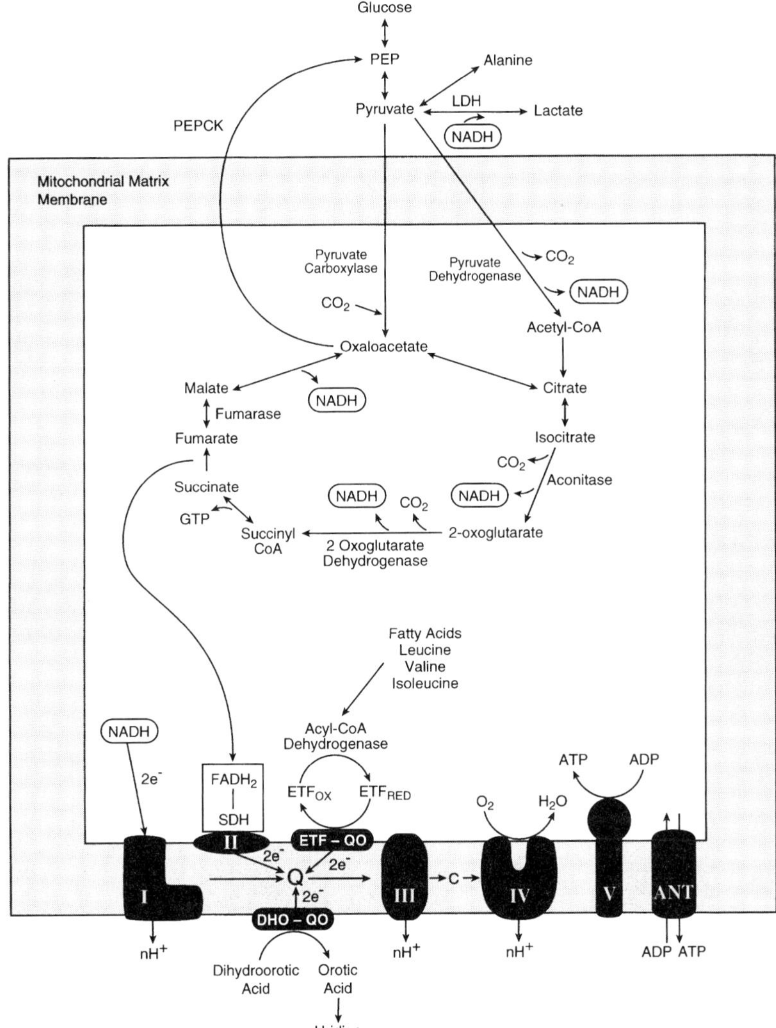

FIGURE 1. An overview of mitochondrial energy pathways. The electron transport chain is imbedded in the inner mitochondrial matrix membrane as is pyruvate dehydrogenase (PDH). Reduced nicotinamide adenine dinucleotide (NADH) is the major high energy product of the citric acid cycle, and electrons from NADH enter the electron transport chain at complex I, passing down the chain to complex IV. FADH = reduced flavine adenine dinucleotide; ETF = electron transfer factor; ETF-QO = electron transfer factor coenzyme Q oxidoreductase; DHO-QO = dihydroorotate coenzyme Q oxidoreductase; complex V = ATPase synthase; ANT = adenine nucleotide transporter; PEP = phosphoenolpyruvate; PEPCK = phosphenolpyruvate carboxykinase; LDH = lactic dehydrogenase; ATP = adenosine triphosphate; ADP = adenosine diphosphate; Q = coenzyme Q.[10]

TABLE 1. Mitochondrial DNA contribution to mammalian electron transport polypeptides

ET complex	Mitochondrial DNA	Nuclear DNA	Total subunits
I	7	36	43
II	0	4	4
III	1	10	11
IV	3	10	13
V	2	13	15

Mitochondrial metabolic defects, particularly, impact cells and organ systems that are dependent on high energy production. Mitochondrial diseases are typically multi-organ system disorders, and because of the great variability of clinical phenotypes, diagnosis may be difficult. The brain, accounting for 2% of body weight, utilizes 20% of oxidative fuel. Central nervous system disease is commonly seen in mitochondrial disorders with symptoms including stroke, dementia, ataxia, seizures, and migraine. The peripheral nervous system is also involved in many mitochondrial diseases, with peripheral neuropathy and sensorineural deafness occurring commonly. Skeletal muscle and cardiac muscle are frequently involved tissues with symptoms including fatigue and muscle weakness, which may be profound. Muscle pain occurs more rarely. Hypertrophic and dilated cardiomyopathies along with conduction disorders and in particular the Wolff-Parkinson-White syndrome may be seen. Pigmentary retinopathy, optic neuropathy, and ophthalmoplegia are seen with mitochondrial DNA point mutations and deletions.

Endocrinopathies commonly occur in mitochondrial disease. In some populations, up to 2% of type 2 diabetics have the A3243G mtDNA mutation, also responsible for the syndrome of mitochondrial encephalomyopathy with lactic acidosis and stroke-like episodes (MELAS).[12,13] Gastroenterological disease includes hepatopathy, pancreatitis, irritable bowel, recurrent vomiting, and pseudoobstruction. Interstitial nephritis, Fanconi's syndrome, and isolated renotubular acidosis may all be manifestations of mitochondrial disease.

COMMON PHENOTYPES OF MITOCHONDRIAL DISEASE

As TABLE 1 details, electron transport protein genes are found in both nuclear and mtDNA. Human diseases can result from nuclear or mtDNA mutations. The decade of the 1990s was a very productive time for the elucidation of mtDNA disorders. Increasingly, research is now focusing on the nuclear genes responsible for mitochondrial disease with recent successes in the discovery of the SURF 1 gene mutations responsible for up to 80% of COX deficiency with the Leigh's phenotype,[14] complex II gene defects leading to ataxia and optic atrophy,[15] and several complex I subunit gene defects in patients with Leigh disease. Currently, mtDNA disorders remain the largest group of identified causes of human oxidative phosphorylative diseases.

Patients with mitochondrial disease often deteriorate with seemingly mild infection, which is frequently viral in nature. Phenotypic variability and multiorgan system disease are two other hallmarks of mitochondrial disease, and this is most marked with the mtDNA disorders. This is in large part because of two phenomena: heteroplasmy, a mixture of mutant and wild-type DNA within cells and tissues that can vary between cells and tissues and over time; and a cellular threshold for percentage of mutation below which a pathogenic mutation may be silent. In the case of nucleoside-induced mtDNA depletion, the threshold for expression of symptoms allows a loss of 70% of mtDNA before symptoms of mitochondrial disease become prominent.

Leigh Disease

Leigh disease is a frequent manifestation of mitochondrial disease in infants and young children. First described in 1951 as a subacute necrotizing encephalomyelopathy, this condition is caused by failure of brain oxidative metabolism during infancy or early childhood. Several biochemical defects in the oxidative metabolic pathway can produce this condition (FIG. 1). Approximately 25% of patients with Leigh disease have complex I deficiency, 25% have PDH deficiency, 25% have complex IV (COX) deficiency, and 15% have defects in complex V (ATP synthase) due to mtDNA mutations, of which the T8993G mutation, first described as the cause of the syndrome of neurogenic weakness, ataxia, and retinitis pigmentosa (NARP), being the most common. FIGURE 2 illustrates the typical course of the infantile presen-

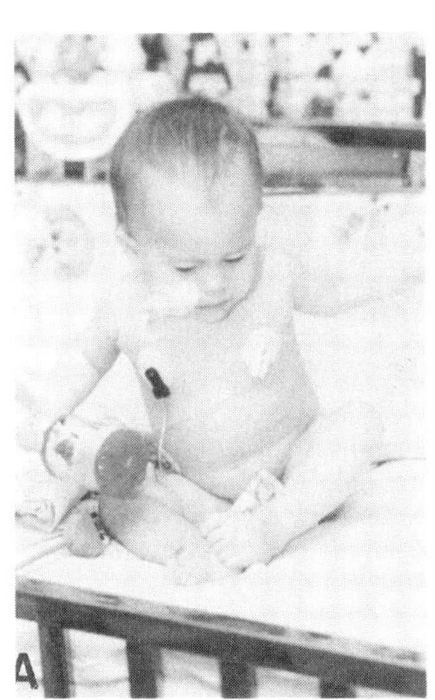

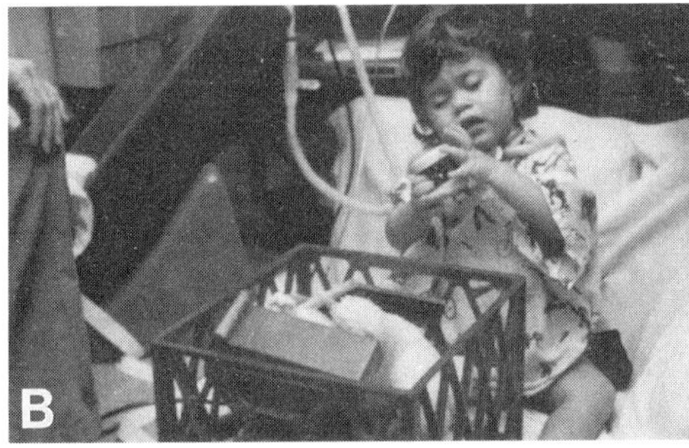

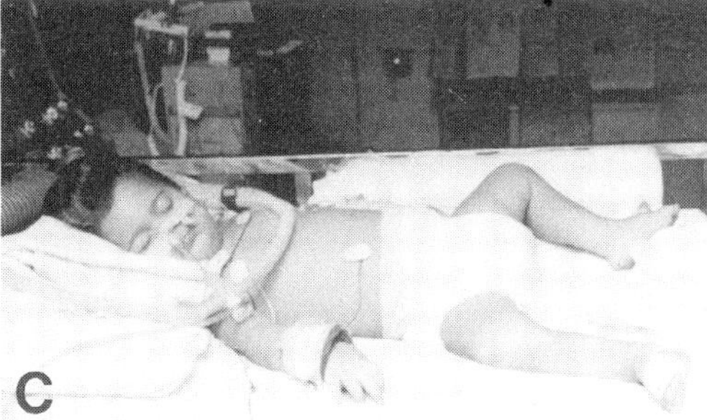

FIGURE 2. Course of a child with Leigh's syndrome. (**A**) At 11 months, playful but failing to thrive with lactic acidosis, diabetes mellitus, and a cardiac conduction defect. (**B**) At age 20 months, ventilator dependent due to central apnea with opthalmoplegia and ptosis. (**C**) At age 25 months, comatose following a mild viral infection that triggered metabolic decompensation and encephalopathy.

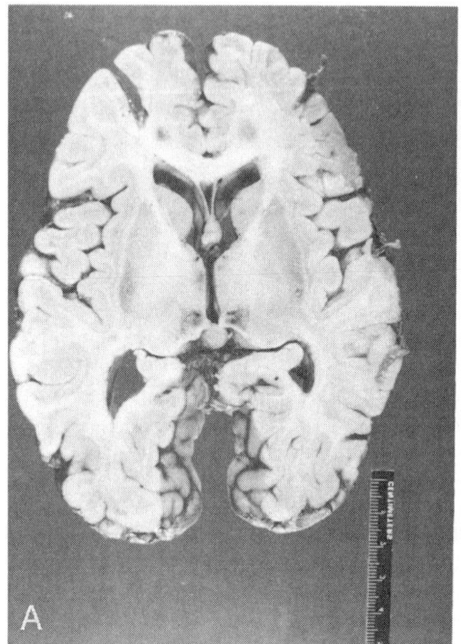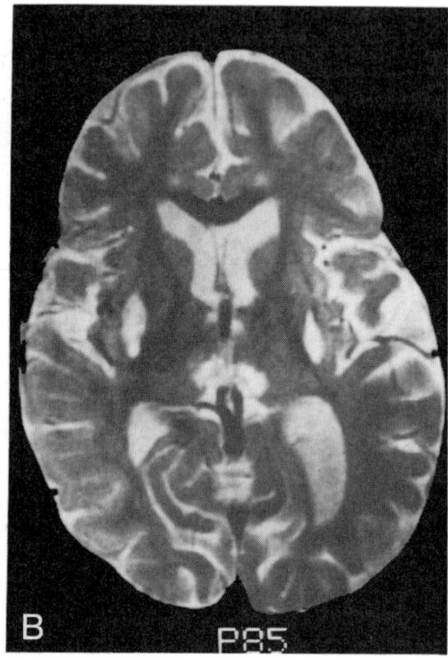

FIGURE 3. Brain of the patient in FIGURE 2. Gross pathology (**A**) shows characteristic necrotic spongiform lesions in the basal ganglia (putamena), thalamus, and frontal white matter. (**B**) Postmortem MR scan shows high T2 signal in the same necrotic areas seen in FIGURE 2A.

tation of Leigh disease. At 11 months the patient presented with failure to thrive, hypotonia, cardiac conduction defects, with the Wolff-Parkinson-White syndrome and lactic acidosis. By 20 months she had had several episodes of encephalopathy associated with mild viral infections, with loss of CNS function at each episode. Brainstem lesions resulted in central apnea and the need for continuous ventilation. At 25 months of age a further episode of viral infection resulted in coma, and this was the terminal illness. In FIGURE 3A, necrotic brain lesions exhibiting typical spongiform change with gliosis and capillary proliferation can be seen with matching abnormal T2 signal hyperintensity on brain magnetic resonance imaging (FIG. 3B).

Myopathy and Cardiomyopathy

Whilst up to 25% of patients with Leigh disease have underlying complex I deficiency, another presentation of this biochemical defect is a myopathy with cardiomyopathy. We recently evaluated a 14-month-old girl at the UCSD Mitochondrial and Metabolic Disease Center who presented with a history of poor weight gain from 6 months of age and plasma lactate levels to 17 mM but normal cerebrospinal fluid lactate. This girl had a normal intellect and no evidence of CNS disease clinically or on MRI. She had gross motor delays due to the myopathy and severe cardiomyopathy that proved fatal within a month of our evaluation. This child had profound complex I deficiency on muscle biopsy. This case illustrates that the same biochemical defect can produce many different phenotypes. Mitochondrial DNA mutations affecting any of the subunit genes for complex I may lower complex I activity. Such disorders include Leber's hereditary optic atrophy including a variant with dystonia.[16] Mitochondrial DNA tRNA defects tend to affect the activities of multiple electron transport complexes. The A3243G tRNA leucine mutation responsible for the syndrome of mitochondrial encephalomyopathy with lactic acidosis and stroke-like episodes (MELAS) often lowers complex I activity significantly.

Leigh Syndrome and Autism

We recently reported a family with the G8363A tRNA lysine point mutation previously reported to produce cardiomyopathy and movement disorder in adults.[17,18] The 6-year-old girl in this family had a typical course of Leigh's syndrome with normal birth history followed by normal development until 15 months of age. She then developed progressive ataxia, myoclonus, and chorea with cardiomyopathy. She had a seizure disorder, and plasma lactate levels were elevated two- to threefold. MRI scan at the age of 4 1/2 years showed bilateral increased T2 signals in the putamena. Muscle biopsy showed nearly complete absence of COX staining on histochemistry. This child had 82% of the G8363A mutation in blood. Her brother, aged 4, also had a normal birth history, and his development appeared normal until at 18 months he developed progressive loss of expressive language and language comprehension. His behavior gradually became more disruptive with hyperkinesis and self-injurious behavior. He developed mild motor clumsiness and partial complex seizures. This boy fulfilled the classical diagnostic criteria for autism. Plasma lactate levels were normal. His blood mutational load was 60%. This family illustrates that mitochondrial phenotypes due to the same molecular defect may appear different even within the same family. In part, this phenomenon arises because of heteroplasmy, producing different loads of mutation in different tissues varying from individual to individual.

Kearns-Sayre Syndrome

This progressive multisystem disorder was identified in 1988 as the first mtDNA disease.[19] The majority of typical cases have large mtDNA deletions, and the cardinal features are a childhood-onset dementing condition with progressive external ophthalmoplegia, cardiac conduction block, and atypical pigmentary retinal degeneration along with a CSF protein greater than 100 mg/dl. A personal case of an 11-year-old girl demonstrates the features. This child had a normal birth and early development apart from observed short stature. At the age of 4 years she presented with hypocalcemic tetany and intermittent ptosis. At the age of 8 she was diagnosed by an ophthalmologist as having the Kearns-Sayre syndrome (KSS) when seen with ophthalmoplegia, ptosis, and retinitis pigmentosa. By this time she also had sensorineural deafness and required a pacemaker for heart block. By the age of 11, she had severe growth retardation, mild lactic acidosis, ataxia, and learning disability. Patients with KSS have ragged-red fiber myopathies due to accumulation of abnormal mitochondria. Some patients with KSS present earlier in life with Pearson syndrome characterized by bone marrow failure with sideroblastic anemia and pancreatic dysfunction. This presentation of mtDNA deletion disease is often fatal in infancy.

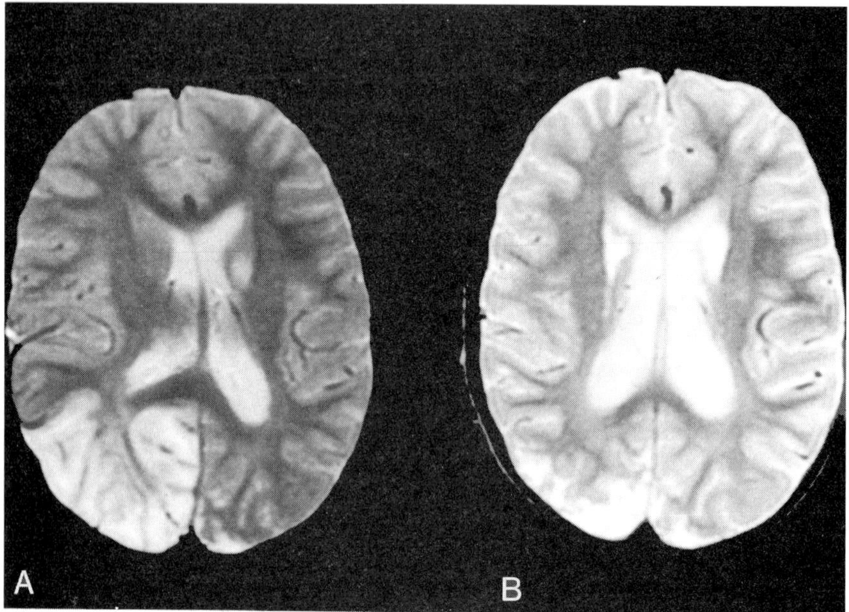

FIGURE 4. MRI scans of 7-year-old boy with the A3243G MELAS mutation who has had two metabolic strokes. Sequential T2 MR images separated by 2 years, showing progression of disease. (**A**) Brain MR at age 5 years showing high T2 signal in the right occipital lobe and left caudate nucleus. There is mild ventriculomegaly. (**B**) MR at age 7 shows the evolution of the right occipital lesion with atrophy and the appearance of a new left occipital bright T2 signal along with a new right caudate lesion.

MELAS Phenotypes

The A3243G mtDNA mutation responsible for the severe phenotype of MELAS is the most common mitochondrial single molecular defect encountered in our center. Approximately 10% of our mitochondrial disease patient population have this mutation. The phenotypes, however, are wide ranging, from the severe form of the disease as exemplified by a prepubertal 19-year-old man who died following a degenerative CNS course with ataxia, dementia, seizures, deafness, and cortical blindness due to recurrent strokes. This patient also had short stature, myopathy, and cardiomyopathy. Plasma lactate was 3.5 mM and CSF lactate 5.5 mM. The other end of the spectrum is illustrated by a 42-year-old asymptomatic mother of a severely affected 14-year-old boy who has lactic acidosis with multiple strokes. The mother's blood mutational load was 1%, and detection of the mutation required high sensitivity end cycle radiolabeled polymerase chain reaction analysis.[20]

FIGURES 4A and B show MRI scans separated by 2 years, showing T2 hyperintensity in the right occipital area at the age of 5 following a stroke-like episode (FIG. 4A), with subsequent atrophy of this occipital lesion and progression of disease with new caudate and left occipital lesions at the age of 7 years (FIG. 4B). This boy was previously healthy until the age of 5 years when he developed right parietal occipital infarction. At the age of 7 he had a second episode, with progression in basal ganglia lesions and left occipital infarction. He had headaches and a seizure disorder. Blood and CSF lactic acid levels were elevated. This patient's mother has the MELAS mutation with insulin-dependent diabetes and deafness; two maternal uncles have diabetes, and a maternal great uncle died at a young age with seizures.

Adults may present with diabetes, deafness, or features of the MELAS syndrome, having been thought normal until their presentation. A common presentation is type 2 diabetes with or without an insulin requirement, often accompanied by deafness[21] which is frequently due to cochlear damage.[22]

We have cared for successful professionals in such fields as banking, nursing, publishing, and investment counseling who first presented with stroke in their late 30s.

Mitochondrial DNA Depletion

The genetic forms of mtDNA depletion are autosomal recessive. This group of disorders usually present with early infantile or juvenile hepatic or myopathic symptoms. The myopathic presentations produce marked ragged-red fiber myopathy, rarely seen in the young child in other mitochondrial diseases. The infantile myopathic presentation is usually fatal by the end of the first year of life, with presentation at 2–4 months due to motor delay and respiratory distress. Muscle mtDNA levels are less than 10% normal. In the juvenile presentation, mtDNA levels are higher but generally less than 30%, and the clinical course is that of a rapidly progressive myopathy with death before the age of 4 years. A hepatic neonatal presentation is seen in small for gestational age infants with hypoglycemia and severe liver disease occurring on the first day of life. Death from hepatic micronodular cirrhosis occurs by 3 months of age. Liver mtDNA levels are less than 10% of normal, but there are no muscle abnormalities. Naviaux *et al.*[23] recently described juvenile combined muscle and liver mtDNA depletion with levels of 30% in muscle and 25% of control in liver. The patient presented as a toddler with truncal ataxia at 19 months of age followed by recurrent encephalopathic episodes, leading to death at 42 months of age from end-stage liver disease and intractable seizures. This is the clinical phenotype of Alpers' syndrome. Mitochondrial DNA polymerase γ activity was undetectable in liver and muscle mitochondria.

AZT-induced mitochondrial myopathy was shown to be associated with mtDNA depletion in muscle in 1991.[4] These patients experienced progressive painful proximal myopathy with prominent wasting and normal or moderately elevated creatine phosphokinase levels. Patients with this complication tended to be on higher doses of AZT, and all had received long-term treatment. Withdrawal of AZT resulted in resolution of myalgia in as little as 3 weeks with continued improvement in muscle weakness over 6 months.[3] Whilst most patients with AZT toxicity have predominant myopathy, other organ systems can be involved with reports of hepatopathy, anemia, and neutropenia. The clinical picture of AZT toxicity with mtDNA depletion is similar to that seen in genetic myopathic mtDNA depletion syndromes. FIAU toxicity is a more striking multisystem phenomenon with prominent hepatopathy similar to the hepatic forms of genetic mtDNA depletion. Inhibition of mitochondrial DNA polymerase γ is the likely mechanism of toxicity in all nucleoside analogue-induced mitochondrial disease.[5]

Mitochondrial Dysfunction Associated with Fetal Nucleoside Analogue Exposure

Eight children were reported by Blanche *et al.*[10] with mitochondrial dysfunction following pre- and postnatal nucleoside analogue treatment. Three of these infants had mitochondrial disease phenotypes similar to the genetic defects just described. Two children died following degenerative neurological disease at 13 and 11 months of age. The first patient had the phenotype of Leigh's syndrome and the second, intractable seizures with spastic quadriparesis and mental retardation. Both children were treated with AZT and 3TC from 32 weeks of gestation until 5 weeks postpartum; the second patient received didanosine in addition. Two other infants received a combination of AZT and 3TC antenatally and postnatally. Both of these infants had lactic acidosis during treatment which persisted on follow-up. One of these infants had an apneic episode at 4 months of age, but both were normal at follow-up. Four other infants received AZT treatment alone starting 14–32 weeks antenatally and continuing 2–6 weeks postnatally. One of these patients had a seizure with fever of 8 months of age, and at 15 months was found to have hypertrophic cardiomyopathy, which later resolved. One other had seizures, quadriparesis, and mental retardation, and the remaining AZT-treated infant was symptom-free throughout. All patients were reported to have abnormal electron transport complex activities based on activity ratio measurements. The patient with Leigh's syndrome had profound complex I deficiency.

We identified a child managed at the University of California, San Diego. This 5 1/2-year-old boy has normal growth with type 1 diabetes and hypothyroidism. He has mild mental retardation, talks in phrases and short sentences, has occasional absence seizures, and shows mild signs of spastic diplegia. He was the product of a term cesarean section for failure to progress. The HIV-positive mother admitted amphetamine use during pregnancy. She was treated with AZT from 24 weeks of gestation, and AZT treatment was continued in the infant until 6 weeks of age. He has remained persistently HIV negative. Presentation was at 6 weeks of age with failure to thrive and insulin-dependent diabetes. Infantile spasms began at 5 months of age. Biochemical testing showed hyperglycemia with hypothyroidism and plasma lactates that have ranged from 1.3–3.6 mM with a normal pyruvate of 0.08 mM. Plasma alanine was elevated at 795 µM (normal range 136–464 µM). Lumbar puncture and muscle biopsy were performed at 4 years 9 months of age. The CSF was normal with a lactate of 1.2 mM, pyruvate 0.04 mM, and a protein of 21 mg/dl. The quadriceps muscle biopsy showed slightly heavy lipid staining and occasional COX negative fibers. Muscle electron microscopy was normal. Measurements of complex I, complex II/III, complex IV, and citrate synthetase in isolated muscle mitochondria were normal. Southern blotting deletion analysis was normal, and a search for the common MELAS, MERRF, and NARP mutations was negative.

Comparison of Inherited and Nucleoside Analogue-Associated Mitochondrial Disease Phenotypes

Reports of nucleoside analogue toxicity in infants could be compared to the phenotypes of the proven mitochondrial disease patients just described. Four of the French cases had persistent lactic acidemia. Of these patients, cases 1, 3, and 7[10] had the most convincing features of mitochondrial disease. Our patient with multiorgan system disease, mild elevation of alanine, and intermittent lactate elevation has suggestive mitochondrial disease features, but cannot be considered a proven case. The CSF and muscle biopsy were obtained at the age of 4 1/2 years, long after biochemical defects from acute exposure would be expected to have disappeared. Detailed biochemical evaluation should be performed as soon after nucleoside analogue treatment as possible.

Another important factor in evaluating reports of mitochondrial toxicity is the background incidence of mitochondrial disease. The total number of nucleoside analogue mother/infant pairs treated in the report by Blanche[10] was 1,754. If the background incidence of metabolic disorders is considered, 1 or 2 cases at most might be expected in such a small sample. The real incidence of genetic mitochondrial disease is unknown, but conservative estimates suggest a prevalence of 1 in 3,000 to 1 in 4,000 in the general population. In Finland, the overall incidence of the A3243G mutation is calculated as 16.3/100,000 in the adult population.[24] Fatty acid oxidation defects alone have a prevalence of 1 in 5,000 to 1 in 10,000 in the general population, medium chain acyl-CoA dehydrogenase deficiency being the most common. Given these estimates of genetic metabolic disease, of which mitochondrial disease is probably the most common, it is disturbing that initial, largely retrospective surveys of perinatally nucleoside analogue-treated infants have failed to detect any metabolic diseases. These studies include the Pediatric Aids Clinical Trials Group, the Women and Infants Transmission Study Group, and the Perinatal Aids Collaborative Transmission Study Group. In total, these studies have followed in excess of 20,000 treated infants. Several cases of genetic disease should have been identified in such a large population, suggesting the possibility of ascertainment bias.

DIAGNOSIS AND EVALUATION OF MITOCHONDRIAL DISEASE

Evaluation of a typical patient presenting with possible mitochondrial disease requires a detailed history, family history, clinical examination, and biochemical studies. A history of chronic and often relapsing multisystem disease should be sought. The examination should confirm the presence of multisystem disease, and organ-specific diagnostic studies such as EKG and echocardiography, EEG and brain MRI scan, nerve conduction studies, and brain stem-evoked responses may be needed. The search for biochemical evidence of mitochondrial failure includes studies of blood and CSF lactate, plasma amino acids, and urine quantitative organic acids. Special diagnostic tests include skin biopsy for fibroblast cultures and biochemistry and muscle biopsy for histochemistry and electronmicroscopy. The study of freshly isolated muscle mitochondria allows the best assessment of electron transport activities. Mitochondrial DNA studies for point mutation analysis and Southern blotting for deletions are best performed on muscle, but can also be studied in blood. Carbohydrate loading tests with glucose and fructose may be needed to show an abnormal lactate response. Patients with mitochondrial disease may be prone to hypoglycemia, and an inpatient fasting study will detect this as well as providing evidence of fatty acid oxidation disorders.

Fetal Nucleoside Analogue Exposure: Predictions

A hypothesis of the likely effects of fetal exposure to nucleoside analogues can be developed, assuming the following facts:

1. Toxicity of nucleoside analogues is due to inhibition of mtDNA synthesis, resulting in depletion.

2. Fetal tissue growth requires rapid mtDNA synthesis.

3. Symptoms of mitochondrial dysfunction occur when levels of mtDNA fall to less than 30% of normal, and this requires chronic treatment.

4. Recovery of mtDNA levels and biochemical abnormalities will occur, following cessation of exposure.

5. Combination nucleoside analogue use may potentiate mitochondrial toxicity.

Treatment Patterns

FIGURE 5 illustrates three possible protocols for nucleoside analogue administration during pregnancy.

Exposure Pattern 1

Whole pregnancy exposure exposes the developing fetus to the longest duration of potential toxicity. Arrest of mtDNA synthesis would likely occur earlier in the pregnancy than with later pregnancy treatment protocols. Given the need for rapid mtDNA synthesis in the developing fetus, a 30% control level of depletion might be reached well before the beginning of the third trimester. This is an important time for organogenesis, particularly for nervous system development. A susceptible fetus might develop an embryopathy with multiorgan disease and signs of mtDNA depletion at birth. With severe disease, spontaneous abortion might occur.

Exposure Pattern 2

Early gestation treatment only might be predicted to damage a susceptible fetus if mtDNA levels fall to less than 30% of normal during treatment. Despite the high mtDNA synthesis requirement in the fetus, levels may not fall low enough, with treatment periods of less than 4.5 months, to reach a threshold for oxidative phosphorylation impairment. Predictably, the shorter the treatment period, the less the likelihood of toxicity. Biochemical features of mtDNA depletion likely will have re-

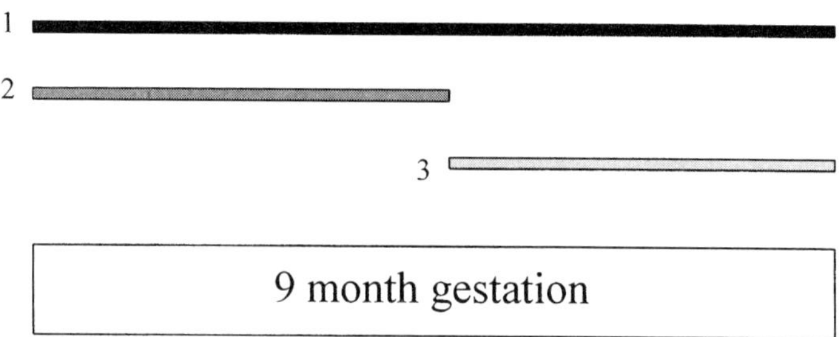

FIGURE 5. Patterns of nucleoside analogue treatment in pregnancy.

TABLE 2. Classification of mitochondrial DNA diseases

mtDNA Defect	Inheritance	Diseases
Protein missense mutation	Maternal or de novo mutation	Leber's hereditary optic atrophy (LHON); dystonia; neurogenic atrophy, ataxia, retinitis pigmentosa (NARP); Leigh's syndrome
Rearrangements; Deletions Duplications	Sporadic generally; multiple deletions may be dominant or recessive	Kearns-Sayre syndrome; Pearson syndrome; Chronic progressive external opthalmoplegia (cpeo); myopathy; cardiomyopathy
tRNA point mutation	Maternal or de novo mutation	MELAS; myoclonic epilepsy with ragged-red fibers (MERRF); CPEO; myopathy; cardiomyopathy; Leigh's syndrome; diabetes and deafness
rRNA point mutation	Maternal or de novo mutation	Aminoglycoside induced deafness; sensorineural deafness
Depletion	Recessive or acquired	Myopathy; cardiomyopathy; Alpers' Syndrome; hepatopathy; pancreatitis; encephalopathy; peripheral neuropathy

solved by the end of gestation. Thus, treatment early in the course of pregnancy might be predicted to have no biochemical markers at birth and may have no discernible effect on the fetus at all, unless the drugs used (like FIAU) are very toxic.

Exposure Pattern 3

Late gestation treatment only might be predicted to arrest mtDNA synthesis in a susceptible fetus after the period of most rapid organogenesis (except for the CNS) is completed. Symptomatic depletion (<30%) may or may not be present depending on the duration of treatment and susceptibility of the infant. Signs of mitochondrial disease may or may not be present at birth.

FUTURE DIRECTIONS

The use of nucleoside analogue treatment in pregnancy to protect the fetus has been a major advance in HIV management. However, given the known toxicity of chronic nucleoside analogue treatment in adults, the possibility of mitochondrial disease in infants exposed prenatally is significant. Assuming that the etiology is similar to that demonstrated in adult humans, animal models, and cell culture mtDNA depletion, this is likely to be a temporary phenomenon, biochemical signs of which may disappear within a few weeks. A search should be made to determine if such depletion is seen in nucleoside analogue-treated newborns. If present, identification of this problem will allow development of optimal treatment regimens to minimize the effect. Changes might be made in drug selection, dosage, drug combinations, and timing of treatment. Studies of mitochondrial toxicity in newborns might include: (1) lactic acid levels, drawn in an optimal manner several days after birth, when acute acidosis related to labor and delivery has resolved; (2) a search for signs of organ damage secondary to mitochondrial disease, which might include myopathy, cardiomyopathy, hepatopathy, and nephropathy as well as multiple CNS symptoms; and (3) measurements of mtDNA content carried out on accessible tissue such as fetal placenta, cord, or cord blood.

ACKNOWLEDGMENTS

This work was supported by the University of California San Diego Mitochondrial and Metabolic Disease Center and by grants from The Kelsey Wright Foundation, The Lennox Foundation, and the General Clinical Research Centers Program, MO1 RR00827, of the National Center for Research Resources, National Institutes of Health.

REFERENCES

1. LANGSTON, J.W. & P. BALLARD. 1983. Chronic parkinsonism in humans due to a product of meperidine-analog synthesis. Science **219:** 979–980.
2. SINGER, T.P., R.R. RAMSAY, K. MCKEOWN *et al.* 1988. Mechanism of the neurotoxicity of 1-methyl-4-phenylpyridinium (MPP+), the toxic bioactivation product of 1-methyl-4-phenyl-1,2, 3,6-tetrahydropyridine (MPTP). Toxicology **49:** 17–23.
3. MHIRI, C., M. BAUDRIMONT, G. BONNE *et al.* 1991. Zidovudine myopathy: a distinctive disorder associated with mitochondrial dysfunction. Ann. Neurol. **29:** 606–614.
4. ARNAUDO, E., M. DALAKAS, S. SHANSKE *et al.* 1991. Depletion of muscle mitochondrial DNA in AIDS patients with zidovudine-induced myopathy. Lancet **337:** 508–510.
5. LEWIS, W. & M.C. DALAKAS. 1995. Mitochondrial toxicity of antiviral drugs. Nat. Med. **1:** 417–422.
6. MCKENZIE, R., M.W. FRIED, R. SALLIE *et al.* 1995. Hepatic failure and lactic acidosis due to fialuridine FIAU, an investigational nucleoside analogue for chronic hepatitis B [see comments]. N. Engl. J. Med. **333:** 1099–1105.
7. CUI, L., S. YOON, R.F. SCHINAZI & J.P. SOMMADOSSI. 1995. Cellular and molecular events leading to mitochondrial toxicity of 1-(2-deoxy-2-fluoro-1-beta-D-arabino-furanosyl)-5-iodouracil in human liver cells. J. Clin. Invest. **95:** 555–563.
8. LEWIS, W., E.S. LEVINE, B. GRINIUVIENE *et al.* 1996. Fialuridine and its metabolites inhibit DNA polymerase gamma at sites of multiple adjacent analog incorporation, decrease mtDNA abundance, and cause mitochondrial structural defects in cultured hepatoblasts. Proc. Natl. Acad. Sci. USA **93:** 3592–3597.
9. LEWIS, W., B. GRINIUVIENE, K.O. TANKERSLEY *et al.* 1997. Depletion of mitochondrial DNA, destruction of mitochondria, and accumulation of lipid droplets result from fialuridine treatment in woodchucks (*Marmota monax*). Lab. Invest. **76:** 77–87.
10. BLANCHE, S., M. TARDIEU, P. RUSTIN *et al.* 1999. Persistant mitochondrial dysfunction and perinatal exposure to antiretroviral nucleoside analogues. Lancet **354:** 1084–1089.
11. GREEN, D.R. & J.C. REED. 1998. Mitochondria and apoptosis. Science **281:** 1309–1312.
12. VIONNET, N., P. PASSA & P. FROGUEL. 1993. Prevalence of mitochondrial gene mutations in families with diabetes mellitus. Lancet (letter 342) : 1429–1430.
13. GERBITZ, K.-D., J.M.W. VAN DEN OUWELAND, J.A. MAASSEN & M. JAKSCH. 1995. Mitochondrial diabetes mellitus: a review. BBA **1271:** 253–260.
14. TIRANTI, V., K. HOERTNAGEL, R. CARROZZO *et al.* 1998. Mutations of SURF-1 in Leigh disease associated with cytochrome c oxidase deficiency [see comments]. Am. J. Hum. Genet. **63:** 1609–1621.
15. TAYLOR, R.W., M.A. BIRCH-MACHIN, J. SCHAEFER *et al.* 1996. Deficiency of complex II of the mitochondrial respiratory chain in late-onset optic atrophy and ataxia. Ann. Neurol. **39:** 224–232.

16. SHOFFNER, J.M., M.D. BROWN, C. STUGARD *et al.* 1995. Leber's hereditary optic neuropathy plus dystonia is caused by a mitochondrial DNA point mutation. Ann. Neurol. **38:** 163–169.
17. SANTORELLI, F.M., S.C. MAK & M.E.A. SCHAHAWI. 1996. Maternally inherited cardiomyopathy and hearing loss associated with a novel point mutation in the mitochondrial tRNA Lys gene (G8363A). Am. J. Hum. Genet. **58:** 933–939.
18. HAAS, R.H, W.D. GRAF, H.G. GAO *et al.* 1999. Autism and Leigh's Syndrome – Widely Differing Phenotypes in Two Siblings with the mtDNA tRNA [lys] G8363A Mutation. Presented at the Society for Inherited Metabolic Disorders, Lake Lanier, Georgia, March 13, 1999.
19. HOLT, I.J., A.E. HARDING & J.A. MORGAN-HUGHES. 1988. Deletions of muscle mitochondrial DNA in patients with mitochondrial myopathies. Nature **331:** 717–719.
20. SMITH, M.L., X.Y. HUA, D.L. MARSDEN *et al.* 1997. Diabetes and mitochondrial encephalomyopathy with lactic acidosis and stroke-like episodes (MELAS): radiolabeled polymerase chain reaction is necessary for accurate detection of low percentages of mutation. J. Clin. Endocrinol. Metab. **82:** 2826–2831.
21. VAN DEN OUWELAND, J.M.W., H.H.P.J. LEMKES, R.C. TREMBATH *et al.* 1994. Maternally Inherited Diabetes and Deafness Is a Distinct Subtype of Diabetes and Associates With a Single Point Mutation in the Mitochondrial tRNA Leu(UUR) Gene. Diabet. **43:** 746–751.
22. SUE, C.M., L.J. LIPSETT, D.S. CRIMMINS *et al.* 1998. Cochlear origin of hearing loss in MELAS syndrome. Ann. Neurol. **43:** 350–359.
23. NAVIAUX, R.K., W.L. NYHAN, B.A. BARSHOP *et al.* 1999. Mitochondrial DNA polymerase gamma deficiency and mtDNA depletion in a child with Alpers' syndrome. Ann. Neurol. **45:** 54–58.
24. MAJAMAA, K., J.S. MOILANEN, S. UIMONEN *et al.* 1998. Epidemiology of A3243G, the mutation for mitochondrial encephalomyopathy, lactic acidosis, and strokelike episodes: prevalence of the mutation in an adult population. Am. J. Hum. Genet. **63:** 447–454.

Incorporation of Zidovudine into Cord Blood DNA of Infants and Peripheral Blood DNA of Their HIV-1–Positive Mothers

OFELIA A. OLIVERO,[a] GENE M. SHEARER,[a] CLAIRE A. CHOUGNET,[a] ANDREA A.S. KOVACS,[b] ROBIN BAKER,[c] ALICE M. STEK,[b] MARGARET M. KHOURY,[b] AND MIRIAM C. POIRIER[a,d]

[a] *Division of Basic Sciences, National Cancer Institute, National Institutes of Health, 37 Convent Drive MSC 4255, Bethesda, Maryland 20892-4255, USA*

[b] *Comprehensive Maternal-Child HIV Management and Research Center, USC School of Medicine, 1640 Marengo St., Los Angeles, California 90033, USA*

[c] *Department of Neonatology, Fairfax Hospital, Falls Church, Virginia 22046, USA*

ABSTRACT: The nucleoside analogue 3′-azido-3′-deoxythymidine (AZT) is a weak carcinogen in adult female mice and a moderately strong carcinogen in the offspring of female mice given the drug during gestation. In addition, incorporation of AZT into DNA was observed in multiple organs of transplacentally exposed newborn mice. Here we investigate the incorporation of AZT into peripheral leukocyte DNA of HIV-1–positive adult pregnant women given AZT for variable times during gestation and cord blood of infants exposed to AZT *in utero*. The length of treatment varied between 10 days and 9 months. High molecular weight DNA was extracted from maternal peripheral blood mononuclear cells (PBMC) and infant cord blood. A specific AZT-DNA radioimmunoassay was used to determine the amount of AZT incorporated into leukocyte DNA. Incorporation of AZT into DNA ranged up to 183.3 and 344.5 molecules of AZT/10^6 nucleotides in the mothers and infants, respectively, and was detected in about 70% of samples. Therefore, AZT-induced mutagenic events are possible in the majority of adults and infants. No correlation was found between level of incorporation and length of AZT treatment, suggesting that the differences observed among the individuals arise from variability in AZT metabolism. These data support previous observations that a high degree of interindividual variability in AZT phosphorylation occurs in primates.

INTRODUCTION

Zidovudine (3′-azido-3′-deoxythymidine, AZT), the first nucleoside analogue approved by the Food and Drug Administration for the therapy of acquired immunodeficiency syndrome (AIDS), is carcinogenic in both adult mice[1,2] and mice exposed to AZT *in utero*.[3,4] In animal and cell culture models, AZT is clastogenic.[5–7] AZT-induced skin tumors have mutagenic H-*ras* activation.[8] AZT-induced HPRT and TK6 mutagenesis has been observed.[9–11] Incorporation of AZT into DNA has been

[d] Address for correspondence: National Cancer Institute, Bldg. 37 Rm. 2A03 NIH, 37 Convent Dr., MSC-4255, Bethesda, MD 20892-4255. Voice: 301-402-1835; fax: 301-402-8230. poirierm@exchange.NIH.gov

demonstrated in multiple cell culture and animal model systems.[3,5,12,13] Offspring of pregnant mice given transplacental AZT exposure at tumorigenic doses and examined at birth were shown to have AZT incorporated into the DNA of multiple organs, some of which were targets for tumorigenicity.[3] Furthermore, AZT-DNA incorporation was observed in nuclear and mitochondrial DNA of brain, lung, liver, kidney, heart, and placenta from fetuses of *Erythrocebus patas* monkeys given ~20% of the human daily dose for the last half of gestation.[3]

In HIV-1–positive pregnant women, administration of AZT during weeks 14–38 of pregnancy reduces maternal-fetal virus transmission approximately three-fold.[14,15] However, studies in monkeys and mice suggest that the human fetus may also sustain AZT-induced DNA damage, which may result in the induction of mutations. We show here that AZT incorporates into peripheral leukocyte DNA of pregnant women receiving AZT therapy and into cord blood leukocyte DNA of infants receiving the drug *in utero*.

MATERIALS AND METHODS

Blood Samples: Source and Processing

Peripheral blood and cord blood samples were obtained from mother-infant pairs at deliveries conducted at the Comprehensive Maternal-Child HIV Management and Research Center, USC, Los Angeles, California. HIV-1–positive patients were treated, not as part of a formal clinical protocol, but using the CDC-recommended AZT treatment comprising 600 mg AZT given in 3 doses daily for the last 14–38 weeks of pregnancy, and infusion of 1 mg AZT/kg body weight/hour (~3 times higher than the daily dose) during labor and delivery. As control for the AZT-exposed infants, cord bloods were obtained from normal pregnancies with no AZT exposure, at Fairfax Hospital, Falls Church, Virginia. Peripheral blood mononuclear cells (PBMC), prepared from all cord blood leukocytes, were separated from whole blood on lymphocyte preparation medium (Lymphoprep, Organon Teknika, Rockville, MD).

DNA Extraction

DNA was isolated following the procedure of Flamm *et al.*[16] To prepare nuclei, PBMC cells were suspended in lysing solution pelleted by centrifugation, suspended in washing solution, and again centrifuged. DNA was prepared from nuclei by $CsCl_2$ buoyant density gradient centrifugation[15] and recovered by fractionation. DNA was dialyzed against water and the concentration determined by A_{260}. Concentrations were adjusted with deionized water to 30 μg DNA/ml.

Quantitation of AZT-DNA Incorporation by AZT Radioimmunoassay

DNA samples were sonicated for 30 seconds and boiled for 5 minutes. Aliquots of DNA were subsequently assayed by competitive anti-AZT radioimmunoassay, as previously described,[3] using a polyclonal anti-AZT antibody (Sigma, St Louis, MO). Briefly, the anti-AZT antibody, reconstituted and diluted 1:7500 in 30 ml of 10 mM TRIS buffer, pH 8.0, was incubated with either standard AZT plus 3 μg of sonicated and boiled carrier calf thymus DNA (Sigma), or 3 μg of sample DNA from

AZT-exposed patients or unexposed patients, for 90 minutes at 37°C in 10 mM TRIS buffer, pH 8.0. One hundred microliters, containing approximately 20,0000 cpm, of [^{3}H]AZT tracer (20 Ci/mmol, Moravek Biochemicals, Mountain View, CA) were added per tube together with 100 µl of the secondary antibody, goat anti-rabbit immunoglobulin G (Sigma) reconstituted in 12 ml of 10 mM TRIS buffer, pH 8.0. The mixture was incubated for 25 minutes at 4°C, and tubes were centrifuged at 2,000 × g for 15 minutes at 4°C. The resulting supernatant was decanted, and the pellets were dissolved in 100 mM NaOH and counted in a liquid scintillation counter. The concentration of standard AZT required to inhibit antibody binding by 50% was 490.0 ± 183.3 fmol AZT (mean ± SD, $n = 20$). The lower limit of detection was 15.2 ± 8.4 molecules AZT/10^6 nucleotides (mean ± SD, $n = 20$). Unless otherwise indicated, each sample was assayed in three separate radioimmunoassays.

RESULTS

Samples of peripheral blood obtained at delivery from 12 HIV-1–positive women given a dose of 600 mg AZT daily during the last 10 days to 9 months of pregnancy exhibited variable values for AZT-DNA incorporation. Four samples were nondetectable, and positive samples ranged from 35.5 to 214.9 AZT molecules/10^6 nucleotides (FIG. 1). For all 12 AZT-treated women, the mean (± SD) AZT-DNA was 79.3 ± 20.3 molecules AZT/10^6 nucleotides. A similar analysis was performed using DNA from cord blood leukocytes obtained at delivery from 22 infants of HIV-1–positive women who were administered 600 mg AZT daily for the last 10 days through 9 months of pregnancy. Cord blood samples from 12 unexposed infants, 11 of HIV-

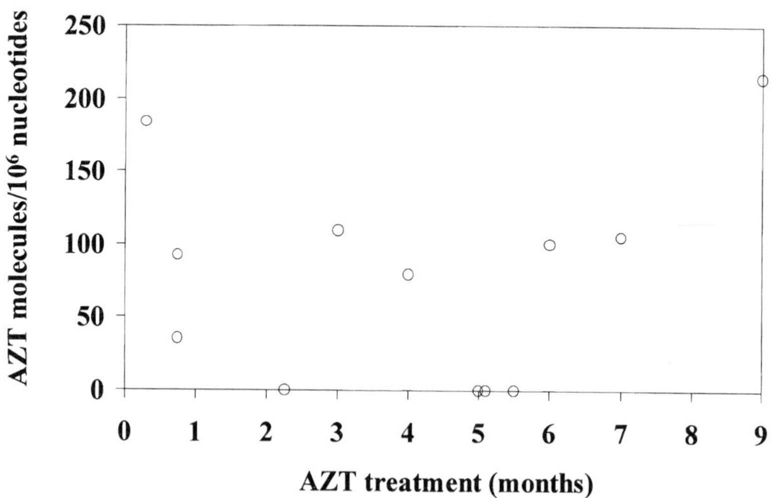

FIGURE 1. Incorporation of AZT (AZT molecules/10^6 nucleotides) into peripheral blood leukocytes of 12 HIV-1–positive mothers who received AZT for variable amounts of time during pregnancy.

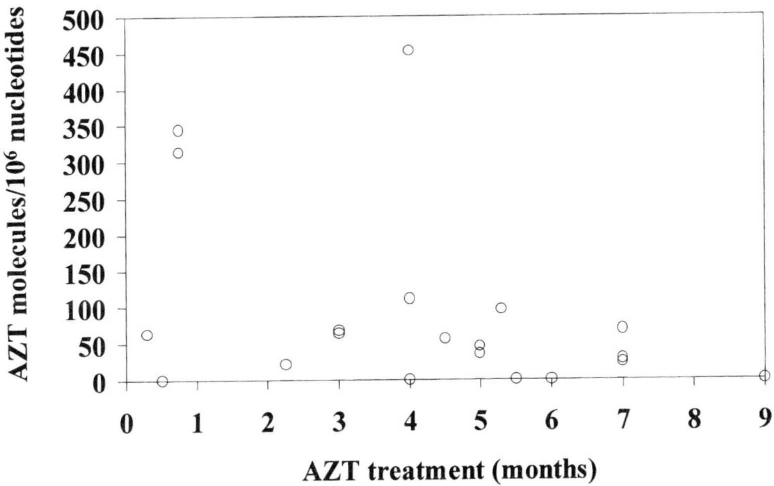

FIGURE 2. Incorporation of AZT (AZT molecules/10^6 nucleotides) into cord blood leukocytes of 22 infants of HIV-positive women who received AZT during pregnancy.

TABLE 1. Incorporation of AZT into maternal and fetal leukocyte of mother–infant pairs DNA

	Molecules of AZT / 10^6 nucleotides	
Time of exposure (mo.)	Mother	Infant
0.3[a]	183.3	22.2
0.75	92.6	344.5
0.75	35.5	313.3
2.25	0	22
3	109.9	68
4	0	0
4.5	0	56.5
5.3	0	95.2
5.5	79.6	0
6	100.4	0
7	105.2	28.7
Mean ± SE	64.2 ± 33.8	86.4 ± 68.3

[a] Mean ± SE of three assays. For calculation of means for each group, the nondetectable samples, designated as "0," were given a value of 7.6 molecules AZT/10^6 nucleotides, the half value between zero and the limit of detection.

1–negative mothers and 1 of an HIV-1–positive mother, were used as untreated controls. For the 22 AZT-exposed infants, the range of AZT incorporation into DNA of the 15 positive samples was 21.8–451.8 molecules AZT/10^6 nucleotides (FIG. 2). No apparent correlation was observed between AZT-DNA incorporation levels and duration of AZT administration during pregnancy (TABLE 1). In addition, TABLE 1 shows that there was no correlation between maternal-fetal levels of AZT-DNA incorporation in each of the 11 mother-infant pairs used for the comparison. Only one pair showed negative values for both members, whereas positive infants with negative mothers and negative infants with positive mothers were found. However, the average number of molecules of $AZT/10^6$ nucleotides ($\pm$ SE) for the 11 infants was 86.4 $\pm$ 68.3, which was not significantly different from the value of 64.2 $\pm$ 33.8 observed for their mothers (TABLE 1).

DISCUSSION

Here we demonstrate that AZT is incorporated into DNA of pregnant women and their infants after therapeutic exposure. A high degree of variability in the level of incorporation was observed. This could be the result of many influences, including metabolic differences in both mother and infant. Although the duration of exposure was different in the 11 mother-infant pairs studied, the daily AZT dose was the same. The extent of AZT infusion during labor and delivery may have been variable, and there might have been individual differences in compliance that influenced AZT-DNA formation. High interindividual variablility in AZT plasma peak levels has been reported in AIDS patients given therapeutic doses.[17] Furthermore, a lack of correlation between AZT pharmacokinetics in the plasma of 41 patients, and clinical effect, measured by CD4 count and HIV p24 antigen levels, has been observed.[18]

Variability in the major metabolic pathways, which results in the formation of AZT-glucuronide (AZTG) and 3'-amino-3'-deoxythymidine (AMT),[17,19] will influence the availability of AZT to become phosphorylated and incorporated into DNA. Theoretically the extent of DNA damage, mutagenesis, and potential carcinogenesis are all related to the phosphorylation of the compound, which results in incorporation of the AZT-triphosphate into DNA in place of thymidine. Once AZT is incorporated into a nascent DNA strand, extension of the DNA chain is not possible and replication is terminated. Numerous reports have documented the mutagenesis induced by AZT,[7–9] and a strong correlation between AZT-DNA incorporation and mutations (mainly large deletions) in the HPRT gene and TK gene has been demonstrated in cultured cells.[10,11]

AZT-DNA incorporation has been demonstrated in mice and monkeys[4,5] exposed transplacentally to AZT during the last third or last half of gestation, respectively. Offspring of pregnant CD-1 mice exposed to AZT during the last week of gestation developed tumors in multiple organs at 1 and 2 years after the initial exposure.[4,5] Besides being a moderately strong transplacental carcinogen in mice, AZT is a weak carcinogen in adult rats and mice exposed for a lifetime.[1,2] Therefore, the finding that fetal AZT-DNA formation can be associated with tumor formation in a mouse transplacental model and the observation that transplacentally exposed fetal monkeys incorporate AZT into the DNA of multiple organs suggest that human infants might also experience genotoxic consequences as a result of transplacental AZT exposure. In the light of this information, long-term followup of AZT-exposed children would appear reasonable.

ACKNOWLEDGMENTS

Our appreciation is extended to Wing Henry Quan and Sara Pietras for technical support.

REFERENCES

1. AYERS, K.M., D. CLIVE, W.E. TUCKER *et al.* 1996. Nonclinical toxicology studies with zidovudine: genetic toxicity tests and carcinogenicity bioassays in mice and rats. Fundam. Appl. Toxicol. **32:** 148–158.
2. NTP. 1996. Toxicology and Carcinogenesis Studies of AZT. National Toxicology Program, Research Triangle Park, NC.
3. OLIVERO, O.A., L.M. ANDERSON, B.A. DIWAN *et al.* 1997. Transplacental effects of 3′-azido-2′,3′-dideoxythymidine (AZT): tumorigenicity in mice and genotoxicity in mice and monkeys. J. Natl. Cancer Inst. **89:** 1602–1608.
4. DIWAN, B.A., C.W. RIGGS, D. LOGSDON *et al.* 1999. Multiorgan transplacental and neonatal carcinogenicity of 3′-azido-3′-deoxythymidine in mice. Toxicol. Appl. Pharmacol. **15:** 82–99.
5. OLIVERO, O.A., F.A. BELAND, N.F. FULLERTON *et al.* 1994. Vaginal epithelial DNA damage and expression of preneoplastic markers in mice during chronic dosing with tumorigenic levels of 3′-azido-2′,3′-dideoxythymidine (AZT). Cancer Res. **54:** 6235–6242.
6. DERTINGER, S.D., D.K. TOROUS & K.R. TOMETSKO. 1996. Induction of micronuclei by low doses of azidothymidine (AZT). Mutat. Res. **368:** 301–307.
7. GONZALEZ, C.M. & I. LARRIPA. 1994. Genotoxicity of azidothymidine (AZT) in *in vitro* systems. Mutat. Res. **321:** 113–118.
8. ZHANG, Z., B.A. DIWAN, L.M. ANDERSON *et al.* 1998. Skin tumorigenesis and K-ras and H-ras mutations in tumors from adult mice exposed *in utero* to 3′-azido-2′,3′-dideoxythymidine (AZT). Mol. Carcinog. **23:** 45–51.
9. GRDINA D.J., P. DALE & R. WEICHSELBAUM. 1992. Protection against AZT-induced mutagenesis at the HGPRT locus in a human cell line by WR-151326. Int. J. Radiation Oncol. Biol. Phys. **22:** 813–815.
10. SUSSMAN, H.E., O.A. OLIVERO, S.M. PIETRAS *et al.* 1999. Genotoxicity of 3′-azido-3′-deoxythymidine (AZT) in the human lymphoblastoid cell line, TK6: relationship between DNA incorporation, mutant frequency, and spectrum of deletions in HPRT. Mutat. Res. **429:** 249–259.
11. MENG, Q., T. SU, O.A. OLIVERO *et al.* 2000. Relationships between DNA incorporation, mutant frequency, and loss of heterozygosity at the *TK* locus in Human Lymphoblastoid cells exposed to 3′-azido-3′deoxythymidine (AZT). Toxicol. Sci. **54:** 322–329.
12. SOMMADOSSI, J.P., R. CARLISLE & Z. ZHOU. 1989. Cellular pharmacology of 3′-azido-3′-deoxythymidine with evidence of incorporation into DNA of human bone marrow cells. Mol. Pharmacol. **36:** 9–14.
13. OLIVERO, O.A., F.A. BELAND & M.C. POIRIER. 1994. Immunofluorescent localization and quantitation of 3′-azido-2′, 3′-dideoxythymidine (AZT) incorporated into chromosomal DNA of human, hamster and mouse cell lines. Int. J. Oncol. **4:** 49–54.
14. CONNOR, E.M., R.S. SPERLING, R. GELBER *et al.* 1994. Reduction of maternal-infant transmission of human immunodeficiency virus type 1 with zidovudine treatment. Pediatric AIDS Clinical Trials Group Protocol 076 Study Group. N. Engl. J. Med. **331:** 1173–1180.
15. SPERLING, R.S., D.E. SHAPIRO, R.W. COOMBS *et al.* 1996. Maternal viral load, zidovudine treatment, and the risk of transmission of human immunodeficiency virus type 1 from mother to infant. Pediatric AIDS Clinical Trials Group Protocol 076 Study Group. N. Engl. J. Med. **335:** 1621–1629.
16. FLAMM, W.G., M.L. BIRNSTIEL & P.M.B. WALKER. 1967. Preparation and fractionation and isolation of single strands of DNA by ultracentrifugation in fixed-angle rotors. *In*

Subcellular Components: Preparation and Fractionation. G.D. Birnie & S.M. Fox, Eds. :126–154. London.
17. ACOSTA, E.P., L.M. PAGE & C.V. FLETCHER. 1996. Clinical pharmacokinetics of zidovudine. An update. Clin. Pharmacokinet. **30:** 251–262.
18. STRETCHER, B.N. 1995. Pharmacokinetic optimization of antiretroviral therapy in patients with HIV infection. Clin. Pharmacokinet. **29:** 46–65.
19. VEAL, G.J. & D.J. BACK. 1995. Metabolism of zidovudine. Gen. Pharmacol. **26:** 1469–1475.
20. OLIVERO, O.A, M.S. SHEARER, C.A. CHOUGNET *et al.* 1999. Incorporation of Zidovudine into peripheral blood DNA of HIV-1 positive adults, cord blood DNA of infants and peripheral blood DNA of their HIV-1 positive mothers. AIDS **13:** 919–925.
21. POIRIER, M.C., T.A. PATTERSON, W. SLIKKER, JR. & O.A. OLIVERO. 1999. Incorporation of 3′-azido-3′-deoxythymidine (AZT) into fetal DNA, and fetal tissue distribution of drug, after infusion of pregnant late-term rhesus macaques with a human-equivalent AZT dose. J. AIDS & Human Retrovirol. **22:** 477–483.

Fetal Patas Monkeys Sustain Mitochondrial Toxicity As a Result of *in Utero* Zidovudine Exposure

MARIANA GERSCHENSON[a] AND MIRIAM C. POIRIER

Division of Basic Sciences, National Cancer Institute, National Institutes of Health, 9000 Rockville Pike, Bethesda, Maryland 20892–4255, USA

ABSTRACT: Mitochondrial toxicity was examined in near-term fetuses of pregnant *Erythrocebus patas* monkeys given human equivalent doses of 3'-azido-3'deoxythymidine (AZT) during the second half of gestation. Pregnant monkeys were dosed daily with 10 or 40 mg AZT, equivalent to about 21% and 86% of the daily AZT dose (500 mg) given to HIV-1-positive pregnant women to prevent maternal-fetal virus transmission. The fetal tissues examined include heart and skeletal muscle, which have high energy requirements, and placenta, which is less dependent on mitochondrial integrity. Slot blot quantitation of mitochondrial DNA (mtDNA) levels showed dose-dependent depletion in heart, skeletal muscle, and placenta from AZT-exposed fetuses compared to unexposed controls. Furthermore, mtDNA degradation, observed by Southern blot analysis, appeared more extensive in AZT-exposed tissues compared to unexposed controls. Mitochondrial functional integrity, as determined by oxidative phosphorylation (OXPHOS) enzyme assays, was also examined in heart, skeletal muscle, and placenta. All three tissues showed strong dose-related decreases in Complex I. In placenta, dose-related increases for Complexes II and IV and a decrease for Complex III were observed. Dose-related increases for Complexes II and IV observed in heart and skeletal muscle have been reported.[1] The increase in Complex IV (cytochrome *c* oxidase) activity in heart and skeletal muscle tissue from patas fetuses exposed to 40 mg AZT/day has been confirmed here by histochemical staining. Overall, data demonstrate that mitochondrial toxicity, evidenced by depletion in mtDNA and OXPHOS enzyme abnormalities, is manifested similarly in heart, skeletal muscle, and placenta of AZT-exposed monkey fetuses. It is therefore possible that the placenta, which is a readily accessible tissue, might be an indicator of potential mitochondrial toxicity in human pregnancies involving nucleoside analog drug exposure.

INTRODUCTION

Treatment with the nucleoside analog drug 3'azido-3'deoxythymidine (AZT) is recommended for pregnant HIV-1–infected women to reduce vertical viral transmission to the fetus.[2] Children exposed *in utero* to AZT do not appear to sustain acute toxicity at birth; however, the long-term effects of this exposure are unclear. Mitochondrial toxicities have been documented in HIV-1–postive adults given long-term (2–12 months) AZT treatment.

[a]Address for correspondence: Dr. Miriam Poirier, National Cancer Institute, 37 Convent Drive, Rm 2A05, NIH, Bethesda, MD 20892-4255. Voice: 301-402-1835; fax: 301-402-8230. poirierm@exchange.nih.gov

Clinical manifestations, which improve when the drug is discontinued, include cardiac and skeletal muscle myopathies as well as lactic acidosis with hepatic steatosis.[3–8] These changes can be documented by elevated serum lactate and creatine kinase levels and by abnormal echocardiogram.[3,7,9] Molecular manifestations of nucleoside analog drug-induced mitochondrial toxicity include a decrease in the quantity of mitochondrial DNA (mtDNA),[10,11] alterations in mitochondrial OXPHOS enzyme activities,[12,13] and visible changes in mitochondrial morphology.[8,12–16]

Recent reports have raised concern that mitochondrial toxicities may occur in children exposed to AZT and other nucleoside analog drugs. Domanski *et al.*[17] demonstrated an 8.4-fold greater odds of abnormal echocardiograms in children treated with AZT compared to untreated children. In addition, several HIV-1–positive children aged 10-18, who received AZT therapy an average of 5.3 years, have presented with abnormal echocardiograms, which improved after drug discontinuation.[18] However, the presence of the HIV-1 infection made it difficult to identify drug-related effects. Recently, Blanche *et al.*[19] reported persistent mitochondrial toxicities in eight HIV-1–negative children, 7 months to 4 years of age, who were exposed *in utero* to either AZT alone or AZT and lamuvidine (3TC) and given one or both drugs for 4–6 weeks after birth. Unfortunately, two children who received the drug combination died at approximately 1 year of age. This may be a chance occurrence or a warning signal of future mitochondrial toxicities in HIV-1–negative children.

In biological systems, mitochondrial toxicity is thought to require AZT phosphorylation to mono-, di-, and triphosphate metabolites and incorporation of the AZT-triphosphate into DNA in the place of thymidine.[5,20,21] AZT incorporation into fetal DNA, as a result of transplacental AZT exposure, has been demonstrated in mice,[22] patas,[22] and rhesus monkeys[23] and newborn humans.[20] Once incorporated, extension of the DNA chain is blocked by the 3'-azido group. Mitochondrial disorders occur both because of chain termination and because the mtDNA replicating enzyme, DNA polymerase-γ, is specifically inhibited by AZT-triphosphate,[21,24] leading to mtDNA depletion.[10,11] Mitochondria constitute the essential source of cellular energy, and mtDNA encodes for 13 polypeptides of oxidative phosphorylation (OXPHOS), 22 transfer RNAs, and 2 ribosomal RNAs necessary for translation of the polypeptides.[25]

The studies described here were designed to examine the fetal mitochondrial consequences of transplacental AZT exposure in tissues with high energy requirements, heart and skeletal muscle, and a tissue less dependent on mitochondria, the placenta. Pregnant patas monkeys were given daily doses of 10 or 40 mg AZT (1.5 or 6.0 mg AZT/kg bw) during the last half of gestation. These doses correspond to 21% and 86% of the daily 500 mg AZT dose given to a 70-kg pregnant woman. In fetuses taken at term, tissues were examined for mtDNA quantity and integrity, mitochondrial OXPHOS enzyme-specific activities, and cytochrome *c* oxidase staining.

METHODS

Monkeys and AZT Exposure

Monkeys were maintained and treated at Bioqual Inc. (Rockville, MD) under conditions approved by the American Association for Accreditation of Laboratory

Animal Care, and treatments were performed in accordance with humane principles for laboratory animal care. Protocols were reviewed by the Animal Care and Use Committee of Bioqual, Inc. Pregnancies were ascertained as described.[26] Pregnant patas monkeys were given 0 ($n = 4$), 10.0 ($n = 3$), or 40 ($n = 3$) mg of AZT (Sigma Chemical Co, St. Louis, MO) per day in a banana, 5 days per week for the last 9.5–10 weeks (final 50%) of a normal 162-day gestation. Daily doses of 10 (1.5 mg/kg) or 40 mg AZT (6 mg/kg) given to the monkeys were about 21% and 86% of the human daily dose, respectively. Cesarean section was performed 24 hours after the last AZT dose, under Telazol and isofluorane anesthesia, on days 153 through 156 of gestation. Mitochondria were isolated immediately from the fetal tissues.

Isolation of Mitochondria

All steps for the isolation of mitochondria were performed at 4°C. Whole heart (3–4 g) or quadricep muscle (3–4 g) were minced using a scalpel blade. Fat and connective tissue were removed. Each tissue was then homogenized for three intervals of 30 seconds in 40 ml of homogenization buffer containing: 210 mM mannitol, 70 mM sucrose, 1 mM EDTA, 20 mM Hepes (pH 7.4), 2 mM dithiothreitol, and 1 mM phenylmethylsulfonyl fluoride using a Polytron tissue processor (Brinkmann Instruments, Westbury, NY). The whole placenta (140–160 g) was cut in pieces and homogenized in Waring commercial blender (Waring, Inc., New Hartford, CT) with 2 liters of homogenization buffer. The tissue homogenate was centrifuged twice in a Beckman centrifuge with a JA-20 rotor at $1,000 \times g$ for 5 minutes to remove cellular debris and nuclei. The mitochondria were collected at $20,000 \times g$ for 20 minutes, gently resuspended in 50–100 µl aliquots in the homogenization buffer, frozen in liquid nitrogen, and stored at −70°C. Mitochondrial protein recovery was consistent in each tissue group regardless of exposure status (data not shown).

Southern and Slot Blot Analyses

MtDNA was isolated from 800 µg of mitochondrial protein. Mitochondria were incubated for 2 hours at 55°C with 0.5% sodium dodecyl sulfate and proteinase K (Roche Molecular Biochemicals, Indianapolis, IN) and then extracted with fresh phenol to minimize oxidative damage and incubated with RNAse for 1 hour at 37°C. The mtDNA was resuspended in 25 µl of 10 mM Tris-EDTA, pH 7.4, and stored at −20°C. Slot blot analysis was performed using 3 µl of mtDNA/slot in a Hoefer Slot blot apparatus (Hoefer Scientific Instruments, San Francisco, CA). Southern blot analysis was performed with 6 µl of mtDNA/well in a 1% agarose gel (FMC Bioproducts, Rockland, ME) and electrophoresed in 1× TBE buffer at 5 V/cm for 3 hours. High stringency hybridizations were performed with nylon membrane filters (Roche Molecular Biochemicals) as previously described.[27] All placental, heart, and skeletal muscle samples were assayed in parallel with known quantities of the patas NADH dehydrogenase subunit 4 (ND4) and tRNA-histidine mtDNA genes.[28] The blots were probed with a 500-bp probe corresponding to the patas ND4 and tRNA-histidine mtDNA genes. The polymerase chain reaction (PCR) primer (Life Technologies, Rockville, MD) sequences were: ND4For: CCT CCT CCA TGC TAT TCT GCT TAG (45-68) and ND4Rev: GCA ATC CTT GCG AGT TTT CTC G (548-527).[28] The reaction parameters were: 94°C for 2 minutes, followed by a two-step amplification of 30 cycles at 94°C for 30 seconds (denaturation) and annealing at 54°C for 3 minutes, with a final extension of 2 minutes at 72°C. The amplification was carried out in 50-μl thin-walled microamp tubes in a 9,600 thermocycler (Perkin Elmer Corporation, Norwalk, CT). The probe was digoxigenin-dUTP labeled by PCR, and chemiluminescence detection was employed (Roche Molecular Biochemicals). Densitometry was performed using Alpha Ease Version 3.24 on an Alpha Imager 2000 (Alpha Innotech Co., San Leandro, CA).

Enzyme and Protein Assays

Specific activities of OXPHOS enzymes Complexes I, II, III, and IV were quantified on a Hewlett Packard diode array spectrophotometer, as previously described.[29] Complex I: NADH-ubiquinone oxidoreductase rotenone sensitive activity was measured by the reduction of decylubiquinone. Complex II: succinate-ubiquinone oxidoreductase activity was measured by the reduction of 2,6-dichlorophenolindophenol (DCPIP) when coupled to Complex II-catalyzed reduction of decylubiquinone. Complex III: ubiquinol: ferricytochrome-c oxidoreductase activity assay monitors the reduction of cytochrome c catalyzed by Complex III in the presence of reduced decylubiquinone. Complex IV: ferrocytochrome-c: oxygen oxidoreductase activity was measured by following the oxidation of reduced cytochrome c. Mitochondrial protein concentrations were measured by the coomassie brilliant blue method using bovine serum albumin as a standard.[30]

Cytochrome c Oxidase Cytochemistry

Heart left ventricle and quadricep muscle were obtained from four untreated fetuses and three fetuses exposed *in utero* to 40 mg AZT/day. Tissues were frozen in isopentane. Cryostat sections, 8 μM thick, were collected on poly (L-lysine)-coated (0.1%) coverslips. Sections were incubated for 1 hour at 37°C in 0.1% 3, 3′-diaminobenzidine (DAB), 0.1% cytochrome c (from horse heart), and 0.2% catalase in 5 mM phosphate buffer, pH 7.4. Sections were rinsed three times with distilled water and mounted on glass slides with warm glycerin gel.[31] (All supplies and chemicals for these experiments were obtained from Sigma Chemical Co.) Cytochrome c oxidase was visualized using the Chromavision Automated Cellular Imaging System (Chromavision Medical Systems, Inc., San Juan Capistrano, CA).

Statistical Analysis

Oxidative phosphorylation enzyme activity assays were measured in triplicate using mitochondria from placenta of each monkey. Results of the OXPHOS enzyme assays expressed as nmol/min/mg were similar and reproducible, and the data are expressed as mean ± SE of three assays. Mean values from the four unexposed monkey fetuses were compared with the mean from the three AZT-exposed fetuses at each dose using a two-tailed Student's *t* test for unpaired variables and a Kruskal-Wallis one-way analysis of variance on ranks (SigmaStat Version 2.0, Jandel Scientific). However, because individual, AZT-exposed monkeys showed considerable variability, mean assay values for each exposed monkey were also compared to the group of four controls by Student's *t* test. MtDNA was quantified densitometrically comparing the average signal strength of each duplicated fetal sample with a standard curve using known amounts of the ND4 probe. Data were compared by Student's *t* test.

RESULTS

MtDNA levels were quantitated by slot blot analysis in fetal monkey heart, skeletal muscle, and placenta to evaluate the effects of AZT exposure (FIG. 1). A dose-dependent decrease of mtDNA was noted in all three tissues. At the 40 mg AZT/day dose, mtDNA levels were decreased by 10% in heart, 70% in skeletal muscle, and 90% in placenta ($p \leq 0.05$). Also, there was threefold more mtDNA in the fetal heart and skeletal muscle than in the placenta.

Mitochondrial genomic integrity was examined by gel electrophoresis and Southern blot analysis on DNA samples adjusted for the same amount of mitochondrial protein. It was possible to distinguish between nicked circular (NC) and linear (L) DNA, with degradation indicated by a decrease in NC DNA and a tail of linear DNA. Among the unexposed animals there was some DNA degradation in all three tissues (FIG. 2A, lane 3; FIG. 2B, lane 1; FIG. 2C, lanes 2 and 3). However, among the AZT-exposed animals the degradation (i.e., linear DNA tailing) was more extensive (FIG. 2A, lanes 6 and 7; FIG. 2B, lane 7; FIG. 2C, lanes 5 and 6.) In addition, decreases in NC DNA appeared more frequently in AZT-treated monkeys than in controls.

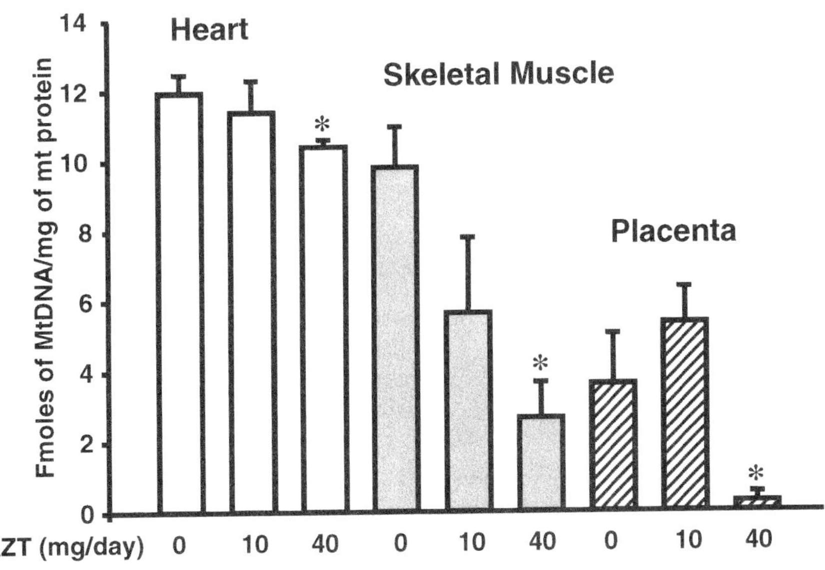

FIGURE 1. Mitochondrial DNA levels are depleted in heart, skeletal muscle, and placentas from fetuses of pregnant patas dams given 0 ($n = 4$), 10 ($n = 3$), or 40 mg ($n = 3$) AZT/day for the last 50% of gestation. MtDNA levels were quantitated by slot blot analysis as described in Materials and Methods. *Asterisk* indicates statistical significance ($p \leq 0.05$) in comparison to unexposed monkeys.

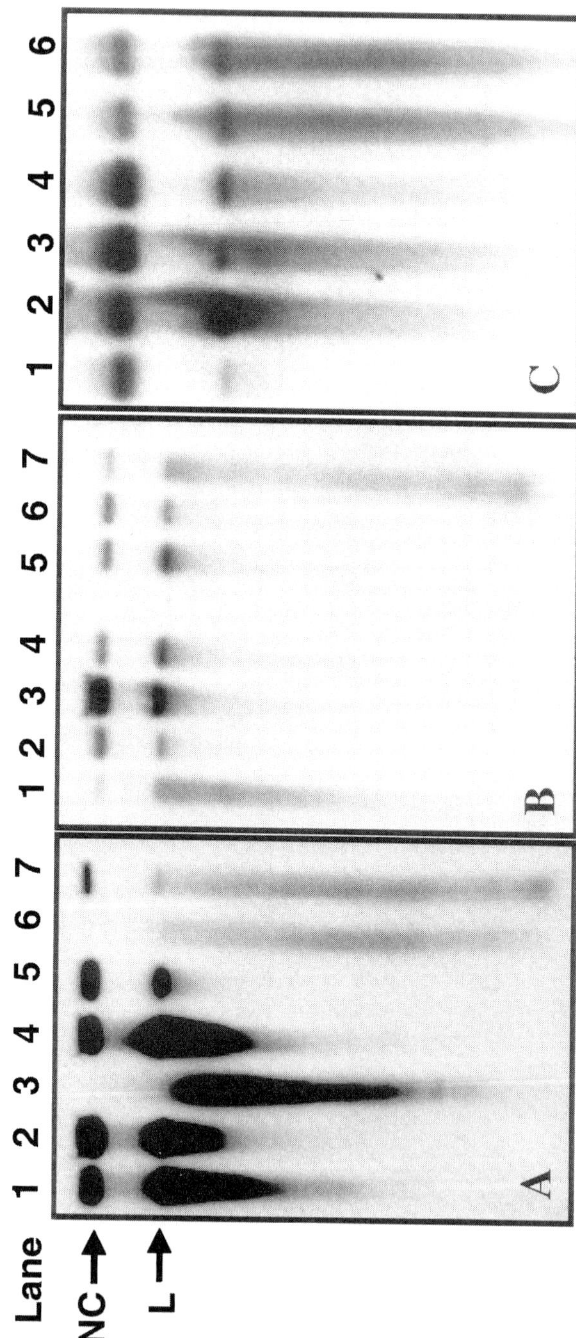

FIGURE 2. Mitochondrial DNA structure of heart (**A**), skeletal muscle (**B**), and placenta (**C**) from fetuses of pregnant patas dams given 0 (**A** and **B**, *lanes 1–4*; **C**, *lanes 1–3*) or 40 mg AZT/day (**A** and **B**, *lanes 5–7*; **C**, *lanes 4–6*) for the last half of gestation. Southern blot analysis was employed as described in Materials and Methods. Mitochondrial DNA is either nicked circular (NC) or linear (L).

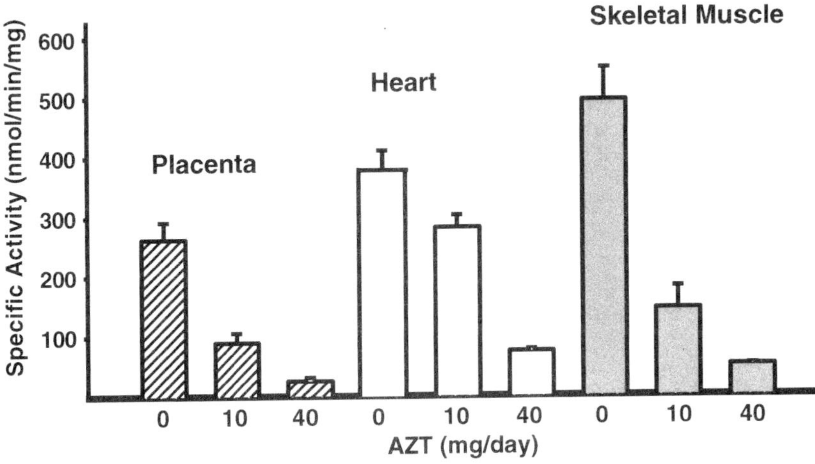

FIGURE 3. Dose-related decreases in Complex I activities in heart, skeletal muscle, and placenta from fetuses of pregnant patas dams given 0 ($n = 4$), 10 ($n = 3$), or 40 mg ($n = 3$) AZT/day for the last 50% of gestation. Each trend analysis was analyzed by Kruskal-Wallis one way analysis of variance on ranks using median values ± SE (Sigma Stat, Version 2.0, Jandel Scientific), and all trends were statistically significant ($p \leq 0.001$).

Specific activities of the OXPHOS enzymes were measured in fetal heart, skeletal muscle, and placenta from four unexposed monkeys and six monkeys exposed transplacentally to AZT at doses of 10 mg/day ($n = 3$) and 40 mg/day ($n = 3$). In all three tissues from AZT-exposed animals, Complex I-specific activities (FIG. 3) were significantly decreased ($\geq 80\%$) (one way ANOVA, $p \leq 0.001$). In contrast, Complex II and Complex IV specific activities were increased significantly in all three tissues. The placenta (FIG. 4B and D) showed two- and fourfold increases for Complexes II and IV, respectively (one way ANOVA, $p \leq 0.001$). Statistically significant increases for Complex II and IV activities have also been observed in heart and skeletal muscle and published previously.[1] Complex III-specific activity was decreased in a dose-dependent fashion in the placenta (FIG. 4C) (one way ANOVA, $p \leq 0.001$), but not in the other organs.[1] In addition, because there can be a high degree of interindividual variability among monkeys, OXPHOS enzyme values for Complexes I–IV for the placentas of all the animals are shown individually in TABLE 1. The OXPHOS values that are significantly different from the mean of the four control animals are indicated by bold text.

Because the increase in Complex IV specific activity is an unusual finding, cytochrome c oxidase activity was visualized histochemically using 3′,3′-diaminobenzidine (DAB) as an electron donor for cytochrome c. The reaction product is the result of oxidation of DAB in the form of a brown pigment. FIGURE 5 shows strong increases in cytochrome c oxidase staining in heart left ventricle (FIG. 5B) and quadricep muscle (FIG. 5D) from patas fetuses exposed transplacentally to 40 mg AZT/day compared to unexposed animals (FIG. 5A and C).

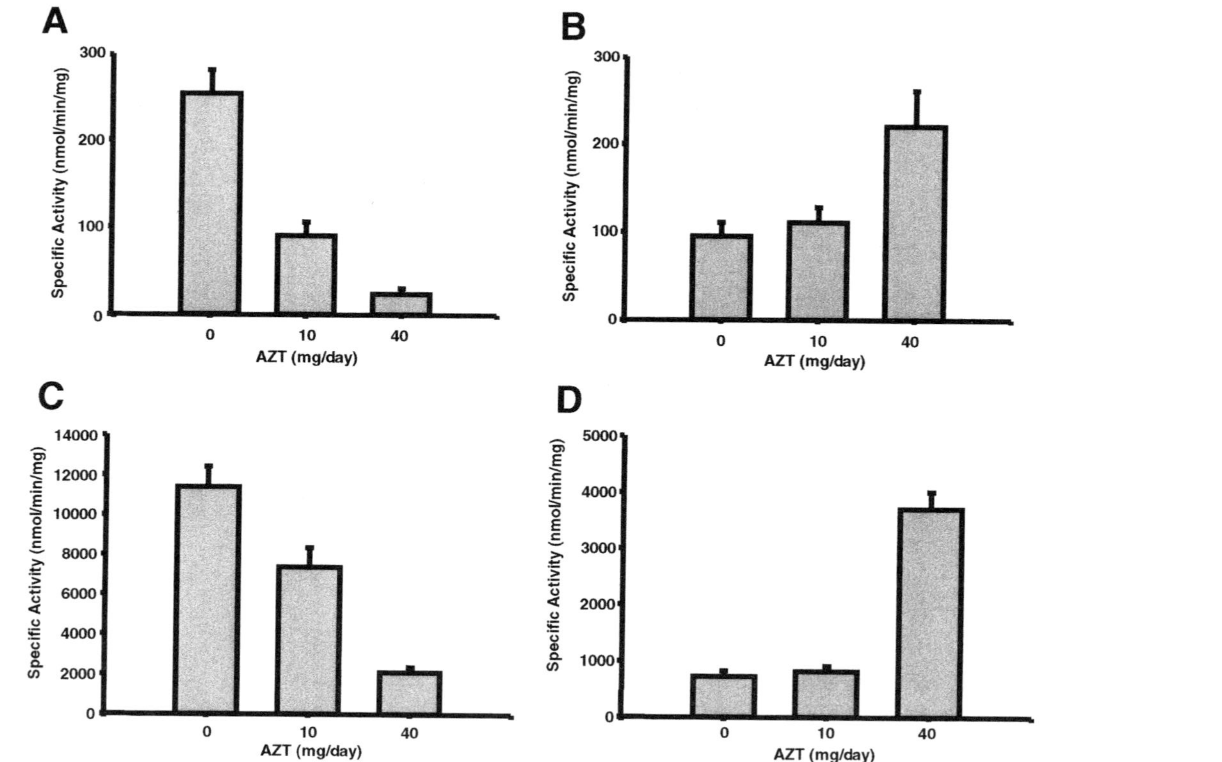

FIGURE 4. Dose-related changes in mitochondrial OXPHOS enzyme-specific activities in placenta from pregnant patas dams given 0, 10, and 40 mg AZT/day for the last 50% of gestation. Trends are for (**A**) Complex I, (**B**) Complex II, (**C**) Complex III, and (**D**) Complex IV. Each trend analysis was analyzed by Kruskal-Wallis one way analysis of variance on ranks using median values ± SE (Sigma Stat, Version 2.0, Jandel Scientific), and all trends were statistically significant ($p \leq 0.001$).

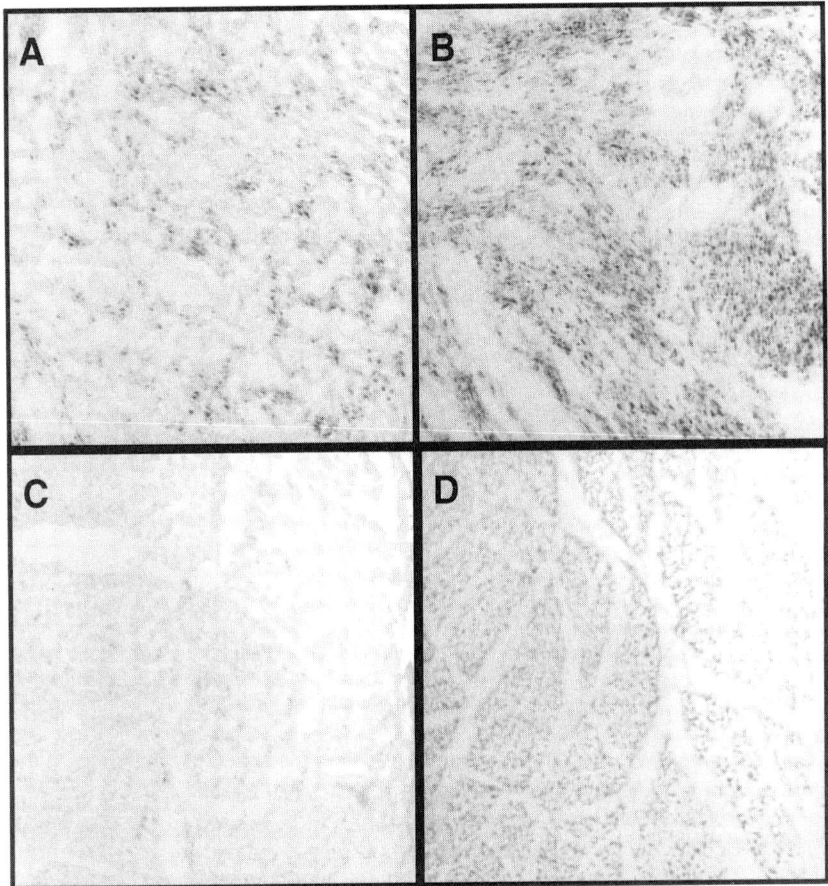

FIGURE 5. Cytochrome *c* oxidase cytochemistry of fetal heart (**A** and **B**) and skeletal muscle (**C** and **D**) from fetuses of patas dams given 0 (**A, C**) or 40 mg AZT/day (**B, D**) for the last half of gestation (10 × magnification).

DISCUSSION

The present study modeled human *in utero* AZT exposure using the patas monkey. The mitochondrial genotoxic and functional consequences of transplacental AZT exposure to the patas placenta, fetal heart, and skeletal muscle were examined. The pattern of mitochondrial toxicity in placenta, an organ with low energy requirements and few mitochondria, was strikingly similar to that in fetal heart and skeletal muscle, tissues with very high energy requirements. All three tissues sustained significant losses in amounts of mtDNA, even though the unexposed placenta had less mtDNA than did the unexposed heart and skeletal muscle. In addition, AZT-induced

TABLE 1. OXPHOS enzyme-specific activities (nmol/min/mg) in placenta from patas dams given AZT daily for the last 10 weeks (50%) of gestation

Monkey numbers	Daily AZT dose (mg)	Sex	Complexes[a]			
			I	II	III	IV
1	0	M	150 ± IS	70 ± 6	12904 ± 1221	877 ± 140
2	0	M	390 ± 37	71 ± 10	9068 ± 892	1227 ± 145
3	0	F	207 ± 32	173 ± 32	7964 ± 592	338 ± 16
4	0	M	319 ± 16	66 ± 6	15583 ± 1526	505 ± 37
5	10	M	**112 ± 7**	56 ± 11	8226 ± 676	712 ± 95
6	10	F	128 ± 11	119 ± 17	10110 ± 382	582 ± 12
7	10	M	**30 ± 2**	156 ± 25	**3719 ± 130**	1159 ± 118
8	40	F	**25 ± 3**	131 ± 19	**1399 ± 243**	**3171 ± 134**
9	40	M	**ND**	158 ± 22	**1906 ± 58**	**3092 ± 88**
10	40	M	**47 ± 3**	**371 ± 46**	**2974 ± 490**	**4858 ± 332**

[a]Complexes I, II, III, and IV were quantitated on a Hewlett Packard diode array spectrophotometer as previously described on male (M) and female (F) fetuses, as described in Materials and Methods. Data are presented as mean ± SE of three assays. ND = nondetectable, <20 nmol/min/mg. For each complex, enzyme-specific activities from each AZT-treated animal were compared to the means of the four unexposed animals (not shown). Significantly different $p \leq 0.05$ values by Student's t test are represented in bold text.

alterations in mitochondrial functional integrity, measured as specific activities of OXPHOS enzymes, were also very similar for all three tissues. Complex I was decreased dramatically in a dose-dependent fashion, whereas Complexes II and IV were increased. The results suggest that the extent of AZT-induced mitochondrial damage incurred after transplacental exposure might be monitored successfully by measuring these parameters in the placental tissue obtained at birth.

The mitochondrial toxicity of *in utero* AZT exposure in the monkeys is most likely due to AZT incorporation into genomic and mtDNA. We previously demonstrated AZT incorporation in the brain cortex, cerebellum, lung, liver, kidney, heart, and placenta of fetal patas monkeys given 10 mg AZT/day, or 21% of the human daily dose. AZT-DNA incorporation in the heart muscle mtDNA ranged from 15–108 molecules AZT/10^6 nucleotides and in the placenta 7–30 molecules AZT/10^6 nucleotides, or 3–18 AZT molecules per mitochondrion.[22] This amount of AZT incorporation into mtDNA would be sufficient to truncate mtDNA replication, leading to mtDNA depletion and decreased mitochondrial OXPHOS polypeptide transcription. In humans, the levels of AZT-DNA incorporation in cord blood leukocyte nuclear DNA from infants of AZT-treated HIV-1–positive pregnant women are similar to those observed in fetal patas monkeys,[20] but sample quantities have been insufficient to measure AZT in human mtDNA.

Mitochondrial OXPHOS enzyme activity alterations and mtDNA depletion have been found in rodent skeletal muscle,[32] cultured human myocytes,[33] and skeletal muscle biopsies of AIDS patients[12,13] as a result of AZT exposure. In adult patients treated with AZT for 2–9 months, cytochrome *c* oxidase (Complex IV) and succinate cytochrome *c* reductase (Complex II–III) activities were reduced, and mtDNA levels were decreased.[10–13] For the eight HIV-1–negative children reported by Blanche *et al.*[19] that had persistent mitochondrial dysfunction after *in utero* AZT or AZT and 3TC exposure, abnormal ratios of Complex IV/Complex I were observed in all of the skeletal muscle, cardiac muscle, and liver homogenates examined. Five of these children had significant decreases in Complex I, and four had significant decreases in Complex IV. Furthermore, six HIV-1–positive children, aged 10.6 ± 4.5 years, treated with a cumulative AZT dose of 35.7 ± 9.0 g/kg body weight for 5.3 years or more have developed cardiac left ventricular dysfunction that was reversible 4–12 weeks after discontinuation of AZT therapy.[18] Since current therapeutic protocols for HIV-1–positive pregnant women and their infants currently include combinations of nucleoside analog drugs, mitochondrial dysfunction may become a more frequent occurrence in HIV-1–negative, exposed children. These data suggest that placenta might be an appropriate indicator tissue for such potential mitochondrial toxicities.

ACKNOWLEDGMENT

We wish to thank Andrea Ceresa, Catherine Paik-Huh, and Kay Huffer for their technical expertise and Marisa C. St. Claire, DVM, Boris Skopets, DVM, Ph.D., Jeffrey W. Harbaugh, and Steven W. Harbaugh from Bioqual Incorporated, Rockville, MD, for veterinary consultation and services. Also, we greatly appreciate the statistical advice of Robert Tarone and the editorial assistance of Bettie Sugar.

REFERENCES

1. GERSCHENSON, M., S.W. ERHART, C.Y. PAIK *et al.* 2000. Fetal mitochondrial heart and skeletal muscle damage in *Erythrocebus patas* monkeys exposed *in utero* to 3′-azido-3′-deoxythymidine (AZT). AIDS Res. Hum. Retrovir. **16:** 635–644.
2. CONNOR, E.M., R.S. SPERLING, R. GELBER *et al.* 1994. Reduction of maternal-infant transmission of human immunodeficiency virus type 1 with zidovudine treatment. N. Engl. J. Med. **331:** 1173–1180.
3. LEWIS, W. 1998. Mitochondrial toxity of antiviral nucleosides used in AIDS: insights derived from toxic changes observed in tissues rich in mitochondria. *In* Cardiology in AIDS. S.E. Lipshultz, Ed. :317– 329. Chapman & Hall. New York, NY.
4. ARKY, R. 1999. Physicians Desk Reference, 53rd Ed. Medical Economics Co., Inc. Montvale, NJ.
5. STYRT, B.A., T.D. PIAZZA-HEPP & G.K. CHIKAMI. 1996. Clinical toxicity of antiretroviral nucleoside analogs. Antiviral Res. **31:** 121–135.
6. GERTNER, E., J.R. THURN, D.N. WILLIAMS *et al.* 1989. Zidovudine-associated myopathy. Am. J. Med. **86:** 814–818.
7. CHARIOT, P., I. DROGOU, I. DE LACROIX-SZMANIA *et al.* 1999. Zidovudine-induced mitochondrial disorder with massive liver steatosis, myopathy, lactic acidosis, and mitochondrial DNA depletion. J. Hepatol. **30:** 156–160.
8. DALAKAS, M.C., I. ILLA, G.H. PEZESHKPOUR *et al.* 1990. Mitochondrial myopathy caused by long-term zidovudine therapy. N. Engl. J. Med. **322:** 1098–1105.
9. D'AMTI, G., W. KWAN & W. LEWIS. 1992. Dilated cardiomyopathy in a zidovudine-treated AIDS patient. Cardiovasc. Pathol. **1:** 317–320.

10. ARNAUDO, E., M. DALAKAS, S. SHANSKE *et al.* 1991. Depletion of muscle mitochondrial DNA in AIDS patients with zidovudine-induced myopathy. Lancet **337**: 508–510.

11. CASADEMONT, J., A. BARRIENTOS, J.M. GRAU *et al.* 1996. The effect of zidovudine on skeletal muscle mtDNA in HIV-1 infected patients with mild or no muscle dysfunction. Brain **119**: 1357–1364.

12. TOMELLERI, G., P. TONIN, M. SPADARO *et al.* 1992. AZT-induced mitochondrial myopathy. Ital. J. Neurol. Sci. **13**: 723–728.

13. MHIRI, C., M. BAUDRIMONT, G. BONNE *et al.* 1991. Zidovudine myopathy: a distinctive disorder associated with mitochondrial dysfunction. Ann. Neurol. **29**: 606–614.

14. CHEN, S.C., S.M. BARKER, D.H. MITCHELL *et al.* 1992. Concurrent zidovudine-induced myopathy and hepatoxicity in patients treated for human immunodeficiency virus (HIV) infection. Pathology **24**: 109–111.

15. CUPLER, E.J., M.J. DANON, C. JAY *et al.* 1995. Early features of zidovudine-associated myopathy: histopathological findings and clinical correlations. Acta Neuropathol. (Berl.) **90**: 1–6.

16. SCHRODER, J.M., M. BERTRAM, R. SCHNABEL & U. PFAFF. 1992. Nuclear and mitochondrial changes of muscle fibers in AIDS after treatment with high doses of zidovudine. Acta Neuropathol. (Berl.) **85**: 39 –47.

17. DOMANSKI, M.J., M.M. SLOAS, D.A. FOLLMANN *et al.* 1995. Effect of zidovudine and didanosine treatment on heart function in children infected with human immunodeficiency virus. J. Pediatr. **127**: 137–146.

18. DRAGAN, T., C. SABLE, P. TAYLOR *et al.* 2000. Reversible cardiac dysfunction associated with zidovudine exposure in HIV-infected children [abstr.]. J. Am. Coll. Cardiol. **35**: 513A.

19. BLANCHE, S., M. TARDIEU, P. RUSTIN *et al.* 1999. Persistent mitochondrial dysfunction and perinatal exposure to antiretroviral nucleoside analogues. Lancet **354**: 1084–1089.

20. OLIVERO, O.A., G.M. SHEARER, C.A. CHOUGNET *et al.* 1999. Incorporation of zidovudine into leukocyte DNA from HIV-1-positive adults and pregnant women, and cord blood from infants exposed *in utero.* AIDS **13**: 919–925.

21. LONGLEY, M.J., P.A. ROPP, S.E. LIM & W.C. COPELAND. 1999. Characterization of the native and recombinant catalytic subunit of human DNA polymerase gamma: identification of residues critical for exonuclease activity and dideoxynucleotide sensitivity. Biochemistry **37**: 10529–10539.

22. OLIVERO, O.A., L.M. ANDERSON, B.A. DIWAN *et al.* 1997. Transplacental effects of 3'-azido-2',3'-dideoxythymidine (AZT): tumorigenicity in mice and genotoxicity in mice and monkeys. J. Natl. Cancer Inst. **89**: 1602–1608.

23. POIRIER, M.C., T.A. PATTERSON, W. SLIKKER, JR. & O.A. OLIVERO. 1999. Incorporation of 3'-azido-3'-deoxythymidine (AZT) into fetal DNA, and fetal tissue distribution of drug, after infusion of pregnant late-term rhesus macaques with a human-equivalent AZT dose. J. AIDS Hum. Retrovirol. **22**: 477–483.

24. LEWIS, W., J.F. SIMPSON & R.R. MEYER. 1994. Cardiac mitochondrial DNA polymerase-gamma is inhibited competitively and noncompetitively by phosphorylated zidovudine. Circ. Res. **74**: 344–348.

25. STRYER, L. 1988. Biochemistry. W.H. Freeman & Co. New York, NY.

26. LU, L.J., L.M. ANDERSON, A.B. JONES *et al.* 1993. Persistence, gestation stage-dependent formation and interrelationship of benzo[a]pyrene-induced DNA adducts in mothers, placentae and fetuses of *Erythrocebus patas* monkeys. Carcinogenesis **14**: 1805–1813.

27. AUSUBEL, F.M. 1999. Current Protocols in Molecular Biology. John Wiley & Sons, Inc. New York, NY.

28. HAYASAKA, K., K. FUJII & S. HORAI. 1996. Molecular phylogeny of macaques: implications of nucleotide sequences from an 896-base pair region of mitochondrial DNA. Mol. Biol. Evol. **13**: 1044–1053.

29. TROUNCE, I.A., Y.L. KIM, A.S. JUN & D.C. WALLACE. 1996. Assessment of mitochondrial oxidative phosphorylation in patient muscle biopsies, lymphoblasts, and trans-mitochondrial cell lines. Methods Enzymol. **264**: 484-509.

30. BRADFORD, M.M. 1976. A rapid and sensitive method for the quantitation of microgram quantities of protein utilizing the principle of protein-dye binding. Anal. Biochem. **72**: 248–254.

31. SCIACCO, M. & E. BONILLA. 1996. Cytochemistry and immunocytochemistry of mitochondria in tissue sections. *In* Methods in Enzymology, Vol. 264. G.M Attardi & A. Chomyn, Eds. :509–521. Academic Press. San Diego, CA.
32. LEWIS, W., B. GONZALEZ, A. CHOMYN & T. PAPOIAN. 1992. Zidovudine induces molecular, biochemical, and ultrastructural changes in rat skeletal muscle mitochondria. J. Clin. Invest. **88:** 1354–1360.
33. BENBRIK, E., P. CHARIOT, S. BONAVAUD *et al.* 1997. Cellular and mitochondrial toxicity of zidovudine (AZT), didanosine (ddI) and zalcitabine (ddC) on cultured human muscle cells. J. Neurol. Sci. **149:** 19–25.

ADVANCES IN PEDIATRIC AIDS

Advances in Pediatric AIDS

Introduction

ARYE RUBINSTEIN[a]

Department of Pediatrics, Microbiology and Immunology, and Centers for AIDS Research, Albert Einstein College of Medicine, Bronx, New York 10461, USA

The Pediatric AIDS Satellite conference is the first one to be linked to the conference on Global Strategies for the Prevention of HIV Transmission from Mothers to Infants. The Pediatric AIDS Satellite was structured to complement the agenda of the "Global Strategies" conference by focusing more attention on basic research.

It is essential that researchers and caregivers from around the world engage in a dialogue to address questions concerning the unprecedented spread of HIV to women and children in developing countries. One of the missions of the satellite conference was to enhance the incorporation of social, economic, ethical, and political issues in developing countries into the ongoing research agenda in resource-rich countries.

The worldwide impact of this epidemic in Africa and Asia was not fully appreciated until recently. Several months after the conference, on January 10, 2000, the UN Security Council dealt for the first time with the AIDS epidemic as a threat to political stability and world peace. In sub-Saharan Africa alone, 23 million people are HIV infected, and over 2 million died in 1 year from AIDS. This region is home to 90% of the world's AIDS orphans, and about 45,000 new cases of HIV infection in children occur in South Africa alone.

What can current research do to arrest this dreadful epidemic affecting women and children? First and foremost, the Pediatric AIDS Satellite conference strived to foster collaboration between health care providers in the front line, researchers, and politicians. It provided a window of opportunity and a forum for international collaboration at all levels of cutting-edge AIDS research. It is to be hoped that this satellite conference will build a momentum to forge new partnerships among all participants for utilizing research advances for the benefit of, and a brighter future for, HIV prevention and treatment in developing countries. We are obligated to work together with our colleagues from developing countries, to educate and persuade governments to take action. This role cannot be left in the hands of politicians; otherwise, the existing debate in some countries such as that concerning the efficacy and risk/benefit ratio of zidovudine and/or nevirapine treatment of pregnant women will continue to the detriment of patients and the general population. In the Pediatric AIDS Satellite Conference we addressed the science and facts documenting the unequivocal benefit of preventive measures. A unanimous call for worldwide action was issued by Dr. Ammann, the Global Strategies Conference Chair. Preventive

[a]Address for correspondence: Albert Einstein College of Medicine, 1300 Morris Park Ave., Bronx, NY 10461. Voice: 718-430-2319.

rubinste@aecom.yu.edu 1

measures have significantly reduced HIV infection in children residing in developed countries. In some cities in the United States and in Europe that in the 1980s had a rapidly growing population of HIV-infected children, there is now only a handful of newly infected children annually. In Berlin, the pediatric center could fortunately be closed for lack of patients. We must achieve similar goals in developing countries. Achieving this lofty goal is not in the realm of an unaccomplishable dream. The complex and expensive zidovudine 076 protocol for mothers and infants designed in the United States has been translated into an effective, shorter and shorter, and less expensive preventive regimen in other countries. There is no reason why other research findings cannot be adjusted to accommodate countries with fewer financial resources. The Pediatric AIDS Satellite Conference also addressed the limitations of optimal antiretroviral therapies in a world in which infections and possible super-infections with newly emerging drug-resistant HIV strains are on the rise. Crossover mutations between different virus clades point to a new era in world epidemics in which no boundaries exist between developing and developed countries. These new HIV forms may evade antiretroviral therapies and immune responses. The "Satellite Conference" has therefore highlighted new findings that broaden our understanding of the protective cellular and humoral immune responses to HIV. These new advances also provide for a higher profile for preventive and therapeutic vaccines. It is now clear that AIDS vaccines must play a more prominent role in the treatment and prevention of HIV infection in women and children. The purpose of this gathering, among others, was to build a momentum for a closer collaboration on the utilization of AIDS vaccines to generate long-term protection against HIV and to stem the burgeoning epidemic.

Antiretroviral Pharmacology in Pregnant Women and Their Newborns

MARK MIROCHNICK[a]

Boston University School of Medicine, Boston Medical Center, One BMC Place, Boston, Massachusetts 02118, USA

ABSTRACT: The physiologic changes of pregnancy have an impact on antiretroviral pharmacokinetic parameters, but the effect is generally not of sufficient magnitude to warrant alterations in dosing. Although administration of oral zidovudine during labor may not provide equivalent serum drug exposure as with continuous intravenous infusion, the clinical relevance of the difference is unknown. Nevirapine is well absorbed during labor, and sufficient drug for prophylaxis against perinatal transmission crosses the placenta if an oral dose is administered to the mother at least 1 hour before delivery. Placental transfer of reverse transcriptase inhibitors is good, whereas preliminary data suggest that protease inhibitors do not cross the placenta well. The use of antiretrovirals during pregnancy is becoming increasingly common, although their safety, toxicity, and teratogencity in pregnancy have not been well described. Normal growth and development have a profound impact on the pharmacokinetics of antiretrovirals in newborns and infants. Washout elimination of transplacentally acquired drug is slow. The pattern of increase in drug clearance over time will depend on the specific elimination pathway for the agent. Dosing regimens must take into account developmental changes in clearance and appropriate scaling for size. Adherence to antiretroviral regimens is a critical factor in determining the success of prophylactic and therapeutic regimens and is made difficult by the inability of infants to swallow pills and capsules.

INTRODUCTION

The use of antiretroviral agents in pregnant women and infants has become increasingly complex. Seventeen antiretroviral drugs are now available in the United States by prescription or through compassionate use protocols (TABLE 1). HIV-infected pregnant women and their newborns may receive antiretroviral therapy for both prophylaxis against mother-child HIV transmission and primary therapy of HIV infection. Combination regimens incorporating multiple antiretroviral agents are becoming more common. The effect on antiretroviral drug disposition of the physiologic changes associated with pregnancy and with growth and development must be understood for these drugs to be safely and effectively used in pregnant women and their infants. Other questions raised by the use of antiretrovirals during pregnancy include whether oral dosing during labor is practical, the nature of placental transfer of these agents, and the short- and long-term risks arising from fetal and postnatal exposure to these agents.

[a]Voice: 617-414-3754; fax: 617-414-7297.
markm@bu.edu

TABLE 1. Antiretroviral agents now approved for use in the United States or available through compassionate use protocols

Reverse transcriptase inhibitors	
Nucleoside analogues	Abacavir, didanosine (ddI), lamivudine (3TC), stavudine (d4T), zalcitabine (ddC), zidovudine (ZDV)
Nucleotides	Adefovir
Nonnucleosides	Delavirdine, efavirenz, nevirapine
Protease inhibitors	Amprenavir, indinavir, nelfinavir ritonavir, saquinavir, lopinavir
Ribonucleotide reductase inhibitors	Hydroxyurea

PREGNANT WOMEN

Effects of Pregnancy on Antiretroviral Drug Disposition

The dramatic physiologic changes of pregnancy impact drug disposition in many ways. Drug disposition is generally divided into drug absorption, distribution, metabolism, and excretion, and pregnancy will affect each. Alteration of gastrointestinal function in pregnancy may impair the absorption of drugs. Increased plasma progesterone is associated with a 30–50% decrease in intestinal motility, resulting in increased gastric emptying time and intestinal transit time.[1] Gastric acid secretion is reduced by 40% and gastric pH increases, affecting the ionization and absorption of weak acids and bases.[2] Nausea and vomiting, especially pronounced in early pregnancy, may also decrease drug absorption. Whereas these physiologic changes would be expected to result in delayed drug absorption and reduced peak maternal blood concentrations, few studies have evaluated the clinical impact of these changes.[3]

The impact of the changes in body composition and protein binding during pregnancy on volume of distribution is significant. During an average pregnancy, total body water increases by 8 liters, plasma volume enlarges by 50%, and body fat stores increase.[4] Protein binding is decreased due to a decrease in serum albumin as well as competitive inhibition from steroid hormones.[5] As a result, volume of distribution increases for both hydrophilic and lipophilic drugs, decreasing peak drug concentrations. The decrease in protein binding also results in an increase in the unbound fraction of drug, which is the pharmacologically active drug as well as the drug available for biotransformation and elimination. The free fraction of many drugs, including theophylline, diazepam, salicylates, and some beta-lactam antibiotics have been shown to increase during pregnancy as a result of changes in protein binding.[6–8]

The effect of pregnancy on drug elimination is variable. Hepatic drug metabolic pathways may be induced by progesterone, as has been shown for phenytoin.[9] Estrogen and progesterone may compete for metabolic binding sites, reducing metabolism of drugs such as theophylline and caffeine.[10] Excretion of drugs and their metabolites by the kidney increases during pregnancy. Pregnancy is associated with a 25–50% increase in renal plasma flow and glomerular filtration rate (GFR), resulting in an increase in clearance of drugs eliminated predominantly by renal clearance, such as ampicillin and gentamicin.[11,12]

While the physiologic changes of pregnancy do result in measurable changes in drug disposition, the magnitude of these changes is generally not sufficient to necessitate adjustment of dosing for most commonly used drugs. Increased volume of distribution and clearance tends to decrease drug exposure, and decreased protein binding leads to a larger free fraction of drug. The net effect for many drugs is a balance, with the change in concentration of the unbound, pharmacologically active drug insufficient to require adjustment in dosing.[2] Monitoring of drugs with narrow therapeutic indices, such as phenytoin and theophylline, may be recommended.[13]

Data are available describing the pharmacokinetics of several antiretrovirals during pregnancy. The greatest amount of data and clinical experience is available for zidovudine. O'Sullivan *et al.*[14] determined zidovudine pharmacokinetics following oral and parenteral dosing in eight women at 28–36 weeks' gestation. All pharmacokinetic parameters were similar to those in nonpregnant adults.[14] In contrast, Watts *et al.*[15] studied three women both during and after pregnancy. These women had a significant increase during pregnancy in Vd/F and Cl/F which balanced out, so there was no change in $t_{1/2}$, whereas AUC decreased by 33%.[15] Standard adult doses of zidovudine are recommended for use in pregnant women.[16]

Pharmacokinetic data from pregnant women are also available for didanosine, nevirapine, and nelfinavir. Wang *et al.*[17] determined didanosine pharmacokinetics in nine women at 31 weeks' gestation and again at 6 weeks postpartum following both iv and oral doses. A significant increase in clearance of intravenous doses was noted during pregnancy compared to postpartum (12.0 ± 2.45 ml/min/kg vs 9.4 ± 3.5 ml/min/kg, $p < 0.05$). Bioavailability averaged 50%, but was very variable, ranging from 15–84%. No significant differences were noted in clearance of oral doses administered during and after pregnancy, as the large variability in absorption masked the modest difference in clearance.[17] Nevirapine pharmacokinetic parameters in pregnant women studied during the late third trimester before the onset of labor were similar to those seen in nonpregnant adult women.[18] Preliminary data from a phase I study of nelfinavir in pregnant women (PACTG 353) suggest a large variability in absorption for this drug as well, along with a trend to a lower AUC during pregnancy.[19] Phase I studies of other protease inhibitors in pregnancy are in progress.

Oral Dosing During Labor

The antepartum/intrapartum/postnatal zidovudine regimen shown to be effective in reducing mother-to-child HIV transmission in the ACTG 076 trial included a continuous zidovudine infusion during labor to maintain a constant serum level of the antiretroviral in mother and fetus.[20] In many parts of the developing world, intravenous access during labor is not routine, and many women and their obstetrical practitioners in the developed world would prefer oral to intravenous administration during labor. There is little experience with oral administration of drugs during labor, and drug absorption and clearance may be diminished by the changes in gastrointestinal activity and hepatic blood flow associated with labor.

Data are available describing zidovudine and nevirapine kinetics following oral administration during labor. In an ongoing study of oral zidovudine dosing in labor (PACTG 324), initial results suggest low trough ZDV concentrations (<0.1 µg/ml) with 300 mg q 3 hours during labor, and a 600 mg initial loading dose is now being investigated.[21] However, target zidovudine blood concentrations during labor have not been established. Zidovudine is metabolized within the cell to its bioactive triphosphorylated form, and it is the concentration of this metabolite within the cell and not the circulating zidovudine concentration that is thought to be of prime importance in its antiretroviral activity.[22] While clinical trials of regimens using zidovudine that begin at 36 weeks' gestation and include oral dosing rather than continuous intravenous infusion during labor have been shown to be effective in reducing mother-to-infant HIV transmission, the reduction is not as great as with the ACTG 076 regimen.[23–25] It is not known to what extent oral dosing during labor contributes to the decrease in effectiveness of these short course regimens.

In the PACTG 250 study, nevirapine pharmacokinetic parameters were determined in a six women dosed during labor and nine women dosed during the late third trimester. The women in labor demonstrated an increase in nevirapine $t_{1/2}$ (72.5 ± 36.2 hours vs 42.6 ± 12.4 hours, $p < 0.05$), a decrease in bioavailability, and an overall increase in the variability of all pharmacokinetic parameters. Median t max was 3.3 hours in both groups.[18]

Placental Transfer of Antiretroviral Agents

Fetal exposure to drugs administered to the mother will be determined by the concentration of drug in the maternal circulation, the kinetics of drug transfer across the placenta, and placental and fetal drug metabolism. Most drugs cross the placenta by passive diffusion, and the rate and extent of transfer are determined by the physicochemical and structural characteristics of the drugs and the physiological characteristics of the maternal-placental-fetal unit.[26] A limitation of studies of human placental drug transfer is that fetal sampling is restricted to cord blood for comparison with a sample from the mother at the time of delivery. Placental transfer of nucleoside reverse transcriptase inhibitors has also been investigated in animal models and with *in vitro* isolated, perfused human placental specimens.[27]

The available data suggest that nucleoside reverse transcriptase inhibitors rapidly cross the placenta. Cord blood concentrations of zidovudine and lamivudine tend to equal or exceed those in the maternal circulation at the time of delivery, whereas cord blood concentrations of didanosine and zalcitabine are approximately 30–50% of maternal concentrations.[27,28] Nevirapine also rapidly crosses the placenta, and concentrations in cord blood are generally equivalent to those in the mother at delivery. Nevirapine absorption during labor is rapid, and if a 200-mg oral dose is administered to the mother at least 1 hour before delivery, sufficient drug reaches the maternal circulation and then crosses the placenta to provide protective concentrations to the infant after birth.[29,30]

In contrast, preliminary data suggest that the protease inhibitors, which are highly protein bound, do not cross the placenta well. Four of 8 infants born to mothers receiving nelfinavir had no detectable nelfinavir in their cord blood samples, and the median ratio of cord blood to maternal serum nelfinavir concentrations was 4.5%, with a maximum of 16.3%.[19] The clinical significance of decreased placental transport of protease inhibitors is unknown. Lower fetal drug concentrations may increase the risk of HIV transmission during pregnancy, labor, and/or the period between birth and postnatal dosing of the infant. However, reduced fetal exposure to an antiretroviral and/or its metabolites may reduce the risk of toxic or teratogenic effects. Another unknown is the role of placental metabolism. The placenta is a highly metabolic organ, and the role of placental metabolism on the transfer of antiretrovirals across the placenta has not been determined.

Safety, Toxicity, and Teratogneicity of Antiretrovirals in Pregnancy

Standard antiretroviral therapy is based on the use of multiple agent combination regimens, frequently including protease inhibitors, and the use of these combination regimens during pregnancy is becoming common. In a report of the first 285 US women enrolling in a study comparing intrapartum/postnatal nevirapine with placebo when added to standard antiretroviral therapy (PACTG 316), only one woman received no antiretroviral therapy during pregnancy. By contrast, 24% received zidovudine alone, 40% received zidovudine and lamivudine, and 31% received a combination including a protease inhibitor.[31] The rate of HIV transmission with the use of combination regimens appears to be low. Two recent abstracts reported that there were no instances of mother-to-child HIV transmission in a combined total of 153 women receiving combination antiretroviral regimens during pregnancy.[32,33]

As the use of combination antiretroviral regimens becomes increasingly common among HIV-infected pregnant women and the rate of transmission goes down, the safety, toxicity, and teratogenicity of the agents used in pregnant HIV-infected women and their infants become of paramount importance. Again, there is the largest amount of data and experience with zidovudine. A common toxicity of zidovudine is bone marrow suppression, and hemoglobin was decreased an average of 1 mg/dl at 3 weeks of age in newborns exposed to zidovudine in ACTG 076 compared to those exposed to placebo. By 12 weeks of age, no differences in hemoglobin were noted between the two groups.[20] Long-term follow-up of the ACTG 076 infants now extends to an average of over 4 years, and no adverse effects of ZDV exposure have been detected.[34]

Few perinatal safety and toxicity data are available for other antiretrovirals. Two drugs are contraindicated during pregnancy or in the newborn period. Efavirenz administration to pregnant monkeys is associated with severe fetal malformations, and this drug should not be used in pregnant women. A common side effect of indinavir is indirect hyperbilirubinemia, and its use in the first weeks of life is contraindicated by its potential for worsening neonatal jaundice. A detailed discussion of the short- and long-term safety of antiretroviral drugs during pregnancy is presented in the section Drug Safety in the Prevention of Perinatal HIV Transmission in this volume.

INFANTS

Effects of Growth and Development on Antiretroviral Drug Disposition

The physiologic changes associated with normal infant growth and development have considerable impact on drug disposition. Drug absorption is often decreased in the newborn, because of prolonged gastric emptying time, increased gastric pH, prolonged intestinal transit time, immaturity in biliary function, and/or variable bacterial colonization of the intestine. There are few studies describing drug absorption in infants and children. The available data suggest that while the extent of absorption is highly variable across the age range and is not related to age, the rate of absorption increases rapidly over the first months of life and it may finally exceed that of older children and adults.[35,36]

Changes in body composition and protein binding will affect drug distribution during infancy and childhood. Total body water and extracellular fluid are increased in the newborn and decrease to adult levels by around 6 months of age. In contrast, total body fat averages about 15% of body weight in the newborn and increases to 20% by 6 months of age.[37] As a result, volume of distribution in newborns is increased for hydrophilic drugs and decreased for lipophilic drugs. Protein binding tends to be decreased in newborns, due to decreased concentrations of albumin and α_1-glycoprotein and increased competitive binding by endogenous substrates, such as free fatty acids and bilirubin.[38] Decreased protein binding will increase the amount of unbound drug available for binding to sites mediating therapeutic and toxic effects as well as for biotransformation and elimination.

Immediately after birth, washout elimination of drug acquired across the placenta following maternal dosing prior to delivery is generally extremely prolonged. Renal and hepatic blood flow and function are low in the immediate newborn period. Drug elimination accelerates as the newborn completes the adaptation to the extrauterine environment over the first days of life, with large increases in renal blood flow and function as well as in hepatic biotransformation and transport activity.[39,40] Drug elimination in the newborn period may also be prolonged from enterohepatic recirculation of glucuronidated drugs, such as zidovudine, due to the high concentrations of β-glucuronidase in the newborn intestine.[40]

Washout elimination data are available for four antiretrovirals (TABLE 2). Washout $t_{1/2}$ is prolonged for all four and is increased four- to fivefold for zidovudine and lamivudine compared to that later during the first weeks of life. Average nevirapine $t_{1/2}$ is 61.0 hours immediately after birth and decreases to 45.8 hours later during the first week of life.[30] As a result of the rapid absorption and placental transfer of nevirapine along with its prolonged neonatal $t_{1/2}$, a dosing regimen limited to a single 200-mg oral dose to the mother during labor and a single oral 2-mg/kg dose to the infant at 48–72 hours of age maintains neonatal serum nevirapine concentrations above 100 ng/ml (10 times the *in vitro* IC_{50} against HIV) throughout the first week of life.[29,30] This regimen has been shown to be more effective in preventing mother-to-child HIV transmission than is a regimen of intrapartum and postpartum ZDV.[41] The success of this peripartum nevirapine regimen in preventing mother-to-child HIV transmission suggests that nevirapine might be effective in protecting against breast milk transmission during the first year of life. However, there are no data available describing nevirapine clearance with chronic dosing during the first months of life, and an appropriate dosing regimen in this age group has not yet been determinded.

The specific elimination pathway for a drug will determine the degree of prolongation of washout elimination and the subsequent pattern of maturation in drug elimination. Zidovudine is rapidly cleared in adults by hepatic conjugation with glucuronide, followed by renal excretion of the conjugated metabolite and some unchanged drug. Low zidovudine clearance in newborns is associated with decreased excretion of zidovudine glucuronide as well as decreased renal function.[42] A recent

TABLE 2. Mean elimination $t_{1/2}$ (hours) of antiretrovirals immediately after birth (washout) and during day 3–10 and week 2–6 of life

	Washout	Day 3–10	Weeks 2–6
Zidovudine (ZDV, AZT)	13.0	3.0	1.96
Nevirapine	61	45.8	NA
Lamivudine (3TC)	14.0	3.0	NA
Didanosine (ddI)	1.7	NA	1.1

NOTE: NA = not available. Data from Refs. 17, 28–30, and 42.

population analysis combining zidovudine pharmacokinetic data from six studies demonstrates a rapid increase in zidovudine clearance over the first weeks of life, reaching adult levels by 4–8 weeks of life.[43] The pattern of increase of zidovudine clearance in the infant parallels that of bilirubin, whose primary route of elimination is also by hepatic glucuronidation. However, although the maturation of clearance of bilirubin and zidovudine are parallel, they are metabolized by different isoenzymes of the UDP-glucuronosyltransferase family.[44,45] Zidovudine clearance is further decreased in premature infants, who require a dosing reduction to avoid the accumulation of potentially toxic serum zidovudine concentrations.[46] The current FDA-approved dosing recommendations for zidovudine in infants are 2 mg/kg qid from birth to 3 months of age and 160 mg/m^2 tid after age 3 months. These recommendations illustrate the difficulty in designing dosing regimens for infants during a period of rapid changes in drug elimination. If these recommendations are followed, the total daily zidovudine dose for an average size infant girl being treated from birth would abruptly increase at 3 months of age over threefold, from a per kilogram dose of 43 mg/day to a meter^2 dose of 136 mg/day.

Maturation of nevirapine clearance follows a different pattern. Nevirapine is metabolized by CYP3A4 and CYP2B6, members of the cytochrome P450 family. Cytochrome P450 enzymes play a major role in drug metabolism, and many drugs used in HIV-infected patients, including the protease inhibitors, dapsone, rifampin, and rifabutin, are metabolized by members of this family of enzymes. Drug-drug interactions involving these enzymes are common and may result in an increase in clearance, due to enzyme induction, or a decrease in clearance, due to inhibition. Nevirapine induces the activity of its own metabolic enzymes, and in adults its clearance roughly doubles over the first weeks of therapy.[47] Drugs metabolized by enzymes of the cytochrome P450 family demonstrate a general pattern of maturation that begins with low clearance in the newborn, followed by an increase over the first years of life to levels that may exceed adult values and a decline to adult levels by the end of puberty.[48] Nevirapine clearance after an initial dose is low in term infants during the first week of life (mean Cl/F = 36.1 ml/kg/hr or 0.6 L/m^2/hr) and in older infants and children (mean Cl/F = 36.8 ml/kg/hr or 0.9 L/m^2/hr).[49,50] In older infants and children, clearance increases dramatically with chronic therapy, averaging around 120 mg/kg/hr in children during the second year of life, and then decreases gradually to about 60 ml/kg/hr by 8–10 years of age.[51] These age-related changes in nevirapine clearance remain even after normalization by body surface area rather than weight and make establishment of a simple pediatric dosing regimen difficult.[50] The FDA-approved regimen of 7 mg/kg below 8 years and 4 mg/kg above 8 years results in an abrupt 43% decrease in dose size when the eighth birthday is reached.

The maturational changes in lamivudine clearance reflect developmental changes in renal function, as lamivudine is eliminated primarily by renal excretion of unchanged drug.[52] Washout of transplacentally acquired lamivudine over the first days of life is prolonged, averaging 14.0 hours. Lamivudine $t_{1/2}$ decreases to around 6 hours by the end of the first week of life and to 2.2 hours in children aged 6 months to 17 years, roughly equivalent to adult values.[28,53] No data are available between 1 week and 6 months of age, so the exact pattern of increase during this period cannot be described. If lamivudine clearance is normalized to body surface area, there is no change in clearance in children over 6 months of age.[53]

Adherence and Formulations

Even the best-designed drug regimen will be ineffective if it is not administered consistently. Adherence is of paramount importance with antiretroviral therapy, where inadequate drug exposure may lead to the failure of a prophylactic regimen or the development of worsening symptoms and viral resistance in infected individuals.[54] There are many ways to assess adherence, including pill/bottle count, questionnaire/interview, and dispensing history. Newer techniques include the administration of a stable isotope-labeled drug and the use of a MEMS cap, a medication cap that contains a microprocessor and records the time and date each time the cap is opened. These tools can be used to learn more about the factors that determine a family's ability to adhere to antiretroviral regimens and how barriers to adherence can be overcome.

In infants and children, who are unable to swallow pills or capsules, adherence is made more difficult by the need for alternative formulations. Liquid preparations of the nucleoside and nonnucleoside reverse transcriptase inhibitors are generally palatable, easy to take, and well absorped, with the exception of didanosine. Absorption of didanosine requires coadministration of an antacid buffer. Even with a buffer, bioavailability averages roughly 50%, and there is considerable interpatient variability.[17] Alternative formulations of the protease inhibitors are much less satisfactory. Liquid formulations, such as for ritonavir, tend to be extremely unpalatable, and powder preparations, such as for nelfinavir, are difficult to deliver consistently. The sick or premature newborn infant who is unable to take enteral feedings or medications presents a special problem. Zidovudine is the only antiretroviral available in a parenteral preparation and is the only treatment option for these infants. The benefits of alternative, potentially more effective agents and the use of combination regimens are denied these infants.

SUMMARY

The physiologic changes of pregnancy have an impact on antiretroviral pharmacokinetic parameters, but the effect is generally not of sufficient magnitude to warrant alterations in dosing. While administration of oral zidovudine during labor may not provide equivalent serum drug exposure as with continuous intravenous infusion, the clinical relevance of the difference is unknown. Nevirapine is well absorbed during labor, and sufficient drug for prophylaxis against perinatal transmission crosses the placenta if an oral dose is administered to the mother at least 1 hour before delivery. Placental transfer of reverse transcriptase inhibitors is good, whereas preliminary data suggest that protease inhibitors do not cross the placenta well. The use of antiretrovirals during pregnancy is becoming increasingly common, although their safety, toxicity, and teratogenicity in pregnancy have not been well described.

Normal growth and development have a profound impact on the pharmacokinetics of antiretrovirals in newborns and infants. Washout elimination of transplacentally acquired drug is slow. The pattern of increase in drug clearance over time will depend on the specific elimination pathway for the agent. Dosing regimens must take into account developmental changes in clearance and appropriate scaling for size. Adherence to antiretroviral regimens is a critical factor in determining the success of prophylactic and therapeutic regimens and is made difficult by the inability of infants to swallow pills and capsules.

REFERENCES

1. MORGAN, D.J. 1997. Drug disposition in mother and foetus. Clin. Exp. Pharmacol. Phys. **24:** 869–873.
2. LOEBSTEIN, R., A. LALKIN & G. KOREN. 1997. Pharmacokinetic changes during pregnancy and their clinical relevance. Clin. Pharmacokinet. **33:** 328–343.
3. WRIGHT, L.L. & C.S. CATZ. 1998. Drug distribution during fetal life. *In* Fetal and Neonatal Physiology. R.A. Polin & W.W. Fox, Eds. :169. W.B. Saunders Co. Philadelphia, PA.
4. KRAUER, B., F. KRAUER & F.E. HYTTEN. 1980. Drug disposition and pharmacokinetics in the maternal-placental-fetal unit. Pharmacol. Ther. **10:** 301–328.
5. KRAUER, B., P. DAYER & R. ANNER. 1984. Changes in serum albumin and "$_1$-acid glycoprotein concentrations during pregnancy: an analysis of fetal-maternal pairs. Br. J.Obstet. Gynecol. **91:** 875–881.
6. CONNELLY, T.J., T.I. RUO, M.C. FREDERIKSEN *et al.* 1990. Characterization of theophylline binding to serum proteins in pregnant and nonpregnant women. Clin. Pharmacol. Ther. **47:** 68–72.
7. DEAN, M., B. STOCK, R.J. PATTERSON *et al.* 1980. Serum protein binding of drugs during and after pregnancy in humans. Clin. Pharmacol. Ther. **28:** 253–261.
8. HEIKKILA, A. & R. ERKKOLA. 1994. Review of beta-lactam antibiotics in pregnancy. The need for adjustment of dosing schedules. Clin. Pharmacokinet. **27:** 49–62.
9. DAVIS, M., C.J. SIMMONS, B. DORDINI *et al.* 1973. Induction of hepatic enzymes during normal pregnancy. J. Obstet. Gynaecol. Br. Common. **80:** 690–694.
10. JUCHAU, M.R., D.L. MIRKIN & P.K. ZACHARIAH. 1976. Interactions of various 19-nor steroids with human placental microsomal cytochrome P-450. Chem. Biol. Interact. **15:** 337–347.
11. PHILLIPSON, A. 1982. Pharmacokinetics of ampicillin in pregnancy. J. Infect. Dis. **136:** 370–376.
12. ZASJE, D.E., R.J. CIPOLLE, R.G. STRATE *et al.* 1980. Rapid gentamicin elimination in obstetric patients. Obstet. Gynecol. **56:** 559–564.
13. BRIGGS, G.G., R.K. FREEMAN & S.J. YAFFE. 1994. Drugs in Pregnancy and Lactation. : 695, 814–815. Williams & Wilkins. Baltimore, MD.
14. O'SULLIVAN, M.J., P.J. BOYER, G.B. SCOTT *et al.* 1993. The pharmacokinetics and safety of zidovudine in the third trimester of pregnancy for women infected with human immunodeficiency virus and their infants: Phase I Acquired Immunodeficiency Syndrome Clinical Trials Group Study (protocol 082). Am. J. Obstet. Gynecol. **168:** 1510–1516.

15. WATTS, H.D., Z.A. BROWN, T. TARTAGLIONE *et al.* 1991. Pharmacokinetic disposition of zidovudine during pregnancy. J. Infect. Dis. **163:** 226–232.
16. CENTERS FOR DISEASE CONTROL AND PREVENTION. 1998. Public Health Service task force recommendations for the use of antiretroviral drugs in pregnant women infected with HIV-1 for maternal health and for reducing perinatal HIV-1 transmission in the United States. MMWR 47(No. RR-2) : 1–30.
17. WANG, Y., E. LIVINGSTON, S. PATIL *et al.* 2000. Pharmacokinetics of didanosine (ddI) in antepartum and postpartum HIV-infected pregnant women and their neonates. J. Infect. Dis. In press.
18. MIROCHNICK, M., S. SIMINSKI, T. FENTON *et al.* 1999. Pharmacokinetics of nevirapine in infants following in utero exposure [abstr.]. Pediatr. Res. **45:** 168A.
19. BRYSON, Y. Unpublished data.
20. CONNOR, E.M., R.S. SPERLING, R. GELBER *et al.* 1994 Reduction of maternal-infant transmission of human immunodeficiency virus type 1 with zidovudine treatment. N. Engl. J. Med. **331:** 1173–1180.
21. DORENBAUM, A., J.H. RODMAN, M. MIROCHNICK, *et al.* 2000. Systemic pharmacokinetics (PK) of oral zivovudine (ZDV) given during labor to HIV-1 infected pregnant women during labor and delivery. Presented at the Seventh Conference on Retroviruses and Opponunistic Infections. San Fransco, CA, Februray 2.
22. FURMAN, P.A., J.A. FYFE, M.H. ST. CLAIR *et al.* 1986. Phosphorylation of 3'-azido-3'-deoxythymidine and selective interaction of the 5'-triphosphate with human immunodeficiency virus reverse transcriptase. Proc. Natl. Acad. Sci. USA **83:** 8333–8337.
23. SHAFFER, N., R. CHUACHOOWONG, P.A. MOCK *et al.* 1999. Short-course zidovudine for perinatal HIV-1 transmission in Bangkok, Thailand: a randomised controlled trial. Lancet **353:** 773–780.
24. WIKTOR, S.Z., E. EKPINI, J.M. KARON *et al.* 1999. Short-course oral zidovudine for prevention of mother-to-child transmission of HIV-1 in Abidjan, Cote d'Ivoire: a randomised trial. Lancet **353:** 781–785.
25. DABIS, F., P. MSELLATI, N. MEDA *et al.* 1999. Six month efficacy, tolerance, and acceptability of a short regimen of oral zidovudine to reduce vertical transmission of HIV in breastfed children in Cote d'Ivoire and Burkina Faso: a double-blind placebo-controlled multicentre trial. Lancet **353:** 786–792.
26. NAU, H. & S.L. PLONAIT. 1992. Physicochemical and structural properties regulating placental drug transfer. *In* Fetal and Neonatal Physiology. R.A. Polin & W.W. Fox, Eds.: 146–160. W.B. Saunders Co. Philadelphia, PA.
27. SANDBERG, J.A. & W. SLIKKER. 1995. Developmental pharmacology and toxicology of anti-HIV therapeutic agents: dideoxynucleosides. FASEB J. **9:** 1157–1163.
28. MOODLEY, J., K. MOODLEY, K. PILLAY *et al.* 1998. Pharmacokinetics and antiretroviral activity of lamivudine alone or when coadministered with zidovudine in human immunodeficiency virus type 1-infected pregnant women and their offspring. J. Infect. Dis. **178:** 1327–1333.
29. MIROCHNICK M., T. FENTON, P. GAGNIER *et al.* 1998. Pharmacokinetics of nevirapine in human immunodeficiency virus type-1 infected pregnant women and their neonates. J. Infect. Dis. **178:** 368–374.
30. MUSOKE, P., L. GUAY, D. BAGENDA *et al.* 1999. A phase I study of the safety and pharmacokinetics of nevirapine in HIV-1 infected pregnant Ugandan women and their neonates. AIDS **13:** 479–486.
31. DORENBAUM, A., J.L. SULLIVAN, Y. BRYSON *et al.* 1998 Antiretroviral Use in Pregnancy in PACTG **316:** a Phase III Randomized, Blinded Study of Single-Dose Intrapartum/Neonatal Nevirapine to Reduce Mother to Infant HIV Transmission [abstr.]. 12th International Conference on AIDS. Geneva, Switzerland.
32. MORRIS, A., C. ZORRILLA, M. VAJARANANT *et al.* 1999. A review of protease inhibitors (PI) use in 89 pregnancies [abstr.]. 6th Conference on Retroviruses and Opportunistic Infections. Chicago, IL.
33. STEK, A., M. KHOURY, F. KRAMER *et al.* 1999. Maternal and infant outcomes with highly active antiretroviral therapy during pregnancy [abstr.]. 6th Conference on Retroviruses and Opportunistic Infections. Chicago, IL.

34. CULNANE, M., M.G. FOWLER, S.S. LEE *et al.* 1999. Lack of long-term effects of in utero exposure to zidovudine among uninfected children born to HIV-infected women. JAMA **281:** 151–157.

35. MORSELLI, P.L., R. FRANCO-MORSELLI & L. BOSSI. 1980. Clinical pharmacokinetics in newborns and infants: age-related differences and therapeutic implications. Clin. Pharmacokinet. **5:** 485–527.

36. HEIMANN, G. 1980. Enteral absorption and bioavailability in children in relation to age. Eur. J. Clin. Pharmacol. **18:** 43–50.

37. REED, M.D. & J.B. BESUNDER. 1989. Developmental pharmacology: ontogenic basis of drug disposition. Pediatr. Clin. North Am. **36:** 1053–1074.

38. NAGOURNEY, B.A. & J.V. ARANDA. 1998. Physiologic differences of clinical significance. *In* Fetal and Neonatal Physiology. R.A. Polin & W.W. Fox, Eds. : 239–249. W.B. Saunders Co. Philadelphia, PA.

39. JOHN, G.J. & J.P. GUIGNARD. 1998 Development of renal excretion of drugs during ontogeny. *In* Fetal and Neonatal Physiology. R.A. Polin & W.W Fox, Eds. : 188–193. W.B. Saunders Co. Philadelphia, PA.

40. GREGUS, Z. & C.D. KLASASEN. 1998. Hepatic disposition of xenobiotics during prenatal and early postnatal development. *In* Fetal and Neonatal Physiology. R.A. Polin & W.W. Fox, Eds. :1472–1493. W.B. Saunders Co. Philadelphia, PA.

41. GUAY, L., P. MUSOKE, T. FLEMING *et al.* 2000. A randomized trial of nevirapine versus azidothymidine for prevention of mother-to-infant transmission of HIV-1 in Kampala, Uganda (HIVNET 012). Lancet. In press.

42. BOUCHER, F.D., J.A. MODLIN, S. WELLER *et al.* 1993. Phase one evaluation of zidovudine administered to infants exposed at birth to the human immunodeficiency virus. J. Pediatr. **122:** 137–144.

43. MIROCHNICK, M., E. CAPPARELLI & J. CONNOR. 2000. Zidovudine pharmacokinetics in infants: a population analysis across studies. Clin. Pharmacol. Ther. In press.

44. RAJAONARISON, J.F., B. LACARELLE, G. DE SOUSA *et al.* 1991. In vitro glucuronidation of 3′azido-3′-deoxythymidine by human liver: role of UDP-gluronyltransferase 2 Form. Drug. Metab. Dispos. **19:** 809–824.

45. HERBER, R., J. MAGDALOU, M. HAUMONT *et al.* 1992. Glucuronidation of 3′-azido-3′-deoxythymidine in human liver microsomes: enzyme inhibition by drugs and steroid hormones. Biochim. Biophys. Acta **1139:** 220–224.

46. MIROCHNICK, M., E. CAPPARELLI, W. DANKNER *et al.* 1998. Zidovudine pharmacokinetics in premature infants exposed to HIV. Antimicrob. Agents Chemother. **42:** 808–812.

47. LAMSON, M.J., S. CORT, J.P. SABO *et al.* 1996. Effects of gender on the single and multiple dose pharmacokinetics of nevirapine 200 mg/day [abstr.]. XI International Conference on AIDS, Vancouver, Canada.

48. LEEDER, J.S. & G.L. KEARNS. 1997. Pharmacogenetics in pediatrics: implications for practice. Pediatr. Clin. North Am. **44:** 55–77.

49. MIROCHNICK, M., T. FENTON, P. GAGNIER *et al.* 1998. Pharmacokinetics of nevirapine in human immunodeficiency virus type-1 infected pregnant women and their neonates. J. Infect. Dis. **178:** 368–374.

50. LUZURIAGA, K., Y. BRYSON, G. MCSHERRY *et al.* 1996. Pharmacokinetics, safety and activity of nevirapine in human immunodeficiency virus type 1-infected children. J. Infect. Dis. **174:** 713–721.

51. LAMSON, M. Unpublished data.

52. HEALD, A.E., P.H. HSYU, G.J. YUEN *et al.* 1996. Pharmacokinetics of lamivudine in human immunodeficiency virus-infected patients with renal dysfunction. Antimicrob. Agents Chemother. **40:** 1514–1519.

53. MUELLER, B.U., L.L. LEWIS, G.J. YUEN *et al.* 1998. Serum and cerebrospinal fluid pharmacokinetics of intravenous and oral lamivudine in human immunodeficiency virus-infected children. Antimicrob. Agents Chemother. **42:** 3187–3192.

54. BANGSBERG, D.R., F.M. HECHT, E.C. CHARLEBOIS *et al.* 1999. Spontaneous adherence (ADH) audits (SAA) predict ciral suppression in the REACH cohort [abstr.]. 6th Conference on Retroviruses and Opportunistic Infections. Chicago, IL.

Evaluation of Immune Survival Factors in Pediatric HIV-1 Infection

WILLIAM T. SHEARER,[a,b] KIRK A. EASLEY,[c] JOHANNA GOLDFARB,[c] HAL B. JENSON,[d] HOWARD M. ROSENBLATT,[b] ANDREA KOVACS,[e] AND KENNETH MCINTOSH[f] FOR THE P²C² HIV STUDY GROUP

[b]Department of Pediatrics, Baylor College of Medicine, Houston, Texas 77030, USA

[c]Cleveland Clinic Foundation, Cleveland, Ohio, USA

[d]University of Texas Health Science Center, San Antonio, Texas, USA

[e]LAC and University of Southern California Medical Center, Los Angeles, California, USA

[f]Boston Children's Hospital/Harvard Medical School, Boston, Massachusetts, USA

ABSTRACT: Peripheral blood CD4⁺ and CD8⁺ T cells, CD19⁺/20⁺ B cells, and serum immunoglobulins (Igs) have been implicated as survival factors for pediatric HIV-1 infection. To determine which of these immune factors might be important in predicting survival, we studied HIV-1 vertically infected (HIV-1⁺) children over a 5-year period. Peripheral blood lymphocytes and Igs were measured in 298 HIV-1⁺ children, who were classified as survivors or nonsurvivors, and in 463 HIV-1 vertically exposed and noninfected (HIV-1⁻) children. Measurements of other possible survival factors were included in this study: albumin, hemoglobin, lactic dehydrogenase (LDH), and HIV-1 RNA levels. Survivors had significantly higher CD4⁺ T-cell, CD8⁺ T-cell, and CD19⁺/CD20⁺ B-cell counts and serum IgG levels, but lower serum IgA and IgM levels than nonsurvivors. Serum albumin and blood hemoglobin levels were higher, but serum LDH and HIV-1 RNA levels were lower in the survivors compared to nonsurvivors. In univariable analysis, factors affecting survival were baseline CD4⁺ T-cell and CD8⁺ T-cell counts, IgG, albumin, hemoglobin, LDH, and HIV-1 RNA (all $p < 0.001$). In multivariable analysis, high baseline CD4⁺ T-cell count, IgG and albumin levels, and low baseline HIV-1 RNA load remained important factors for survival. Serum IgG level has been identified as an immune factor that independently predicts survival, in addition to the already established CD4⁺ T-cell count. The HIV-1 RNA and serum albumin levels also predicted survival.

INTRODUCTION

A preliminary report of the immune function of the children enrolled in the National Institutes of Health National Heart, Lung and Blood Institute P²C² HIV-1 Study recorded the measurements of CD4⁺ (helper) T cells and CD8⁺ (cytotoxic) T cells in HIV-1⁺ children followed for less than 24 months of the 60-month study.[1]

[a]Address for correspondence: William T. Shearer, M.D., Ph.D., Texas Children's Hospital, 6621 Fannin Street (MC 1-3291), Houston, TX 77030. Voice: 713-770-1274; fax: 713-770-7131. wshearer@bcm.tmc.edu

Results of this study showed an early and continuing loss of $CD4^+$ T cells through 17 months of age in HIV-1$^+$ children and an early rise at 2–4 months followed by a decline of $CD4^+$ T cells in HIV-1$^-$ children, although at 17 months the mean cell count was higher by 1,200 cells/µl. There was an expansion of the $CD8^+$ T-cell population, beginning as early as 2 months of age in some HIV-1-infected children and rising to 50% of the peripheral blood mononuclear cell population. There was 70% mortality in HIV-1$^+$ children with fewer than 200 $CD4^+$ T cells/µl.[1]

Several large-scale, multicenter studies have identified the peripheral blood $CD4^+$ T-cell count, and plasma or serum HIV-1 RNA level as important predictors of survival in HIV-1$^+$ children.[2–4] Earlier studies of antibody function demonstrated the extraordinarily elevated serum concentrations of IgG, IgA, and IgM.[5–7] Measurements of antibody responses to T-cell-dependent recall antigens (e.g., diphtheria and tetanus toxoid) or neoantigen (e.g., bacteriophage φX174) demonstrated mostly weak primary antibody (IgM) responses and severely reduced secondary antibody (IgG) responses.[8–11] This failure to switch from an IgM to an IgG antibody (long-lived, high-affinity, memory antibody) is probably due to the lack of $CD4^+$ (helper) T cells, which generate a second signal to B cells upon cognate recognition of antigen.[12]

This report of the peripheral blood immune cells and serum immunoglobulins in the completed P^2C^2 HIV Study cohort will evaluate the importance of these immune survival factors identified in studies of HIV-1$^+$ children.[13–18]

METHODS

Study Population and Informed Consent

The P^2C^2 HIV Study population has been described fully elsewhere, with explanations of recruitment, examinations, laboratory and clinical tests, quality assessment, and data analysis.[19] Briefly, a group of 600 study subjects born to HIV-1$^+$ women were enrolled at birth or by 28 days of life (birth cohort) beginning in 1990 and followed prospectively for up to 6 years. This group comprised 93 HIV-1$^+$, 463 HIV-1$^-$, and 44 HIV-1-indeterminate infants. Another group of 205 infants and children with HIV-1 infection were enrolled at greater than 28 days of life (older cohort) between 1990 and 1993 and were similarly followed for up to 6 years. Infants and children in both cohorts were examined at regular intervals of 3–6 months.

Definitions of HIV-1 Disease Survival

A survivor was defined as a child who survived for 5 years after enrollment into study or a child who was alive when lost to follow-up. A nonsurvivor was defined as a child who died during the course of this study.

Examinations of Subjects

Study subjects had periodic physical examinations and laboratory tests, including complete blood count, lymphocyte counts ($CD4^+$, $CD8^+$, $CD19^+/20^+$ lymphocytes), serum Ig measurements (IgG, IgA, IgM), serum albumin, blood hemoglobin, LDH, and HIV-1 RNA. Laboratory tests and interpretation of physical measurements were quality-controlled.[19] Serum Ig data from children who had IgG replacement therapy within 90 days (≥ 4 half-lives of IgG) were excluded from analysis. CD4$^+$ and CD8$^+$ T cells and CD19$^+$/20$^+$ B cells were determined by two- or three-color fluorescence-activated flow cytometry in laboratories certified by the National Institute of Allergy and Infectious Diseases Division of AIDS Quality Assurance Program. Absolute numbers of lymphocyte subsets were determined arithmetically on the basis of complete blood counts performed on the same blood sample. Serum was analyzed for immunoglobulin concentrations by laser nephelometry. Hemoglobin concentrations were measured by local hematology laboratories as part of the complete blood count, and serum albumin and LDH levels were measured by local chemistry laboratories. Serum (81% of the subjects) was frozen at $-70°C$, stored in a central repository, thawed once, and analyzed for HIV-1 RNA concentration by quantitative HIV-1 RNA polymerase chain reaction (PCR) using the Amplicor HIV-1 Monitor Test (Roche Diagnostic Systems, Branchburg, NJ).[2,18]

Statistical Analysis

Because the cumulative 5-year survival was similar for the two HIV-1-infected cohorts (65.6% for the older cohort after 5 years of follow-up and 67.3% for the birth cohort at 5 years of age), they were combined across the overlapping ages (1 month to 5 years) for data analysis (168 from the older cohort and 91 from the birth cohort). This was done to ensure reasonable sample sizes across the 5-year period for survivors and nonsurvivors.

Repeated-measures analyses of lymphocyte phenotypes (cube-root transformation of counts), serum Ig (natural log), serum albumin, hemoglobin, LDH (natural log), and HIV-1 RNA ($\log_{10}$) were performed using the SAS mixed linear models procedure, which provided estimates of the mean and 95% confidence intervals at each age by HIV-1 status and by survivorship. Reported p values are two-sided and are considered significant at $p \leq 0.05$.

Cumulative survival was estimated with the Kaplan-Meier method. Log-rank tests were used to compare survival according to the baseline measurements of lymphocyte counts, serum Ig levels, serum proteins, and HIV-1 RNA viral burden, with groups defined as above or below the median value for each covariate.

To assess the simultaneous effect of baseline factors on survival time, Cox's proportional-hazards regression model was used. Forward and backward stepwise selections were used to choose variables for the multivariable model. Only factors that were significant at $p \leq 0.05$ in the univariable analyses were included in the multivariable analyses. The relative risk and 95% confidence interval were calculated for each factor in the presence of the others in the final model.

RESULTS

Patient Study Groups

The demographic and clinical characteristics of the children in this study are given in TABLE 1. Most children (87%) were members of minority groups, and the distributions of races in the survival categories were roughly equal. Similarly, the sex distribution of children in the disease categories was approximately equal. Over 60%

TABLE 1. Demographic and clinical characteristics of children born to HIV-1–infected women

Characteristic	Children enrolled from birth and up to 28 days of age (birth cohort)				Children enrolled after 28 days of age (older cohort) HIV-1[+] (n = 205)			
	HIV-1[+] (n = 93)		HIV-1[−] (n = 463)		Survivors[a] (n = 134)		Nonsurvivors[a] (n = 71)	
Race								
African-American	41	(44.1)	245	(52.9)	59	(44.0)	30	(42.3)
Hispanic	32	(34.4)	138	(29.8)	48	(35.8)	34	(47.9)
White	15	(16.1)	54	(11.7)	22	(16.4)	6	(8.5)
Other	5	(5.4)	26	(5.6)	5	(3.7)	1	(1.4)
Sex								
Male	44	(47.3)	249	(53.8)	60	(44.8)	34	(47.9)
Female	49	(52.7)	214	(46.2)	74	(55.2)	37	(52.1)
CDC Pediatric Disease Classification (1994)[b]								
Asymptomatic	59	(63.4)			20	(14.9)	5	(7.0)
Mild (Category A)	16	(17.2)			31	(23.1)	4	(5.6)
Moderate (Category B)	11	(11.8)			25	(18.7)	10	(14.1)
Severe (Category C)	7	(7.5)			58	(43.3)	52	(73.2)

NOTE: Figures given represent frequency with percent given in parentheses.
[a]Defined at end of 5-year study regardless of age at enrollment.
[b]Most severe symptom status by 3 months of age for HIV-1[+] children followed from birth and at the time of enrollment for the older HIV-1[+] cohort (median enrollment age = 23 months).[20]

of the HIV-1[+] birth cohort was asymptomatic at 3 months of age, but only 12.2% of the HIV-1[+] older cohort was asymptomatic at enrollment (median ages of survivors and nonsurvivors were 22 and 26 months, respectively). By 2 years of age, only 10.5% of the birth cohort remained asymptomatic; cumulative mortality was 16.3%; and 46.8% had died or reached Centers for Disease Control and Prevention category C.[20] Virtually all study children (over 90%) took antiretroviral medications (principally zidovudine and dideoxyinosine) at some time during the study period; 29 HIV-1[+] children (9.7%) took protease inhibitors (ritonavir, nelfinavir, saquinavir, or indinavir) when they were over 2 years of age; 38% of study subjects received intravenous IgG at some time during the study period.

Lymphocyte Subsets

At all ages the survivors had significantly higher CD4[+] T-cell counts compared to the nonsurvivors ($p < 0.001$) but their CD4[+] T-cell counts were lower than those of the HIV-1[−] controls values (FIG. 1A).

Mean CD8[+] T-cell numbers in survivors were always higher than those of the nonsurvivors ($p \leq 0.001$) (FIG. 1B). Nonsurvivors and HIV-1[−] controls had similar CD8[+] T-cell counts at the earliest ages ($p = 0.21$ at <1 year) but then nonsurvivors

1A.

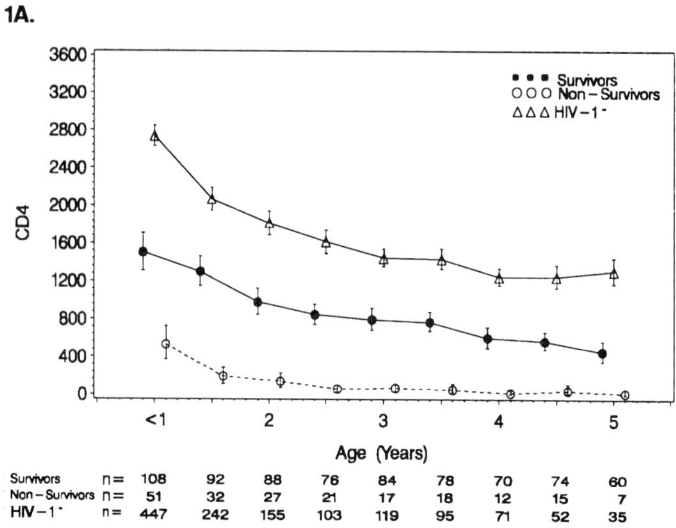

1B.

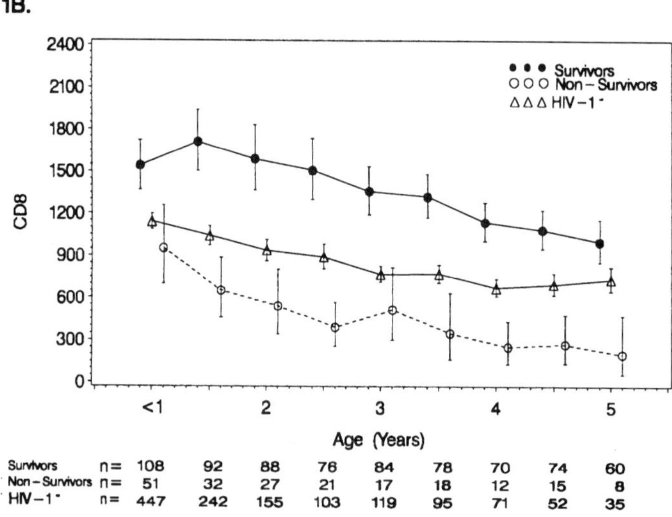

FIGURE 1A,B. Longitudinal changes in mean peripheral blood lymphocyte counts (cells/μl) and serum Igs (mg/dl) in children born to HIV-1-infected women. The lines represent the model-based means and 95% confidence intervals. The mean age of the infants at the time of first immunological study was 8.6 months (range 1.0–12.0 months). **(A)** CD4[+] T-cell counts ($n = 174$ survivors, $n = 81$ nonsurvivors, and 453 HIV-1⁻ controls). **(B)** CD8[+] T-cell counts ($n = 174$ survivors, $n = 81$ nonsurvivors, and $n = 453$ HIV-1⁻ controls).

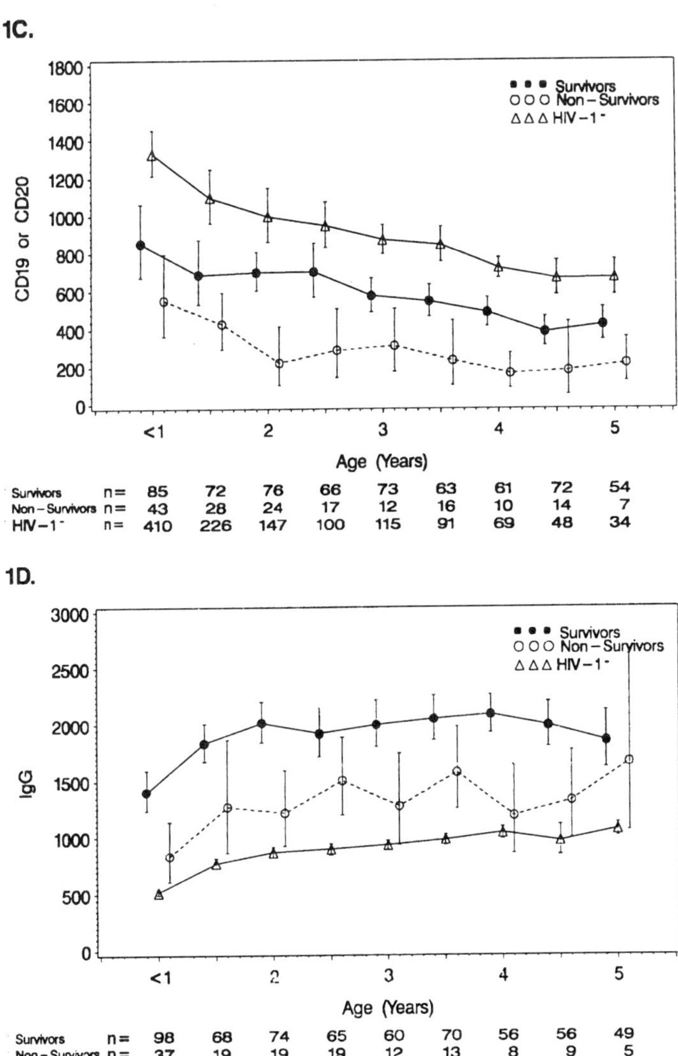

FIGURE 1C,D. See FIGURE 1A,B legend. **(C)** CD19$^+$ or CD20$^+$ B-cell counts ($n = 164$ survivors, $n = 72$ nonsurvivors, and $n = 435$ HIV-1$^-$ controls). **(D)** Serum IgG ($n = 159$ survivors, $n = 63$ nonsurvivors, and $n = 447$ HIV-1$^-$ controls).

1E.

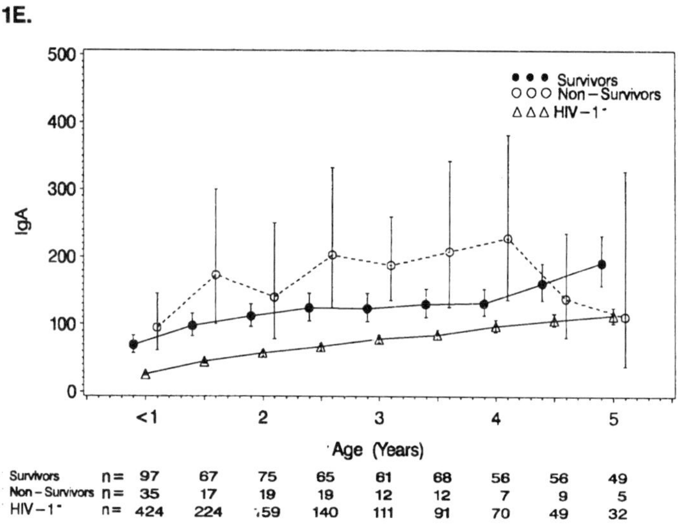

1F.

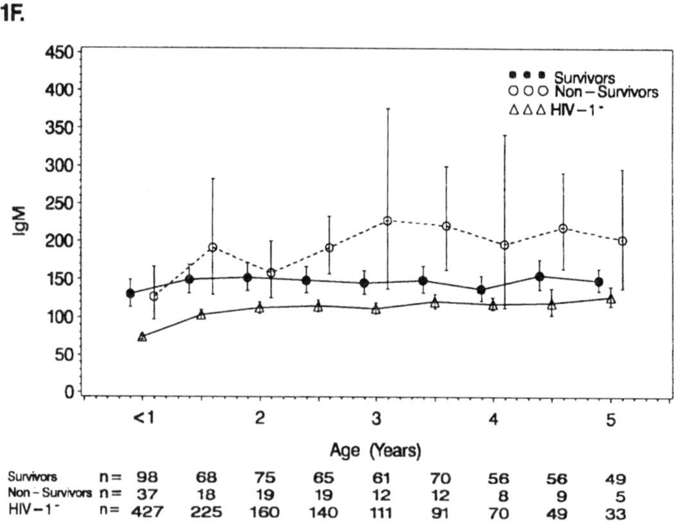

FIGURE 1E,F. See FIGURE 1A,B legend. (**E**) Serum IgA ($n = 159$ survivors, $n = 62$ nonsurvivors, and $n = 445$ HIV-1⁻ controls). (**F**) Serum IgM ($n = 159$ survivors, $n = 62$ nonsurvivors, and $n = 445$ HIV-1⁻ controls).

began to lose $CD8^+$ T cells as they grew older and demonstrated $CD8^+$ T-cell values lower than those of the $HIV-1^-$ controls (all p values ≤ 0.007 except at 2.5–3.0 years $[p = 0.10]$).

Survivors had significantly higher mean $CD19^+/20^+$ B-cell counts than did the nonsurvivors at most ages (< 1 year $[p = 0.05]$, 1.0–1.5 years $[p = 0.03]$, 1.5–2.0 years $[p < 0.001]$, 2.0–2.5 years $[p = 0.003]$, 2.5–3.0 years $[p = 0.02]$, 3.0–3.5 years $[p = 0.01]$, 3.5–4.0 years $[p < 0.001]$, 4.0–4.5 years $[p = 0.11]$ and 4.5–5.0 years $[p = 0.01]$ (FIG. 1C). Both suvivors and nonsurvivors had values well below those of the $HIV-1^-$ controls with nonsurvivors being the lowest category.

Serum Immunoglobulin Concentrations

Survivors had higher mean serum IgG values than nonsurvivors (< 1 year $[p = 0.003]$, 1.0–1.5 years $[p = 0.07]$, 1.5–2.0 years $[p < 0.001]$, 2.0–2.5 years $[p = 0.06]$, 2.5–3.0 years $[p = 0.008]$, 3.0–3.5 years $[p = 0.04]$, 3.5–4.0 years $[p < 0.001]$, 4.0–4.5 years $[p = 0.009]$, and 4.5–5.0 years $[p = 0.66]$ (FIG. 1D). Both survivor and nonsurvivor IgG mean values were extremely elevated compared to the $HIV-1^-$ controls, with the survivor values being highest.

The survivors, in general, had lower mean serum IgA concentrations than the nonsurvivors through 4 years of age (1.0–1.5 years $[p = 0.05]$, 2.5–3.0 years $[p = 0.03]$, and 3.5–4.0 years $[p = 0.04]$) (FIG. 1E). Both survivors and nonsurvivors had mean values of serum IgA above the $HIV-1^-$ controls, with the survivor values being closer to the controls.

Survivors generally had lower mean serum IgM concentrations than the nonsurvivors (2.0–2.5 years $[p = 0.03]$, 3.0–3.5 years $[p = 0.02]$, and 4.0–5.0 years $[p = 0.03]$) (FIG. 1F). The $HIV-1^-$ controls had mean IgM values below both other groups, but were closer to the survivors.

Albumin, Hemoglobin, and LDH

We also studied serum albumin, blood hemoglobin, and serum LDH levels (FIG. 2). Survivors had higher mean albumin ($p \leq 0.007$ at all ages, FIG. 2A), higher mean hemoglobin (< 1 year $[p = 0.03]$ and $p \leq 0.002$ at all other ages, FIG. 2B), but lower LDH mean levels ($p \leq 0.003$ at all ages, FIG. 2C). The $HIV-1^-$ controls exhibited mean values of serum albumin and blood hemoglobin that were higher than the other two groups but closest to the survivors, whereas the $HIV-1^-$ controls had lower mean LDH levels than both $HIV-1^+$ groups but very close to the survivors before age two.

HIV-1 RNA Viral Burden of Infected Children

Mean levels of HIV-1 RNA were lower at all but one age for surviving children compared to nonsurvivors (< 1 year–2.5 years $[p \leq 0.002]$, 2.5–3.0 years $[p = 0.28]$, and 3.0–5.0 years $[p \leq 0.02]$, FIG. 2D). For infants less than 1 year of age, mean HIV-1 RNA levels were significantly higher in nonsurvivors (geometric mean = 243,355 copies/ml) compared to survivors (geometric mean = 39,196 copies/ml, $p < 0.001$).

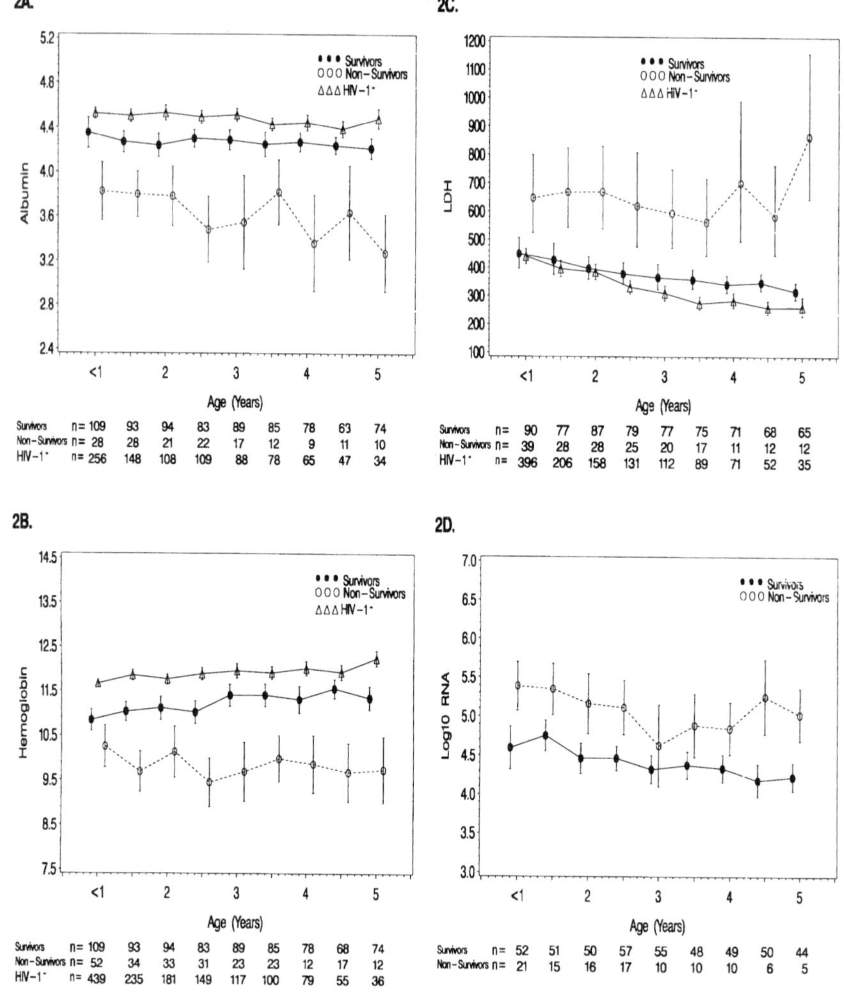

FIGURE 2. Longitudinal changes in proteins and HIV-1 RNA in children born to HIV-1-infected women. The lines represent the model-based means and 95% confidence intervals. (**A**) Albumin (g/dl) ($n = 168$ survivors, $n = 66$ nonsurvivors, and $n = 323$ HIV-1$^-$ controls). (**B**) Hemoglobin (g/dl) ($n = 176$ survivors, $n = 81$ nonsurvivors, and $n = 449$ HIV-1$^-$ controls). (**C**) Lactic dehydrogenase (international units [IU]/l) ($n = 170$ survivors, $n = 76$ nonsurvivors, and $n = 439$ HIV-1$^-$ controls). (**D**) Log$_{10}$ HIV-1 RNA (copies/ml) ($n = 142$ survivors and $n = 47$ nonsurvivors).

TABLE 2. Cumulative survival among 259 HIV-1-infected children according to baseline laboratory measurements

Measurement		Total n	Deaths n	(%)	5-year cumulative survival $\pm$ SE	p Value
CD4 cell count	$\geq$ Median	128	13	(10.2)	89.8 $\pm$ 2.8	
	< Median	127	68	(53.5)	57.4 $\pm$ 4.5	<0.001
CD8 cell count	$\geq$ Median	127	25	(19.7)	85.2 $\pm$ 3.4	
	< Median	128	56	(43.8)	61.9 $\pm$ 4.4	<0.001
CD19 or CD20 cell count	$\geq$ Median	118	27	(22.9)	80.3 $\pm$ 3.8	
	< Median	118	45	(38.1)	69.0 $\pm$ 4.4	0.07
IgG	$\geq$ Median	111	23	(20.7)	89.5 $\pm$ 3.0	
	< Median	111	40	(36.0)	61.5 $\pm$ 4.9	<0.001
IgA	$\geq$ Median	112	35	(31.3)	70.3 $\pm$ 4.5	
	< Median	109	28	(25.7)	82.4 $\pm$ 3.8	0.07
IgM	$\geq$ Median	108	36	(33.3)	75.5 $\pm$ 4.3	
	< Median	113	26	(23.0)	76.8 $\pm$ 4.2	0.47
Albumin	$\geq$ Median	132	16	(12.1)	91.1 $\pm$ 2.6	
	< Median	102	50	(49.0)	56.4 $\pm$ 5.1	<0.001
Hemoglobin	$\geq$ Median	138	31	(22.5)	83.1 $\pm$ 3.2	
	< Median	119	50	(42.0)	61.3 $\pm$ 4.9	<0.001
LDH	$\geq$ Median	123	51	(41.5)	62.8 $\pm$ 4.7	
	< Median	123	25	(20.3)	86.5 $\pm$ 3.2	<0.001
HIV-1 RNA	$\geq$ Median	94	32	(34.0)	68.5 $\pm$ 5.1	
	< Median	95	15	(15.8)	89.9 $\pm$ 3.2	<0.001

NOTE: The median age of the children at the first available test was 9.8 months.

Survival Analysis

Univariable Survival

There was a 5-year cumulative survival rate of 72.3% in the 259 HIV-1[+] children (83 deaths). Survival was associated with higher baseline CD4[+] T-cell counts and higher baseline CD8[+] T-cell counts by univariable analysis (TABLE 2). Children with higher baseline CD19[+] or CD20[+] B-cell counts also tended to have higher survival ($p = 0.07$). Survival was also associated with higher baseline levels of albumin, hemoglobin, and lower LDH. Higher baseline levels of IgG predicted better 5-year survival than lower baseline levels of IgG (89.5% and 61.5%, respectively). Lower baseline HIV-1 RNA levels also predicted 5-year survival.

TABLE 3. Multivariable analysis of factors associated with survival for children infected with HIV-1

Effect	Relative risk of death	95% CI	*p* Value
3A			
CD4 cell count (per 500 cells/μl decrease)	1.76	1.35–2.28	<0.001
Serum IgG (per 500 mg/dl decrease)	1.44	1.20–1.74	<0.001
Albumin (per 0.5 g/dl decrease)	1.53	1.25–1.86	<0.001
3B			
CD4 cell count (per 500 cells/μl decrease)	1.45	1.11–1.91	0.007
Serum IgG (per 500 mg/dl decrease)	1.52	1.20–1.52	<0.001
Albumin (per 0.5 g/dl decrease)	2.20	1.52–3.19	<0.001
HIV-1 RNA (per 0.5 log10 unit increase)	1.27	1.02–1.57	0.03

Multivariable Modeling of Survival

Multivariable analyses were affected by missing data and the correlation among the laboratory measurements. The sample sizes for the laboratory measurements were 257 for hemoglobin, 255 for CD4[+] and CD8[+] T-cell counts, 249 for LDH, 236 for CD19[+] or CD20[+] B-cell counts, 234 for albumin, 222 for IgG, 221 for IgA and IgM, and 189 for HIV-1 RNA. The correlation between CD4[+] T-cell counts and CD8[+] T-cell counts (Spearman's rho = 0.59, $p < 0.001$) and between albumin and hemoglobin (Spearman's rho = 0.52, $p < 0.001$) was high. Based on these relationships and the results from Cox regression analyses, CD4[+] T-cell count, IgG, albumin, and HIV-1 RNA appear to be the best predictors of survival among the 10 laboratory measurements.

TABLE 3 summarizes the Cox regression analyses. In the final model (205 children, 52 deaths, TABLE 3A), CD4[+] T-cell count, IgG, and albumin were independent prognostic factors of survival after adjusting for baseline age. Factors that did not remain significant included C19[+] or CD20[+] B-cell counts, CD8[+] T-cell count, and LDH. Higher baseline levels of both albumin (adjusted relative risk = 1.67 per 0.5 g/dl decrease) and IgG (adjusted relative risk = 1.48 per 500 mg/dl decrease) thus appeared to provide independent markers of survival after adjustment for CD4[+] T-cell count and age in HIV-1-infected children that may be clinically useful. In a subset analysis of 160 children for whom HIV-1 RNA copy number was available, CD4[+] T-cell count, IgG, and albumin remained associated with survival, as well as HIV-1 RNA copy number ($p = 0.03$, TABLE 3B).

DISCUSSION

This new analysis of the immune factors in the 5-year P[2]C[2] HIV-1 Study has confirmed the projections of the early report.[1] In that report, lower CD4[+] T-cell and higher CD8[+] T-cell counts appeared to be associated with advanced disease in several age categories, as well as with increased morbidity. Here, we extend these findings to demonstrate that the survivor children had a unique age profile of peripheral blood CD4$^+$ T-cells, thus adding useful information about lymphocyte subset counts in various stages of HIV-1 infection. Higher CD4$^+$ T-cell counts were found in survivor children at every age, emphasizing the central role of this T-cell subset in protection from HIV-1 disease progression. At all ages, the CD8$^+$ T-cell counts were higher in survivors than nonsurvivors. At early ages, the numbers of CD8$^+$ T-cells in nonsurvivor children were similar to those of HIV-1$^-$ controls but later fell to lower levels, suggesting the protective role these cells play in HIV-1 infection. Polyclonal stimulation by Epstein-Barr virus and possibly cytomegalovirus may be responsible for the increased number of CD8$^+$ T cells in survivor children.[22,23] Coinfection with Epstein-Barr virus has been associated with increased survival.[13,14,16,17]

In addition to observations on T cells, an interesting finding concerning B-cell regulation of IgG has emerged from univariable analysis, indicating that higher concentration of serum IgG was associated with predicted survival of HIV-1$^+$ children. This discovery was Ig class specific, since serum IgA and IgM concentrations of the survivors were generally lower than those of the nonsurvivors. These observations are consistent with the early reports of lack of immunoglobulin class switching from IgM to IgG production in HIV-1$^+$ patients.[8–10] Thus, nonsurvivors are likely those that can only mount IgM (primary) antibody responses due to lack of adequate T-cell help to switch from IgM to IgG production. Although this report did not find that higher numbers of B cells were important in 5-year survival, other reports have documented decreases in the following: (a) CD19$^+$/CD5$^+$ B-cell compartment in 7- to 12-month-old HIV-1$^+$ infants,[24] (b) CD19+ B-cell numbers in more symptomatic HIV$^+$ children,[25] and (c) functionally active B cells in HIV$^+$-1 patients with low p24 antibody serum titers.[26] Moreover, increased CD19$^+$ B-cell subsets have been described in pediatric HIV-1$^+$ patients given the protease inhibitor ritonavir.[27,28] Both CD19$^+$/CD20$^+$ B-cell counts and serum IgG measurements have been recently shown to be important in the prediction of bacterial infections.[29] The mechanism of elevation of serum Igs in HIV-1 infection may have been partially clarified by the *in vitro* evidence that HIV-1 glycoprotein 120 acts as a superantigen and produces stimulation of several human B-cell functions, including the increased production of Igs.[30] All of these observations indicate the need to re-evaluate the role of B cells and IgG in HIV-1 disease progression and survival.

This update of the P^{2}C^2 HIV-1 Study has examined the measurements of blood T-cell and B-cell counts, Ig, albumin, hemoglobin, LDH, and HIV-1 RNA concentrations in a 5-year study of 298 HIV-1$^+$ children. Serum IgG was discovered to have predictive power for survival, in addition to CD4$^+$ T-cells, HIV-RNA, and serum albumin.

ACKNOWLEDGMENTS

We are grateful to the investigators, the study staff, and the families who participated in the P^{2}C^2 HIV Study. This work was supported by National Heart, Lung, and Blood Institute Grants N01-HR-96037, N01-HR-96038, N01-HR-96039, N01-HR-96040, N01-HR-96041, N01-HR-96042, and N01-HR-960043 and in part by NIH General Clinical Research Center Grants RR-00071, RR-00188, RR-00533, RR-00643, RR-00645, RR-00865, and RR-02172.

REFERENCES

1. SHEARER, W.T., H.M. ROSENBLATT, M.D. SCHLUCHTER, *et al.* 1993. Immunologic targets of HIV infection: T-cells. NICHD IVIG Clinical Trial Group, and the NHLBI P^2C^2 Pediatric Pulmonary and Cardiac Complications of HIV Infection Study Group. Ann. N.Y. Acad. Sci. **693:** 35–51.
2. SHEARER, W.T., T.C. QUINN, P. LaRUSSA, *et al.* 1997. Women and Infants Transmission Study Group. Viral load and disease progression in infants infected with human immunodeficiency virus type 1. N. Engl. J. Med. **336(19):** 1337–1342.
3. PALUMBO, P.E., C. RASKINO, S. FISCUS, *et al.* 1998. Predictive value of quantitative plasma HIV RNA and $CD4^+$ lymphocyte count in HIV-infected infants and children. JAMA **279:** 756–761.
4. MOFENSON, L.M., D.R. HARRIS, K. RICH, *et al.* 1996. Serum HIV-1 p24 antibody, HIV-1 RNA copy number and CD4 lymphocyte percentage are independently associated with risk of mortality in HIV-1 infected children. AIDS **13:** 31–39.
5. BERNSTEIN, L.J., B.Z. KRIEGER, B. NOVICK, *et al.* 1985. Bacterial infection in the acquired immunodeficiency syndrome of children. Pediatr. Infect. Dis. **4:** 472–475.
6. BLANCHE, S., F. LE DEIST, A. FISCHER, *et al.* 1986. Longitudinal study of 18 children with perinatal LAV/HTLV III infection: attempt at prognostic evaluation. J. Pediatr. **109:** 965–970.
7. KRASINSKI, K., W. BORKOWSKY, S. BONK, *et al.* 1988. Bacterial infections in human immunodeficiency virus-infected children. Pediatr. Infect. Dis. J. **7:** 323–328.
8. BERNSTEIN, L.J., H.D. OCHS, R.J. WEDGWOOD, *et al.* 1985. Defective humoral immunity in pediatric acquired immune deficiency syndrome. J. Pediatr. **107:** 352–357.
9. BORKOWSKY, W., C.J. STEELE, S. GRUBMAN, *et al.* 1987. Antibody responses to bacterial toxoids in children infected with human immunodeficiency virus. J. Pediatr. **110:** 563–566.
10. PAHWA, S., S. FIKRIG, R. MENEZ, *et al.* 1986. Pediatric acquired immunodeficiency syndrome: demonstration of B lymphocyte defects in vitro. Diagn. Immunol. **4:** 24–30.
11. RUBINSTEIN, A., Y. MIZRACHI, L. BERNSTEIN, *et al.* 2000. Progressive specific immune attrition after primary, secondary and tertiary immunizations with bacteriophage ϕX174 in asymptomatic HIV-1 infected patients. AIDS **14:** F55–F62.
12. FULEIHAN, R.L. & R.S. GEHA. 1997. X-linked hyper IgM. The immunologist **5:** 133–136.
13. POLLACK, H., M.X. ZHAN, J.T. SAFRIT, *et al.* 1997. $CD8^+$ T-cell-mediated suppression of HIV replication in the first year of life: association with lower viral load and favorable early survival. AIDS **11:** F9–F13.
14. KRASINSKI, K., W. BORKOWSKY, R.S. HOLZMAN, *et al.* 1989. Prognosis of human immunodeficiency virus infection in children and adolescents. Pediatr. Infect. Dis. **8:** 216–220.
15. TOVO, P.A., M. DE MARTINO, C. GABIANO, *et al.* 1992. Prognostic factors and survival in children with perinatal HIV-1 infection. Lancet **339:** 1249–1253.
16. ITALIAN REGISTER FOR HIV INFECTION IN CHILDREN. 1994. Features of children perinatally infected with HIV-1 surviving longer than 5 years. Lancet **343:** 191–195.
17. KLINE, M.W., M.E. PAUL, B. BOHANNON, *et al.* 1995. Characteristics of children surviving to five years of age or older with vertically acquired human immune deficiency infection. Pediatr. AIDS HIV Infect. **6:** 350–353.
18. SHEARER, W.T., S.E. LIPSHULTZ, K.A. EASLEY, *et al.*, for the Pediatric Pulmonary and Cardiovascular Complications of Vertically Transmitted Human Immunodeficiency Virus Study Group. 2000. Alterations in cardiac and pulmonary function in pediatric rapid HIV-1 disease progressors. Pediatrics **105:** e9.
19. THE P2C2 HIV STUDY GROUP. 1996. The Pediatric Pulmonary and Cardiovascular Complications of Vertically Transmitted Human Immunodeficiency Virus (P^2C^2 HIV) Infection Study: design and methods. J. Clin. Epidemiol. **49:** 1285–1294.
20. CENTERS FOR DISEASE CONTROL AND PREVENTION. 1994. 1994 revised classification system for human immunodeficiency virus infection in children less than 13 years of age. Morbid. Mortal. Wkly. Rep. **43(RR-12):** 1–20.

21. LIPSHULTZ, S.E., K.A. EASLEY, E.J. ORAV, *et al.*, for the Pediatric Pulmonary and Cardiac Complications of Vertically Transmitted HIV Infection (P^2C^2 HIV) Study Group. 2000. Cardiac dysfunction and mortality in HIV-infected children: The prospective P^2C^2 HIV multicenter study. Circulation **102:** in press.
22. JENSON, H., K. MCINTOSH, J. PITT, *et al.* 1999. Natural history of primary Epstein-Barr virus infection in children of mothers infected with human immunodeficiency virus type 1. J. Infect. Dis. **179:** 1395–1404.
23. KOVACS, A., M. SCHLUCHTER, K. EASLEY, *et al.* 1999. Cytomegalovirus infection and HIV-1 disease progression in infants born to HIV-1-infected women. Pediatric Pulmonary and Cardiovascular Complications of Vertically Transmitted HIV Infection Study Group. N. Engl. J. Med. **341:** 77–84.
24. IBEGBU, C.H., T.J. SPIRA, S. NESHEIM, *et al.* 1994. Subpopulations of T and B cells in perinatally infected and non-infected age-matched children compared to those in adults. Clin. Immunol. Immunopathol. **71:** 27–32.
25. RODRIGUEZ, C., E.R. STIEHM & S. PLAEGER-MARSHALL. 1993. Peripheral B-cell activation and immaturity in HIV-infected children. Ann. NY. Acad. Sci. **693:** 291–294.
26. TEEUWSEN, V.J., J.M. LANGE, R. KEET, *et al.* 1991. Low number of functionally active B lymphocytes in the peripheral blood of HIV-1-seropositive individuals with low p24-specific serum antibody titers. AIDS **5:** 971–979.
27. SLEASMAN, J.W., R.P. NELSON, M.M. GOODENOW, *et al.* 1999. Immunoreconstitution after ritonavir therapy in children with human immunodeficiency virus infection involves multiple lymphocyte lineages. Pediatrics **134:** 597–606.
28. BORKOWSKY, W., K. STANLEY, S.D. DOUGLAS, *et al.*, and the Pediatric AIDS Clinical Trials Group 338 Study Team. 2000. Immunologic response to combination nucleoside analogue plus protease inhibitor therapy in stable antiretroviral therapy-experienced HIV-infected children. J. Infec. Dis. **182:** 96–103.
29. BETENSKY, R.A., T. CALVELLI & S. PAHWA. 1999. Predictive value of CD19 measurements for bacterial infections in children infected with human immunodeficiency virus. Clin. Diag. Lab. Immunol. **6:** 247–253.
30. PATKE, C.L. & W.T. SHEARER. 2000. gp120- and tumor necrosis factor-α-induced modulation of human B-cell function: proliferation, cAMP generation, immunoglobulin production, and B-cell receptor expression. J. Allergy Clin. Immunol. **105:** 975–982.

Appendix

A complete list of study participants can be found in reference #19.

NATIONAL HEART, LUNG AND BLOOD INSTITUTE

Hannah Peavy, M.D., (Project Officer), Anthony Kalica, Ph.D., Elaine Sloand, M.D., George Sopko, M.D., M.P.H., Margaret Wu, Ph.D.
Chairman of the Steering Committee: Robert Mellins, M.D.

Clinical Centers

Baylor College of Medicine, Houston, TX: William Shearer, M.D., Ph.D.,* Nancy Ayres, M.D., J. Timothy Bricker, M.D., Arthur Garson, Jr., M.D., Peter Hiatt,

*Principal Investigator.

M.D., Debra Kearney, M.D., Howard M. Rosenblatt, M.D., Linda Davis, R.N., B.S.N., Paula Feinman, Mary Beth Mauer, R.N., B.S.N., Ruth McConnell, R.N., B.S.N., Debra Mooneyham, R.N., Teresa Tonsberg, R.N.

The Children's Hospital, Boston/Harvard Medical School, Boston, MA: Steven Lipshultz, M.D.,* Steven Colan, M.D., Andrew Colin, M.D., Ellen Cooper, M.D., Lisa Hornberger, M.D., Kenneth McIntosh, M.D., Marcy Schwartz, M.D., Suzanne Steinbach, M.D., Mary Ellen Wohl, M.D., Helen Donovan, Janice Hunter, M.S., R.N., Karen Lewis, R.N., Ellen McAuliffe, B.S.N., Patricia Ray, B.S., Sonia Sharma, B.S.

Mount Sinai School of Medicine, New York, NY: Meyer Kattan, M.D.,* Stephen Heaton, M.D., David Hodes, M.D., Wyman Lai, M.D., Andrew Ting, M.D., Debbie Benes, M.S., R.N., Diane Carp, M.S.N., R.N., Donna Lewis, Sue Mone, M.S., Mary Ann Worth, R.N.

Presbyterian Hospital in the City of New York/Columbia University, New York, NY: Robert Mellins, M.D.,* Anastossios Koumbourlis, M.D., Jane Pitt, M.D., Thomas Starc, M.D., Anthony Brown, Margaret Challenger, Kim Geromanos, M.S., R.N.

UCLA School of Medicine, Los Angeles, CA: Samuel Kaplan, M.D.,* Yvonne Bryson, M.D., Joseph Church, M.D., Arno Hohn, M.D., Andrea Kovacs, M.D., Barry Marcus, M.D., Arnold Platzker, M.D., Helene Cohen, P.N.P., R.N., Lynn Fukushima, M.S.N., R.N., Audrey Gardner, B.S., Sharon Golden, R.D.M.S., Lucy Kunzman, R.N., M.S., C.P.N.P., Karen Simandle, R.D.M.S., Ah-Lin Wong, R.D.M.S., Toni Ziolkowski, R.N., M.S.N.

Clinical Coordinating Center

The Cleveland Clinic Foundation, Cleveland, OH: Kirk Easley, M.S.,* Michael Kutner, Ph.D. (through 12/99),* Mark Schluchter, Ph.D. (through 4/98),* Richard Martin, M.D. (Case Western Reserve University), Johanna Goldfarb, M.D., Douglas Moodie, M.D., Cindy Chen, M.S., Scott Husak, B.S., Victoria Konig, ART, Sunil Rao, Ph.D., Paul Sartori, B.S., Lori Schnur, B.S., Amrik Shah, Sc.D., Sharayu Shanbhag, B.Sc, Susan Sunkle, B.A., C.C.R.A.

Policy, Data, and Safety Monitoring Board

Henrique Rigatto, M.D., (Chairman), Edward B. Clark, M.D., Robert B. Cotton, M.D., Vijay V. Joshi, M.D., Paul S. Levy, Sc.D., Norman S. Talner, M.D., Patricia Taylor, Ph.D., Robert Tepper, M.D., Ph.D., Janet Wittes, Ph.D., Robert H. Yolken, M.D., Peter E. Vink, M.D.

Immunotherapy for Pregnant Women and Newborns

WILLIAM BORKOWSKY[a]

New York University Medical School, Bellevue Hospital Center, 550 First Avenue, New York, New York 10016, USA

THE CHALLENGE

Transmission of HIV from an infected women to her offspring is a multifactorial process wherein virus can presumably be passed to her fetus (as evidenced by finding HIV DNA in occasional abortuses and in 30% of infected newborns at the time of birth) as well as postpartum at the time of delivery. Critical factors that are determinates of infection are (1) maternal HIV load (whether cell-free or cell-associated), and (2) duration and extent of exposure of the fetus/newborn to maternal blood or vaginal HIV (modified to increased infection by excessive length of ruptured membranes in vaginal delivery, the presence of disruptions in vaginal mucosal integrity, the presence of untreated sexually transmitted diseases such as syphilis and chorioamnionitis, and vitamin A deficiency, or modified to decreased infection by the likelihood of elective cesarean section or antiretroviral therapy). In addition, exposure to breast milk constitutes an ongoing postnatal risk for infection.

STRATEGIES TO MEET THE CHALLENGE

"How to Handle the Women"

Various immunologic approaches have been considered in an attempt to modify or prevent the chances of HIV transmission. Attempts to prevent *in utero* infection would be aimed at reducing maternal viremia at all times during pregnancy, inducing active production and transfer of maternal antibodies to the fetus during the last trimester (which might neutralize), or supplying this antibody passively with hyperimmune immunoglobulin, HIV-specific monoclonal antibodies, or a combination of both. Because there is also an increased risk of transmitting HIV in pregnant women who demonstrate decreased CD8 cell-mediated viral suppression of HIV,[1] a vaccination that augments CD8 anti-HIV responses might also be desirable.

Any strategy aimed at the pregnant women must be proven safe for mother and child. A limited number of vaccine studies demonstrating safety in the mother have been described.[2,3] These include tetanus, influenza, *Hemophilus influenza b*, and hepatitis B vaccination. Other vaccines in the process of being evaluated include vaccines to protect children against group B streptococcal infection, pneumococcal infection, and respiratory syncytial infection.[4,5]

[a]borkow01@gcrc.med.nyu.edu

A vaccine delivered to a pregnant women would obviously need to be immunogenic as a minimal requirement. The fact that even non-HIV–infected pregnant women have some degree of immunodeficiency poses an obstacle to optimal immunization. If possible, any successful vaccination might also result in "vaccination" of the fetus. Maternal infection with rubella virus, cytomegalovirus, and *Toxoplasma gondii* has been shown to induce IgM production in the fetus. The immunization of baboon fetuses with hepatitis B surface antigen during the last trimester also produces antigen-specific IgG in the fetus without inducing immunization of the mother.[6] Early studies in humans suggested that antigen might be available to the fetus when IgM to tetanus toxoid was found in children born to mothers who sometimes received two immunizations during pregnancy.[7,8] A more recent evaluation of tetanus responses (as well as influenza vaccine) after immunization of pregnant women in their last trimester confirmed that the vaccines were immunogenic in women, but no evidence was found that the child was vaccinated in the process.[9]

Only one HIV-specific vaccine study has been performed in pregnant women. This study utilized a recombinant gp120 vaccine (in an alum adjuvant) produced by VaxGen, and it targeted a small number of individuals with more than 400 CD4 cells/mm^3 during the latter half of their pregnancy. Although the vaccine was considered safe, little evidence of an effect on maternal CD4 cell counts, HIV viral titer, or anti-HIV neutralizing antibody was seen in the vaccinees.[10] A recent report[11] of the results of a trial of HIV immunotherapy using this vaccine in an immunologically comparable group of HIV-infected nonpregnant adults suggested that the performance of this vaccine was not related to the state of pregnancy. Clinical findings, CD4 count, and both virological and immunological parameters were followed. No significant differences were observed in the treatment and placebo control groups in the rate of CD4 T-cell decline, time to initiation of antiretroviral therapy, incidence of opportunistic infections, HIV RNA plasma viremia, HIV viral infectivity as measured by quantitative HIV coculture assay, and death.

These findings suggest that a different vaccine might be a better candidate for immunotherapy. A group using a gp160 construct together with zidovudine for 6 months demonstrated some improvement in HIV-specific immune responses.[12] Some have suggested that an HIV gag construct would perform better than an envelope-expressing immunogen. Among the vaccines tested with this in mind was a viral-like particle (VLP-24), an envelope-depleted inactivated whole viral particle (Remune, Agouron Pharmaceuticals), and a DNA-based vaccine (Wyeth-Lederle). The VLP vaccine appears to have limited therapeutic effects in the absence of concurrent antiretroviral therapy.[13] Remune has boosted some cell-mediated and humoral immune responses, but evidence of CD8-mediated antiviral augmentation has not been presented.[14] The DNA vaccine appears to boost some humoral and cell-mediated immune responses, including CD8-mediated cytotoxicity against HIV expressing targets, but no change in CD4 or CD8 counts was seen.[15]

The largely nondramatic effects of active immunotherapy in HIV-infected adults have caused many to focus on passive immunotherapy of pregnant women. A pediatric AIDS Clinical Trials study (ACTG 185) was initiated to test this hypothesis. In this study, infected women with a median of 200 CD4 T cells per cubic millimeter of blood were treated with zidovudine and either standard monthly infusions of gamma globulin or a preparation of hyperimmune gamma globulin with broad neutralizing capability. Unfortunately, this study was terminated because of very low HIV transmission rates in the participants, indicating the need to enroll an excessively large population of pregnant women to attain any statistical confidence in the conclusions. At the end of the study, although the therapies were shown to be safe, there was no significant difference in the transmission rate between the two groups (4.1% in the hyperimmune globulin group [95% confidence interval of 1.6–6.5%] and 6.0% in the standard gamma globulin cohort [95% confidence interval of 2.9–9.0%]; $p = 0.34$).[16] Although this study does not rule out the potential efficacy of a passive immunotherapeutic approach to preventing transmission, the cost of producing and administering either hyperimmune immunoglobulin or monoclonal antibodies to an adult (pregnant woman) is prohibitive in less developed countries than the United States or Europe, where the HIV transmission rate is sufficiently high for a definitive study of efficacy. No HIV-specific monoclonal antibody has yet been tested in pregnant women. However, a recombinant molecule that binds to the CD4 binding site of the virus (CD4-IgG) has been tested in pregnant women and found to be safe and transmitted across the placenta.[17] This molecule can neutralize different strains of virus and consequently has the theoretic potential to perform as well as any monoclonal antibody. Moreover, its ability to neutralize cross-clade make it an attractive prophylactic for use in different parts of the world. A modified molecule, CD4-IgG2, with a longer half-life than that of the monovalent form, is currently being evaluated in phase I studies. In addition, the CD4-IgG2 was designed with four gp120 binding sites in order to have a higher avidity for HIV-1 virions or infected cells than monomeric sCD4 or dimeric CD4-heavy chain constructs.

Pediatric Interventions

The small size of the neonate makes passive immunotherapy an economic reality. The administration of a truly neutralizing anti-HIV antibody shortly after birth could possibly abort HIV infection in those 70% of children who are first exposed to the virus during labor and delivery. Moreover, the timing of HIV transmission also lends itself to a "hepatitis B strategy" of active-passive therapy with an antibody-delaying viral replication, while an incipient cell-mediated immune response provides for "clean-up" and longer-lasting protection (possibly long enough to abort or prevent any breastfeeding-associated transmission. Early sensitization to HIV envelope epitopes might succeed in preventing infection only if such immunization were proven to be immunogenic. Thus far, only hepatitis B vaccine, vaccinia, polio, and BCG have proven to be immunogenic when given at birth. Other vaccines such as tetanus and diphtheria toxoid need to be delayed 1–2 months in order to elicit an immune response.

Beginning in 1994, as part of an ACTG protocol (ACTG 230), children born to HIV-1–infected mothers were immunized at birth and at 1, 3, and 5 months of age with recombinant gp120 vaccines prepared from either SF-2 (Chiron/Biocine [CB]) or MN (VaxGen [VG]) strains of HIV-1. Three concentrations of each immunogen were tested. Of the 126 children who proved to be HIV-uninfected, 21 received adjuvant only. Production of HIV-binding antibody was seen in those uninfected children who received vaccine only. No significant difference in titer was found among the different dosage recipient groups. Vaccine recipients were more likely to develop stimulation indices greater than 3 on two or more occasions (assays performed 1 month after each vaccination and at 52, 76, and 104 weeks) to homologous HIV-1 antigens than were adjuvant recipients (56% vs 14%, p <0.001). Responses could be appreciated at 2 months of age, after two immunizations, and were maintained for more than 84 weeks after the last immunization. An accelerated immunization schedule (birth, 2 weeks, 2 months, and 5 months) was devised to see whether immunization with optimal doses of vaccine could result in earlier responses. Immunization with the lowest dose of CB vaccine resulted in good responses in all 11 vaccinees at as early as 4 weeks of age. Responses to heterologous HIV-1 envelope antigens were also detected. Thus, cell-mediated immune responses to vaccination with this dose of gp120 in MF59 adjuvant are readily achievable at an age when some infection (perinatal infection and that from breast milk exposure) may be prevented. The vaccine proved to be safe, with side effects occurring no more often in those who received vaccine compared to those in the placebo group. Fourteen of the vaccinated children proved to be infected, three *in utero* prior to vaccination. Of the 125 infants reported to have received zidovudine (ZDV) in the first week of life, 9 (7.2%) were HIV infected. No ZDV use in the first week was reported for 58 infants, and 5 (8.6%) of these infants were HIV infected.

Recent studies of second-generation HIV vaccines in newborns are ongoing (ACTG 326). Thus far, vaccination with a canarypox vector expressing gp160 and p24, given at birth and at 3 subsequent monthly intervals, has proven to be safe and to produce lymphoproliferative and cytotoxic T-cell responses to HIV antigens in 20–50% of the vaccinees (J. Lambert and D. Johnson, personal communication). This strategy is being supplemented with a "prime-boost" approach, wherein the vaccinee first receives 2 avipox vaccinations and then 2 recombinant protein immunizations. Studies in seronegative adults who receive a regimen of vaccinia or avipox vaccines followed by gp120 boost appear to make good CTL responses as well as humoral immunity to HIV.[18,19] A newer avipox vaccine (vCP300, Pasteur Merieux), which incorporates HIV nonstructural gene epitopes (pol and nef) with its structural genes, when given together with rgp 120 (Chiron), produced neutralizing antibody to HIV in almost all vaccine recipients after their third dose. In addition, it evoked CD8 CTL in 70% of vaccinees at one of the three study points (3, 4, and 12 months).[20] It is anticipated that vaccination of the newborn with these newer vaccines, including prime boost strategies will be the next generation of vaccines to be tested. However, looming in the background are vaccines based on naked DNA immunogens capable of eliciting CTL[21] and possibly also fusion-competent vaccines, capable of producing broad neutralization of primary isolates of HIV.[22]

REFERENCES

1. PLAEGER, S., S. BERMUDEZ, Y. MIKYAS *et al.* 1999. Decreased CD8 cell-mediated viral suppression and other immunologic characteristics of women who transmit Human Immunodeficiency Virus to their infants. J. Infect. Dis. **179:** 1388–1394.
2. AMERICAN COLLEGE OF OBSTETRICIANS AND GYNECOLOGISTS. 1991. Immunization during pregnancy. Tech. Bull. 160.
3. GLEZEN, W.P., J.A. ENGLUND, G.R. SIBER *et al.* 1992. Maternal immunization with vaccines for *H. influenza* type b. J. Infect. Dis. **165**(suppl): S134–136.
4. ENGLUND, J., W.P. GLEZEN & P.A. PIEDRA. 1998. Maternal immunization against viral disease. Vaccine **16:** 1456–1463.

5. MULHOLLAND, K. 1998. Maternal immunization for the prevention of bacterial infection in young infants. Vaccine **16:** 1464–1467.
6. WATTS, A.M. J.R. STANLEY, M.H. SHEARER *et al.* 1999. Fetal immunization of baboons induces a fetal-specific antibody response. Nature Med. **5:** 427–430.
7. GILL, T.J., C.F. REPETTI, L.A. METLAY *et al.* 1983. Transplacental immunization of the human fetus to tetanus by immunization of the mother. J. Clin. Invest. **72:** 987–996.
8. VANDERBEEKEN, Y., M. SARVATI, R. BOSE *et al.* 1991. *In utero* immunization of the fetus to tetanus by maternal vaccination during pregnancy. Am. J. Reprod. Immunol. **25:** 69–71.
9. ENGLUND, J.A., I.N. MBAWUIKE, H. HAMMILL *et al.* 1993. Maternal immunization with influenza or tetanus toxoid vaccine for passive antibody protection in young infants. J. Infect. Dis. **168:** 647–656.
10. WRIGHT, P.F., J.S. LAMBERT, G.J. GORSE *et al.* 1999. Immunization with envelope MN rgp 120 vaccine in human immunodeficiency virus-infected pregnant women. J. Infect. Dis. **180:** 1080–1085.
11. Tsoukas, C.M., J. Raboud, N.F. Bernard *et al.* 1998l. Active immunization of patients with HIV infection: a study of the effect of VaxSyn, a recombinant HIV envelope subunit vaccine, on progression of immunodeficiency. AIDS Res. & Human Retroviruses **14:** 483–490.
12. LEANDERSSON, A.C., G. BRATT, J. HINKULA et al. 1998. Induction of specific T-cell responses in HIV infection. AIDS **12:** 157–166.
13. KELLEHER, A.D., M. ROGGENSACK, A.B. JARAMILLO *et al.* 1998. Safety and immunogenicity of a candidate therapeutic vaccine, p24 virus-like particle, combined with zidovudine, in asymptomatic subjects. Community HIV Research Network Investigators. AIDS **12:** 175–182.
14. LIMSUWAN, A., V. CHURDBOONCHART, R.B. MOSS *et al.* 1998. Safety and immunogenicity of REMUNE in HIV-infected Thai subjects. Vaccine **16:** 142–149.
15. MACGREGOR, R.R., J.D. BOYER, K.E. UGEN *et al.* 1998. First human trial of a DNA-based vaccine for treatment of human immunodeficiency virus type 1 infection: safety and host response. J. Infect. Dis. **178:** 92–100.
16. STIEHM, E.R., J.S. LAMBERT, L.M. MOFENSON *et al.* 1999. Eficacy of zidovudine and human immunodeficiency virus (HIV) hyperimmune immunoglobulin for reducing perinatal HIV transmission from HIV-infected women with advanced disease: results of Pediatric AIDS Clinical Trials Group Protocol 185. J. Infect. Dis. **179:** 567–575.
17. SHEARER, W.T., A.M. DULIEGE, M.W. KLINE *et al.* 1995. Transport of recombinant human CD4-immunoglobulin G across the human placenta: pharmacokinetics and safety in six mother-infant pairs in AIDS clinical trial group protocol 146. Clin. Diag. Lab. Immunol. **2:** 281–285.
18. COREY, L., M.J. MCELRATH, K. WEINHOLD *et al.* 1998. Cytotoxic T cells and neutralizing antibody responses to human immunodeficiency virus type 1 envelope with a combination vaccine regimen. AIDS Vaccine Evaluation Group. J. Infect. Dis. **177:** 301–309.
19. CLEMENTS-MANN, M.L., K. WEINHOLD, T.J. MATTHEWS *et al.* 1998. Immune response to human immunodeficiency virus (HIV) type 1 induced by canarypox expressing HIV-1 MN gp120, HIV-1 SF2 recombinant gp120, or both vaccines in seronegative adults. NIAID AIDS Vaccine Evaluation Group. J. Infect. Dis. **177:** 1230–1246.
20. EVANS, T.G., M.C. KEEFER, K.J. WEINHOD *et al.* 1999. A canarypox vaccine expressing multiple HIV type 1 genes given alone or with Rgp120 elicits broad and durable CD8+ cytotoxic T lymphocyte responses in seronegative volunteers. J. Infect. Dis. **180:** 290–298.
21. BAGARAZZI, M.L., J.D. BOYER, K.E. UGEN *et al.* 1998. Safety and immunogenicity of HIV-1 DNA constructs in chimpanzees. Vaccine **16:** 1836-1841.
22. LACASSE, R.A., K.E. FOLLIS, M. TRAHEY *et al.* 1999. Fusion-competent vaccines: broad neutralization of primary isolates of HIV. Science **283:** 357–362.

Gene Therapy for Pediatric AIDS

GERHARD BAUER, DAVID SELANDER, BARBARA ENGEL,
DENISE CARBONARO, SUSIE CSIK, STEVE RAWLINGS,
JOSEPH CHURCH, AND DONALD B. KOHN[a]

*Division of Research Immunology/Bone Marrow Transplantation,
Childrens Hospital Los Angeles, Departments of Pediatrics and
Molecular Microbiology & Immunology, University of Southern California
School of Medicine, Los Angeles, California 90027, USA*

ABSTRACT: Gene therapy is an experimental treatment modality under investigation for applications to HIV-1 infection. We have developed retroviral vectors carrying anti-HIV-1 genes, demonstrated that these genes cause significant suppression of HIV-1 replication in cultures of primary hematopoietic cells, and performed a clinical trial in pediatric AIDS patients. Four HIV-1–infected children and adolescents underwent bone marrow harvest from which CD34+ cells were isolated and transduced by a retroviral vector carrying an RRE decoy gene. The cells were re-infused into the subjects, without complications, showing that gene transfer in pediatric AIDS patients is safe and feasible. However, gene-containing leukocytes in the peripheral blood were seen only at a low level and only in the first months following cell infusion. To attain some degree of efficacy, it will be necessary to achieve a higher level of gene transfer and to obtain sustained gene expression. We are currently developing new gene transfer methods and vectors designed to improve the results in future trials. If it becomes possible to reach the ideal goal of producing high percentages of T lymphocytes and monocytic cells that are resistant to HIV-1 infection, gene therapy could serve as a complement to antiretroviral drug therapy and help to sustain immunologic function.

INTRODUCTION

Gene therapy is an experimental treatment modality under investigation for applications to HIV-1 infection. The predominant approach, dubbed intracellular immunization (Baltimore), is to introduce "anti–HIV-1 genes," which confer relative resistance to HIV-1 infection or replication into HIV-1–susceptible cells. The target cells for gene transfer may be either pluripotent hematopoietic stem cells or mature peripheral blood T lymphocytes. Hematopoietic stem cells are attractive targets because they produce essentially all of the cells involved in HIV-1 pathogenesis, and therefore genetically modified hematopoietic stem cells could produce T lymphocytes and monocytes, microglial cells, and dendritic cells that would be resistant to HIV-1 replication.

[a]Address for correspondence: Division of Research Immunology/B.M.T., Mailstop #62, Childrens Hospital Los Angeles, 4650 Sunset Blvd., Los Angeles, CA 90027. Voice: 323-669-4617; fax: 323-667-1021.
dkohn@chla.usc.edu

Many anti–HIV-1 genes have been developed, with some now being studied in phase 1 trials. These include antisense, ribozymes, dominant–negative mutants, RNA decoys, intracellular antibodies, inhibitors of expression of cellular receptors, and HIV-1–inducible cytotoxic genes. Studies by Nabel and co-workers have shown that T lymphocytes expressing a dominant-negative *rev* gene (revM10)[2] have prolonged survival *in vivo,* providing excellent support for further studies.[3]

We have developed retroviral vectors carrying anti–HIV-1 genes, evaluated these genes in cultures of primary hematopoietic cells, and performed a clinical trial in pediatric AIDS patients. The results of these studies will be described, followed by discussion of our future directions.

We have focused on three classes of anti-HIV-1 genes: (1) dominant–negative mutants of the HIV-1 regulatory genes tat and rev,[4] (2) a small synthetic portion of the *rev*-responsive element (RRE) to serve as a decoy to sequester REV protein,[5] and (3) hammerhead ribozymes, designed by John Rossi and co-workers to cleave HIV-1 mRNA.[6] These genes were inserted into retroviral vectors based on the Moloney murine leukemia virus (MLV) and used to transduce human T lymphocytes and CD34+ hematopoietic progenitor cells. Cells expressing these genes showed significant inhibition of HIV-1 replication (>95–99.5%) compared to control cells.[5–7] No adverse effects on cellular growth and proliferation were observed. Based on these findings, the vectors have been studied in clinical trials.

A CLINICAL TRIAL OF GENE TRANSFER INTO BONE MARROW CELLS OF PEDIATRIC AIDS PATIENTS

Beginning in August 1997, we performed a clinical trial to transfer the RRE decoy gene into CD34+ cells from the bone marrow of HIV-1–infected pediatric AIDS subjects.[8] This was a phase 1 study to evaluate the safety and potential adverse effects from the gene transfer procedure. Feasibility was defined as the ability to obtain adequate numbers of bone marrow cells, using the ranges of cell numbers thought to be necessary for allogeneic bone marrow transplantation. Efficacy was assessed by determining whether the manipulated bone marrow cells would engraft and produce peripheral blood leukocytes containing and expressing the introduced gene. To test the hypothesis that cells expressing an anti–HIV-1 gene would be protected from HIV-1–induced cytopathicity, a comparative marking approach was used to assess whether cells expressing the RRE decoy vector (L-RRE-neo) would preferentially accumulate, compared to cells marked by the control vector (LN).

The four study subjects were patients followed by the Pediatric AIDS Program at Childrens Hospital Los Angeles. They were between 8 and 18 years of age, had been HIV-1–positive for 8–17 years, and had moderately to severely advanced AIDS; two of the subjects had absolute CD4+ T-lymphocyte counts of only 2 and 6/mm^3. All were on multiple antiretroviral medications, but had plasma HIV-1 RNA levels between 15,000 and 95,000/ml. Each subject underwent bone marrow harvest under general anesthesia. The bone marrow was processed to isolate CD34+ cells that were subsequently transduced with the retroviral vectors. The cells were then re-infused intravenously, without any preparative cytoreduction conditioning. Peripheral blood samples were obtained for up to 2 years afterwards, to evaluate toxicities and to quantify the presence of gene-containing peripheral blood leukocytes.

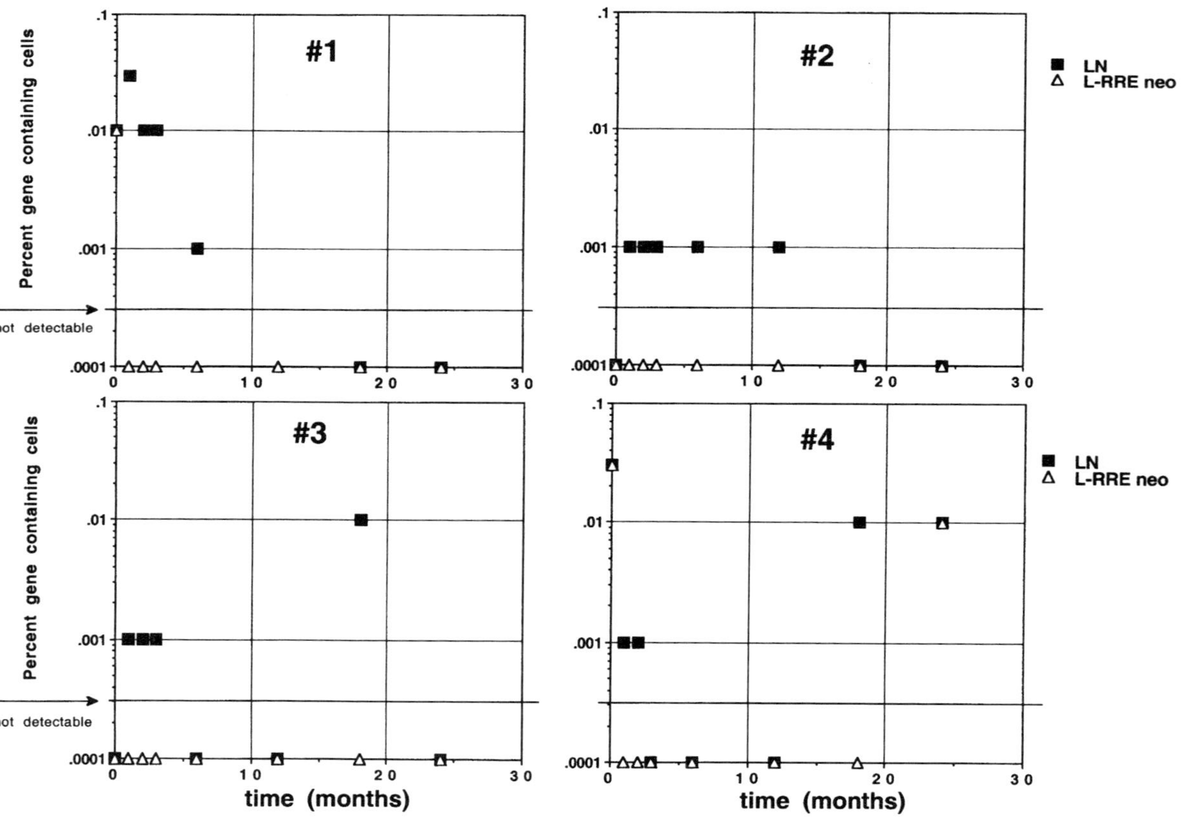

FIGURE 1. Level of gene marking in peripheral blood leukocytes after infusion of gene-transduced CD34+ cells.

In fact, no adverse effects were noted. Subjects tolerated cell infusions without difficulties and were discharged within a day. No changes were noted in hematologic parameters, blood chemistries, or plasma HIV-1 RNA levels, and there was no evidence that the subjects had been exposed to replication-competent retrovirus. We also determined that it was possible to obtain the target numbers of bone marrow CD34+ cells from these patients, despite the advanced state of their illness.

The level of gene-marking in peripheral blood leukocytes has been low (FIG. 1). Peripheral blood samples taken days and weeks after cell infusion showed the presence of gene-containing leukocytes at frequencies of 0.10–0.003%. However, most blood samples taken over the subsequent months did not have detectable gene-containing cells above the sensitivity limit of 0.001%.

The short-term production of gene-containing cells is consistent with previous findings in gene-marking studies in oncology patients.[9,10] MLV-based retroviral vectors only transduce cells that are actively replicating. In bone marrow, the majority of the cycling cells are short-term, lineage-committed progenitor cells; most long-lived pluripotent stem cells are quiescent. Gene transduction of the progenitor cells would lead to transient production of gene-containing leukocytes, which would then be replaced by unmarked cells arising from the more primitive stem cells.

The low level of gene-marking precluded determination of whether the RRE decoy gene was being expressed in any cells. In a study of gene transfer into the CD34+ cells from the umbilical cord blood of adenosine deaminase (ADA)-deficient severe combined immunodeficient neonates, expression from the MLV retroviral LTR was absent in resting peripheral blood lymphocytes, but could be induced on *ex vivo* stimulation with phytohemagglutinin (PHA) and interleukin (IL)-2.[11]

This study thus showed that gene transfer in pediatric AIDS patients is safe and feasible. To attempt to attain some degree of efficacy, it will be necessary to achieve higher levels of gene transfer and to obtain sustained gene expression. We are currently developing new gene transfer methods and vectors designed to improve the results in future trials.

EVALUATION OF NEW RETROVIRAL VECTORS CARRYING ANTI–HIV-1 GENES

Whereas the anti–HIV-1 genes that have been developed do confer significant resistance to HIV-1, this resistance is relative. Using increased MOI of HIV-1 for the *in vitro* challenges typically overwhelms the protection and leads to HIV-1 replication in "protected" cells. Therefore, we performed studies to evaluate the anti–HIV-1 genes under conditions of increased stringency. We used the human AA2 cell line, which readily forms syncytia with infection by HIV-1IIIb. The AA2 cells were transduced with a series of retroviral vectors and then selected in G418 or by FACS for vectors carrying the neomycin resistance gene or the green fluorescent gene (eGFP), respectively (FIG. 2). The transduced cells were inoculated with HIV-1 at MOI over a five order-of-magnitude range. Syncytia formation and release of reverse transcriptase were measured after 7–10 days. Positive controls were provided by infection of mock-transduced cells in the presence of the non-nucleoside reverse transcriptase (RT) inhibitor delaviridine at 0.1 and 1.0 mM.

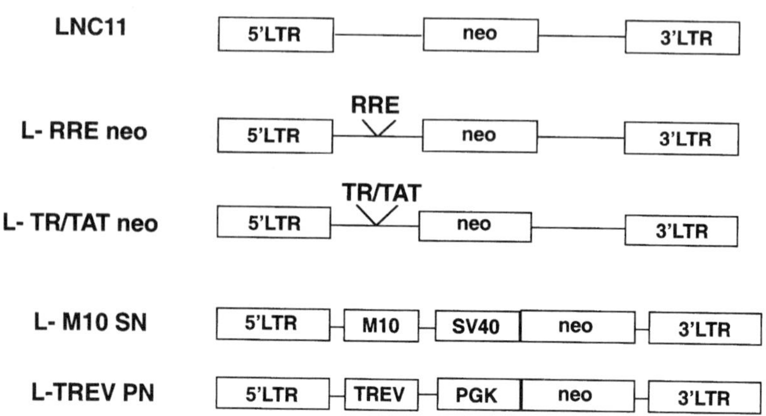

FIGURE 2. Diagram of retroviral vectors with anti–HIV-1 genes evaluated in AA2 cells.

Using this model, we again found that cells carrying anti–HIV-1 genes showed reduced growth of HIV-1, compared to mock-transduced cells (FIG. 3A). Whereas inhibition of HIV-1 by anti–HIV-1 genes was overcome at higher MOI of HIV-1, so was inhibition by 0.1 mM delaviridine. As seen in this experiment, we reproducibly found that the vector expressing the dominant–negative revM10 gene[2] was most consistently inhibitory, compared to the more variable protection from either the RRE decoy or the hammerhead ribozymes (FIG. 3B).

Based on findings of the apparent superiority of the revM10 gene over the other anti–HIV-1 genes that we have studied, we have developed new retroviral vectors, designed to yield improved expression of revM10. These vectors were based on a modified MLV vector backbone that we developed, named MND.[12] The MND vector, like the MSCV vector, has modifications in the *cis*-acting transcriptional elements that lead to expression in a higher percentage of hematopoietic and lymphoid cells, at higher levels and with greater persistence over time, compared to the standard MLV vectors.[13–15]

Additionally, we have included the Woodchuck Hepatitis Virus posttranscriptional regulatory element (WPRE) in some vectors, because of its ability to increase the levels of vector-derived transcripts, which leads to improved titers and gene expression.[16] Prior efforts to produce high-titer revM10 vector preparations led to the observation that vectors capable of expressing revM10 were produced consistently at lower titers than were similar vectors that did not contain a translatable revM10 reading frame (G. Nabel, personal communication). We have also produced similar vectors carrying a fusion gene, *trev*, consisting of a dominant–negative *tat* and a dominant negative *rev*, which has shown superior activity compared to a dominant-negative *rev* alone.[17] For the research vectors, the eGFP reporter gene was inserted downstream of the anti–HIV-1 gene, linked by an IRES to allow translation of the reporter gene from the same transcript as the anti–HIV-1 gene (FIG. 4). Vectors for possible clinical applications do not have the eGFP gene, because of the likely immunogenicity of this protein *in vivo*.[18]

The vectors have been produced by transient transfection into 293T cells of the vector plasmids with plasmids expressing the MLV gag/pol proteins and the VSV-G

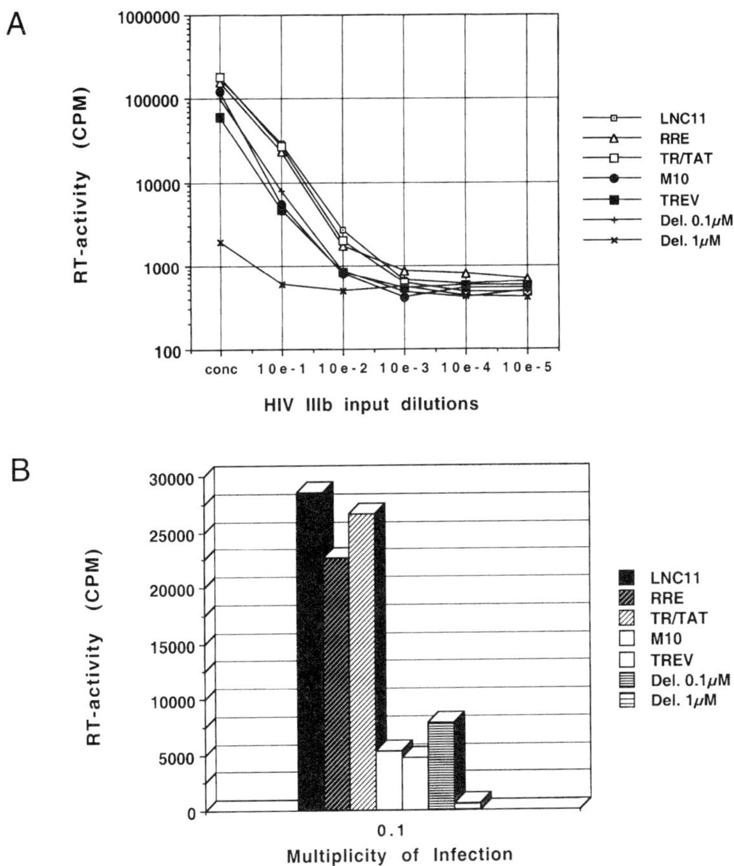

FIGURE 3. Challenge of gene-transduced AA2 cells with HIV-1 IIIb. (**A**) Response to increasing MOI of HIV-1. (**B**) Relative inhibition of HIV-1 (MOI = 0.01).

surface protein. Expression levels by vectors in the 293T cells were monitored by measuring the fluorescence of the eGFP reporter. As seen in FIGURE 5, the presence of the *trev* gene (MND-trev-IRES-eGFP) inhibits expression, compared to the control vector lacking *trev* (MND-X-IRES-eGFP). The presence of the WPRE improves the expression level to meet or exceed that of the control vector.

The vector supernatants were titered by transducing 293A cells with serial dilutions of the vector and determining the numbers of cells transduced by FACS analysis. The titers of the vectors correlated with the expression intensity seen in the transient transfections, suggesting that the levels of vector transcripts produced in the transfected cells are the limiting factor in the titers of the vectors produced (TABLE 1). These vectors are being used to transduce human T cells and CD34+ progenitor cells, which will then be challenged with HIV-1.

Based on the findings, we will derive high-titer packaging cell clones, making the most effective vectors (lacking eGFP) for study in future clinical trials. These clinical

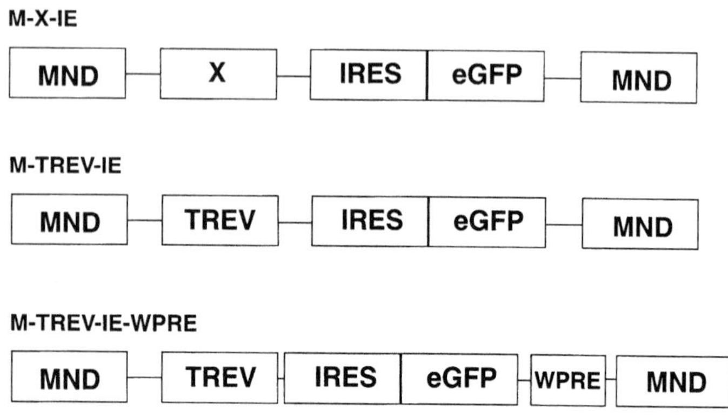

FIGURE 4. Diagram of MND-based retroviral vectors with trev.

TABLE 1. Expression and titers of MND-based retroviral vectors with trev

Vector	Expression[a]	Titers[b]
MND-IRES-eGFP	16.2	$2.4 \times 10e5$/ml
MND-trev-IRES-eGFP	13.4	$0.4 \times 10e5$/ml
MND-trev-IRES-eGFP-WPRE	29.7	$1.7 \times 10e5$/ml

[a]Geometric mean fluorescence of eGFP expression in transfected 293T cells, gating only on the transfected cells with fluorescence above the nontransduced control background.

[b]The vectors were packaged by cotransfection into 293T cells with plasmids expressing MLV gag/pol {pHIT60} and the VSV-G protein as described.[24] Supernatants were collected 36 hours after transfection and titered by using serial dilutions to transduce 293A. The percentages of 293A cells expressing eGFP were determined by FACS.

studies will also evaluate the efficacy of improvements in the conditions for retroviral-mediated gene transfer into hematopoietic stem cells, which have been identified in recent years. These include the use of serum-free conditions, recombinant cytokines with the capacity to support survival and proliferation of primitive hematopoietic stem cells (e.g., c-kit ligand, flt-3 ligand , thrombopoietin), and support matrices, such as recombinant fibronectin CH-296, which increase gene transfer by colocalizing vector particles and stem cells.[20] These conditions have been found to produce increased levels of gene-marked cells in primate gene transfer/BMT models.[21,22]

LENTIVIRAL VECTORS TO TRANSDUCE QUIESCENT HEMATOPOIETIC STEM CELLS WITH ANTI–HIV-1 GENES

A major limitation of retroviral vectors remains their requirement for target cell replication for gene transduction. The majority of primitive human hematopoietic stem cells are quiescent, in the Go state, and therefore are poorly transduced by MLV vectors. In recent years, vectors have been produced based on HIV-1 itself, because

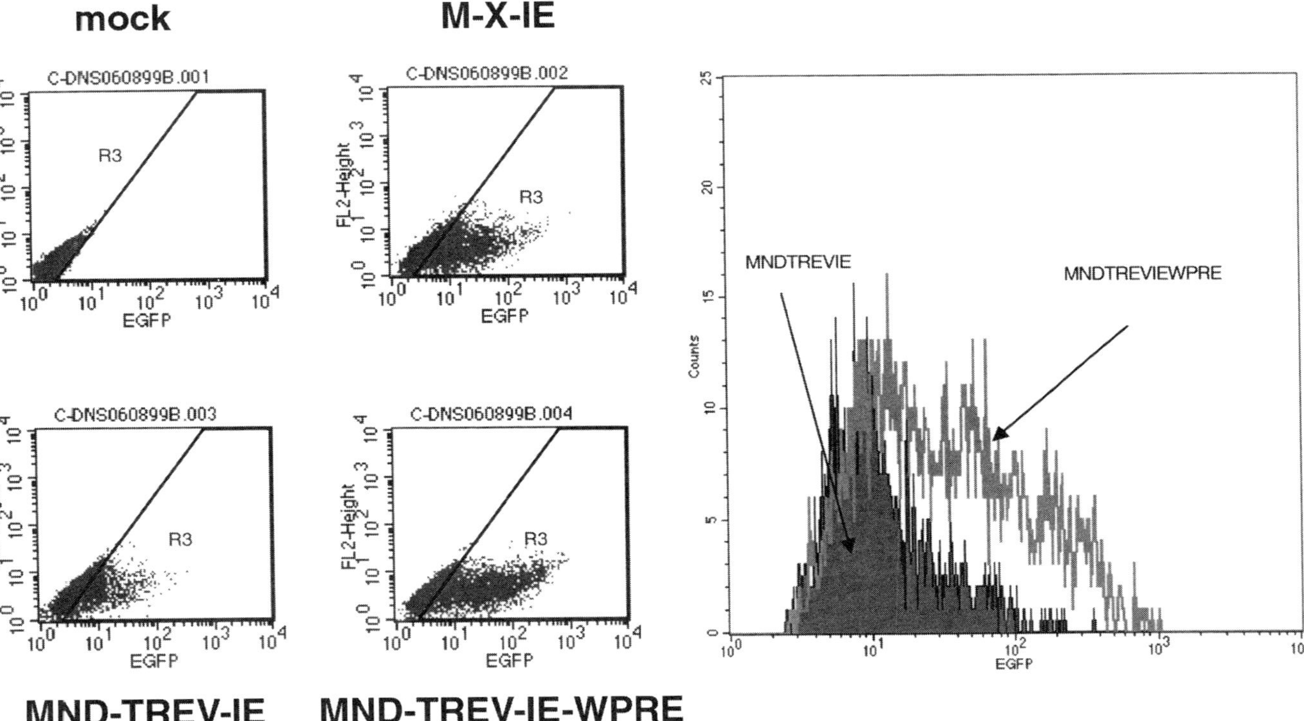

FIGURE 5. FACS analysis of vector expression: effects of trev and WPRE.

of the known ability of lentiviruses to infect nondividing cells, such as macrophages.[23] These vectors have been developed to lack any HIV-1 protein-coding regions and therefore are not immunogenic in transduced cells. The necessary HIV-1 virion and regulatory proteins can be produced during vector production from other plasmids, and the VSV-G protein provides a stable, broadly targeted pseudotype.

Studies by our group and others have shown that the HIV-1–based lentiviral vectors are capable of transducing primitive human hematopoietic stem cells, which are poorly transduced by MLV vectors.[24–27] However, the demonstration of sustained gene transduction of human hematopoietic cells in long-term culture and NOD/SCID xenograft models still may not be sufficiently stringent to guarantee that transduction has been attained in pluripotent stem cells capable of long-term engraftment and cell production after transplantation. Results have not yet been reported in canine or monkey models which confirm the superiority of lentiviral vectors over MLV-based retroviral vectors. Ultimately, clinical trials will need to be performed to examine transduction of human stem cells *in vivo*, after appropriate pharmacology/toxicity studies have been performed in preclinical models.

We have developed lentiviral vectors to carry the *rev* and *trev* dominant–negative genes. One potential problem with using these anti–HIV-1 genes in lentiviral vectors is that they may inhibit the achievable titers, because the vectors are derived from HIV-1 and expression of vector transcripts in the packaging cells is dependent on *rev* and *tat* function. Recently, so-called "3rd generation" HIV-1 vectors have been developed with additional modifications to maximize safety, such as deletion of the enhancer and promoter from the LTR to obviate LTR-driven transcription.[23,29] In 3rd generation constructs, the 5′ HIV-1 LTR is replaced by either the CMV promoter or the RSV LTR, alleviating the dependence on *tat* for transcription. Thus, 3rd generation vectors should not be inhibited by genes that interfere with tat function.

Potential means to overcome the interference from revM10 with REV-mediated nuclear export of vector genomes include the addition of other RNA export elements (e.g., the constitutive transport element [CTE] of the Mason-Pfizer Monkey Virus-MPMV), the overexpression of wild-type REV by the addition of a *rev* expression plasmid to the cotransfection for vector production, or the arrangement of the revM10 gene in a reversed orientation in the 3′ LTR so that it comes under transcriptional control of an antisense-oriented promoter only following reverse transcription in a target cell. We have constructed lentiviral vectors containing revM10 (and an IRES-linked eGFP reporter to facilitate measurement of vector transcription and titers) using each of these approaches to compare their effectiveness (FIG. 6).

We have begun to evaluate these lentiviral vector designs for the titers that can be produced and their abilities to inhibit HIV-1. The vector plasmids were transfected into 293T cells and expression of transcripts was measured by FACS. We found that the presence of revM10 did decrease the level of vector transcripts in the 293T cells (TABLE 2). The MPMV CTE or additional wild-type REV had no significant enhancement of expression (TABLE 2 and FIG. 7). Measurement of the titers of these vectors showed parallel reduction of the vector titers by revM10, with no improvements by inclusion of the CTE or by overexpression of wild-type REV (TABLE 2 and FIG. 7).

The vectors are currently being evaluated for their ability to inhibit HIV-1 in cell lines and primary cell models. We are also exploring other strategies to overcome the

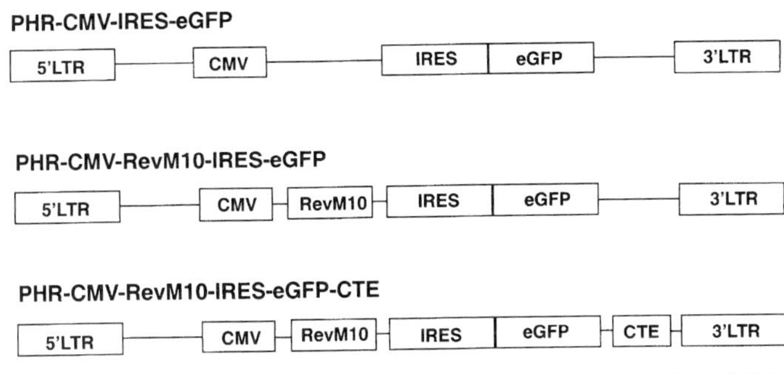

FIGURE 6. Diagram of HIV-1–based lentiviral vectors with revM10.

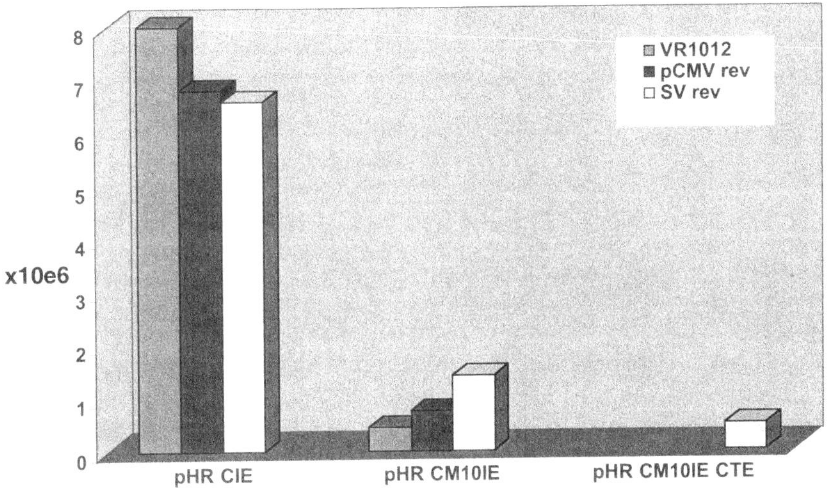

FIGURE 7. Titers of HIV-1–based lentiviral vectors: effects of CTE and rev expression.

TABLE 2. Expression and titers of HIV-1–based lentiviral vectors with revM10

Vector	Expression[a]	Titer[b]
pHR-CMV-IRES-eGFP	116.6	$9.0 \times 10e6$/ml
pHR-CMV-M10-IRES-eGFP	44.1	$0.89 \times 10e6$/ml
pHR-CMV-M10-IRES-eGFP-CTE	27.1	$0.76 \times 10e6$/ml

[a]Geometric mean fluorescence of eGFP expression in transfected 293T cells, gating only on the transfected cells with fluorescence above the nontransduced control background.

[b]The vectors were packaged by cotransfection into 293T cells with plasmids expressing HIV 1 gag/pol/tat/rev {$p\Delta8.9$} and the VSV-G protein as described.[24] Supernatants were collected 36 hours after transfection and titered by using serial dilutions to transduce 293A. The percentages of 293A cells expressing eGFP were determined by FACS.

inhibitory effects of revM10 and trev in the vector titers. If these are not successful, it may be necessary to only use anti–HIV-1 genes which do not interfere with the HIV-1 genes needed for vector production, such as targeting HIV-1 gp120 envelope, co-receptors, etc.

CONCLUSION

The role of gene therapy in the treatment of pediatric AIDS is largely speculative at the present time. The ideal of producing high percentages of T lymphocytes and monocytic cells that are resistant to HIV-1 infection is currently not attainable. More effective methods for transfer and expression of anti–HIV-1 genes that confer more complete protection need to be identified. If it becomes possible to reach this goal, gene therapy could serve as a complement to antiretroviral drug therapy; the global reduction of virus produced from cells achieved by the combination therapy plus the relative inhibition of HIV-1 growth in genetically modified cells could allow sustained immunologic function.

ACKNOWLEDGMENTS

This work was supported by grants from the National Institute of Allergy and Infectious Diseases (AI #1U19AI36606) and the T.J. Martell Foundation. D.B.K. is the recipient of an Elizabeth Glaser Scientist Award from the Elizabeth Glaser Pediatric AIDS Foundation.

REFERENCES

1. BALTIMORE, D. 1988. Intracellular immunization. Nature (Lond.) **335:** 395–396.
2. MALIM, M.H., S. BOHNLEIN, J. HAUBER & B.R. CULLEN. 1989. Functional dissection of the HIV-1-1 *rev trans*-activator--derivation of a *trans*-dominant repressor of *rev* function. Cell **58:** 205–214.
3. WOFFENDIN, C., U. RANGA, Z.-Y. YANG & G.J. NABEL. 1996. Expression of a protective gene prolongs survival of T cells in human immunodeficiency virus-infected patients. Proc. Natl. Acad. Sci. **93:** 2889–2894.
4. BAHNER, I., C. ZHOU, X.-J. YU *et al.* 1993. Comparison of *trans*-dominant Inhibitory mutant human immunodeficiency virus type 1 genes expressed by retroviral vectors in human T lymphocytes. J. Virol. **67:** 3199–3207.
5. BAHNER, I., K. KEARNS, Q.L. HAO *et al.* 1996. Transduction of human CD34+ hematopoietic progenitor cells by a retroviral vector expressing an RRE decoy inhibits HIV-1 replication in the myelomonocytic cells produced in long-term culture. J. Virol. **70:** 4352–4360.
6. ZHOU, C., I. BAHNER, G. LARSON *et al.* 1994. Anti-HIV-1 hammerhead ribozymes transduced by retroviral vectors inhibit HIV-1 replication in human T lymphocytes. Gene **149:** 33–39.
7. BAUER, G., P. VALDEZ, K. KEARNS *et al.* 1997. Inhibition of HIV-1 replication after transduction of G-CSF-mobilized CD34+ cells from HIV-1-infected donors using retroviral vectors containing anti-HIV-1 genes. Blood **89:** 2259–2267.
8. KOHN, D.B., G.H. BAUER, P. VALDEZ *et al.* 1999. A clinical trial of retroviral-mediated transfer of an RRE decoy gene into CD34+ cells from the bone marrow of HIV-1 infected children. Blood **94:** 368–371.

9. CORNETTA, K., E.F. SROUR, A. MOORE *et al.* 1996. Retroviral gene transfer in autologous bone marrow transplantation for adult acute leukemia. Hum. Gene Ther. **7:** 1323–1329.

10. DUNBAR, C.E., M. COTTLER-FOX, J.A. O'SHAUGHNESSY *et al.* 1995. Retrovirally marked CD34-enriched peripheral blood and bone marrow cells contribute to long-term engraftment after autologous transplantation. Blood **85:** 3048–3057.

11. KOHN, D.B., M.S. HERSHFIELD, D. CARBONARO *et al.* 1998. T lymphocytes with a normal ADA gene accumulate after transplantation of transduced autologous umbilical cord blood CD34+ cells in ADA-deficient SCID neonates. Nature Med. **4:** 775–780.

12. CHALLITA, P.M., D. SKELTON, A. EL-KHOUEIRY *et al.* 1995. Multiple modifications in *cis*-elements of the LTR of retroviral vectors lead to increased expression and decreased DNA methylation in embryonic carcinoma (EC) cells. J. Virol. **69:** 748–755.

13. ROBBINS, P.B., D.M. SKELTON, X.J. YU *et al.* 1998. Consistent, persistent expression from modified retroviral vectors in murine hematopoietic stem cells. Proc. Natl. Acad. Sci. USA **95:** 10182–10187.

14. HALENE, S., L. WANG, R. COOPER *et al.* 1999. Improved expression in murine hematopoietic and lymphoid cells after transplantation of bone marrow transduced with a modified retroviral vector. Blood **94:** 3349–3357.

15. HAWLEY, R.G., F.H. LIEU, A.Z. FONG & T.S. HAWLEY. 1994. Versatile retroviral vectors for potential use in gene therapy. Gene Ther. **1:** 136–138.

16. ZUFFEREY, R., J.E. DONELLO, D. TRONO & T.J. HOPE. 1999. Woodchuck hepatitis virus posttranscriptional regulatory element enhances expression of transgenes delivered by retroviral vectors. J. Virol. **73:** 2886–2892.

17. AGUILAR-CORDOVA, E., J. CHINEN, L.A. DONEHOWER *et al.* 1995. Inhibition of HIV-1 by a double transdominant fusion gene. Gene Ther. **2:** 181–186.

18. STRIPECKE, R., M.D.C. VILLACRES, D. SKELTON *et al.* 1999. Immune response to green fluorescent protein: implications for gene therapy. Gene Ther. **6:** 1305–1312.

19. KOHN, D.B. 1999. Gene therapy using hematopoietic stem cells. Curr. Opin. Mol. Ther. **1:** 437–442.

20. HANENBERG, H., X.L. XIAO, D. DILLOO *et al.* 1996. Colocalization of retrovirus and target cells on specific fibronectin fragments increases genetic transduction of mammalian cells. Nature Med. **2:** 876–882.

21. TISDALE, J.F., Y. HANAZONO, S.E. SELLERS *et al.* 1998. Ex vivo expansion of genetically marked rhesus peripheral blood progenitor cells results in diminished long-term repopulating ability. Blood **92:** 1131–1141.

22. KIEM, H.-P., R.G. ANDREWS, J. MORRIS *et al.* 1998. Improved gene transfer into baboon marrow repopulating cells using recombinant human fibronectin fragment CH-296 in combination with interleukin-6, stem cell factor, FLT-3 ligand, and megakaryocyte growth and development factor. Blood **92:** 1878–1886.

23. NALDINI, L., U. BLOMER, P. GALLAY *et al.* 1996. In vivo gene delivery and stable transduction of nondividing cells by a lentiviral vector. Science **272:** 263–267.

24. CASE, S.S., M.A. PRICE, C.T. JORDAN *et al.* 1999. Stable transduction of quiescent CD34(+)CD38(-) human hematopoietic cells by HIV-1 based lentiviral vectors. Proc. Natl. Acad. Sci. USA **96:** 2988–2993.

25. MIYOSHI, H., K.A. SMITH, D.E. MOSIER *et al.* 1999. Efficient transduction of human CD34+ cells that mediaste long-term engraftment of NOD/SCID mice by HIV vectors. Science **283:** 682–686.

26. SUTTON, R.E., H.T.M. WU, R. RIGG *et al.* 1998. Human immunodeficiency virus Type 1 vectors efficiently transduce human hematopoietic stem cells. J. Virol. **72:** 5781–5788.

27. UCHIDA, N., R.E. SUTTON, A.M. FRIERA *et al.* 1998. HIV, but not murine leukemia virus, vectors mediate high efficiency gene transfer into freshly isolated G_0/G_1 human hematopoietic stem cells. Proc. Natl. Acad. Sci. USA **95:** 11939–11944.

28. MIYOSHI, H., U. BLÖMER, M. TAKAHASHI *et al.* 1998. Development of a self-inactivating lentivirus vector. J. Virol. **72:** 8150–8157.

29. DULL, T., R. ZUFFEREY, M. KELLY *et al.* 1998. A third-generation lentivirus vector with a conditional packaging system. J. Virol. **72:** 8463–8471.

Rapid Characterization of HIV Clade C-Specific Cytotoxic T Lymphocyte Responses in Infected African Children and Adults

PHILIP J. R. GOULDER[a,b,c]

[a]*Partners AIDS Research Center, Massachusetts General Hospital, Charlestown, Massachusetts 02129, USA*

[b]*Division of Infectious Diseases, The Children's Hospital, Boston, Massachusetts 02115, USA*

ABSTRACT: Cytotoxic T lymphocytes (CTL) play a central role in successful control of HIV. Induction of effective CTL responses may therefore be an essential requirement of HIV vaccines. Knowledge of CTL epitopes targeted either in natural infection or following vaccination will be critical to understanding the anti-HIV immune response. Until recently, epitope definition was a slow and laborious process that could only be undertaken in laboratories specialized in this work. Recent incremental advances in the technologies that may be applied to this field have transformed what is possible, so that within 48 hours of receipt of a blood sample, novel epitopes may be optimized and the HLA restriction defined. Moreover, these technologies can now be applied in nonspecialized laboratories, so that new epitopes can be characterized locally in sites where the epidemic is most severe. Sub-Saharan Africans and C clade infection have been relatively neglected in terms of the HIV-specific CTL epitopes that have been defined to date. This review summarizes the evidence that cellular immunity is important in successful containment of HIV and describes the novel methods of epitope detection, illustrating their ready application to the study of C-clade infected persons in sub-Saharan Africa.

INTRODUCTION

After almost two decades of intensive research directed towards understanding the correlates of protective immunity against HIV, it is now established beyond reasonable doubt that HIV-specific cellular immunity plays a central part in controlling viral replication. Recent dramatic advances in the way that cytotoxic T lymphocytes (CTL) and T helper cells can be detected have contributed significantly towards this appreciation of their role in determining the level of virus in infected persons. However, perhaps the most exciting aspect of these new technologies available is in their application to the study of HIV-specific CTL and T helper responses in the developing countries that are worst affected by the global epidemic, but that have been relatively neglected in terms of the focus of research.

[c]Address for correspondence: Dr. Philip J.R. Goulder, Partners AIDS Research Center, Massachusetts General Hospital, 13th Street, Bldg 149, Rm 5218, Charlestown, MA 02129. Voice: 617-726-5787; fax: 617-726-5411.

goulder@helix.mgh.harvard.edu

This review briefly summarizes the evidence that anti-HIV CTL and T helper responses are critically effective components of the immune response that would be important to incorporate into vaccine design. The advantages and limitations of the new methodologies now available for detecting and measuring these cells are outlined. The application of these novel techniques to understanding the cellular immune responses generated in clade-C infected Africans in Durban, South Africa and in clade-B infected African Americans is described and illustrated. Possible approaches to improving further the rapid definition of novel CTL and T helper epitopes are discussed. Finally, future directions that urgently need to be explored in this exciting area of research will be considered.

IMPORTANCE OF CYTOTOXIC T LYMPHOCYTES IN CONTROL OF HIV

Early studies identified the very high levels of virus-specific CTL detectable in chronic HIV infection,[1] but the significance of these CTL responses was difficult to interpret in view of the fact that an inexorable decline towards AIDS appeared to occur irrespective of their presence.[2] One possible interpretation[3,4] was that HIV-specific CTL were detectable at very high levels, not because virus was limited by CTL, but because CTL were driven by a very high viral turnover.[5,6] Even though three studies demonstrated the temporal association of initial control of viremia in acute AIDS virus infection with the emergence of virus-specific CTL, in both HIV[7,8] and the SIV-macaque model,[9] it was argued that these data might simply reflect saturation of target cells available for infection by virus[10] and that the immune response could be irrelevant.

Most directly, the argument was resolved in the SIV model by infusion of anti-CD8 monoclonal antibodies (mAb) into infected animals in both acute and chronic infection.[11,12] Animals in whom these infusions had resulted in long-term depletion of CD8+ T cells showed no initial control of viremia following acute infection, and progression to simian AIDS and death occurred very rapidly. Short-term CD8+ T-cell–depleted animals showed the reduction in viremia that normally occurs in acute infection only when the CD8+ T cells started to emerge. In chronically infected animals, anti-CD8 mAb infusions brought about immediate reductions in CTL levels and simultaneous increases in viral load. Work by Mellors et al.[13] had already demonstrated with crystal clarity the relation between plasma HIV viral load and rate of progression to disease. In chronic HIV infection, a strong negative association was demonstrated between CTL numbers and viral load.[14] Although a potential role of CD8+ CD3- natural killer cells cannot be excluded, these anti-CD8 mAb infusion experiments, taken together with the other studies just described, are among the most compelling to show that CTL not only affect the initial control of viremia in acute infection, but also critically determine the level of AIDS virus in chronic infection.

A somewhat different approach to the problem of understanding the role of CTL in AIDS virus infection has been to look for evidence of CTL "escape," that is, evasion of the CTL response by mutation within the virus sequences specifically encoding for the CTL epitopes targeted. Evidence of CTL-mediated selection pressure on the virus would imply that the virus was constrained by CTL, as opposed to CTL activity merely following ineffectively in the virus' wake. The best examples of CTL escape in HIV infection have come from studies of acute infection[15,16] and also of late infection,[17,18] where escape occurred in association with progression to disease. However, these examples are relatively sparse, mainly because of the considerable challenges to demonstrating escape in HIV infection,[19,20] and it is still a matter of discussion how important escape really is in HIV infection. Recent studies in SIV infection, however, have spectacularly demonstrated that CTL escape is strongly associated with progression to disease in infected macaques[21] and also that escape occurs *universally* in acute infection.[22] These data clearly show that CTL are controlling virus to some extent. What is of greatest interest from these data is why certain epitopes appear to show escape in early infection, whereas others show escape late, and what is the significance of these differences. Qualitative differences between CTL will be discussed in the final section of this review.

IMPORTANCE OF T HELPER CELLS IN CONTROL OF HIV

Perhaps the most glaring immune defect in HIV infection is the characteristic CD4 T-cell loss that occurs throughout the course of infection. HIV-specific T helper responses, in contrast to virus-specific CTL, are difficult to detect in most chronically infected persons, but their potential importance in underpinning an effective immune response was first revealed by Rosenberg *et al.*[23] in a study showing a strong negative association between viral load and p24 Gag-specific helper activity. Similar studies subsequently were consistent with these findings.[24]

There remained the paradox of CTL being clearly vital for control of HIV, and yet, in most infected persons, being unable to prevent progression to AIDS. This problem was resolved by Kalams *et al.*[25] who showed that Gag-specific CTL activity is only associated with control of viremia in the presence of Gag-specific T helper responses. These data are reminiscent of similar studies in LCMV-infected mice, in which the role of virus-specific T helper responses was clearly shown as a prerequisite for control of chronic viral infection.[26–28]

METHODOLOGICAL ADVANCES IN DETECTION OF CYTOTOXIC T LYMPHOCYTES AND T HELPER CELLS

The means by which CTL and T helper cells can now be studied have genuinely been transformed over the course of the last 3–4 years, and these incremental changes are still incomplete. When previously it would have taken several months of dedicated work, not to mention large volumes of blood from dedicated donors, in order to reach an unsatisfactorily incomplete picture of the anti-HIV CTL response of each subject studied, it now takes a matter of hours to obtain vast amounts of much more accurate data. The two main advances have been the use of the interferon (IFN)-gamma Elispot (enzyme-linked immunospot) assay[29] and detection of antigen-specific T cells by flow cytometry using peptide-MHC class I tetrameric complexes[30] or by intracellular cytokine staining.[24,31,32]

The chief advantage of the Elispot assay is the huge number of peptides that can readily be tested for recognition in assays using freshly separated (or thawed cryopreserved) peripheral blood mononuclear cells (PBMC). Crucially, this requires no knowledge of the subject's HLA type, there is no need for an *in vitro* stage of cell expansion, and no autologous or HLA-matched EBV-transformed B lymphoblastoid cell line (BCL) is involved. For example, we aim to screen responses effectively using 300 overlapping 15–20 mer peptides spanning p17 Gag, p24 Gag, Nef, RT, gp41, gp120, Rev, and Tat in a single overnight assay that uses only 5–10 million PBMC. The result is that large numbers of infected persons can be screened for CTL responses extremely conveniently and rapidly. Furthermore, very little in the way of sophisticated equipment is needed to undertake these assays. The advantages to performing these assays on site in laboratories in developing countries situated in the midst of the global epidemic are self-evident. Finally, the small number of cells required for these assays enables pediatric CTL responses to be characterized comprehensively for the first time.

The flow cytometric equivalent of the IFN-gamma Elispot assay is in many ways a perfect complement to the screening Elispot assay. Intracellular IFN-gamma staining (ICS) of cells that have been stimulated with particular peptides allows the CD8 or CD4 dependence of the responding cells to be determined. In addition, precise quantification of the responder cells can be made that is readily verifiable objectively. Peptide-MHC class I tetramers are the most sensitive of all these methods, but the synthesis of each complex is labor-intensive and the shelf-life of each is somewhat variable; no information regarding functional aspects of cells that can bind tetramers is available from such assays; and, most significantly, each tetramer is specific for only a single CTL response out of hundreds or even thousands of possible responses. Thus, the tetramer assay on its own may provide only very limited information about the total CTL response.

In the comparisons we have made,[31] the tetramer assay is 3.5-fold more sensitive than the Elispot assay ($r = 0.90$) and 1.4-fold more sensitive than the IFN-gamma ICS assay ($r = 0.98$) (FIG. 1A and B). Thus, at least in the chronically infected subjects that we have studied, the ICS assay is far more flexible than the tetramer assay and provides access to almost the same information. Thus, other than to study CTL specificities that occur very commonly within a given population being studied, the value of tetramer assays on their own may be limited.

For study of T helper responses, no data are yet published regarding the value of class II tetramers in HIV infection. The challenges to refolding peptide-MHC complexes are clearly greater for class II, and ICS may already provide as dramatic data as one could wish for (FIG. 1C). Although direct comparisons of ICS helper assays versus the gold standard proliferation assay have yet to be published, ICS clearly is more sensitive than the proliferation assay[33,34] for detection of T helper responses.

We have utilized the Elispot assay not only to characterize rapidly the total anti-HIV CTL response by screening for CTL responses to different regions of HIV proteins, but also to fine-map novel epitopes.[35] The established method of generating CTL clones to determine the optimal epitope and HLA restriction of a response in chromium release assays was compared to a method developed using the Elispot assay. The Elispot assay was demonstrably as effective and clearly much more rapid and less labor-intensive an approach. Determination of the HLA restriction of the responses was hindered by the (presumed) EBV-specific background activity when using peptide-pulsed HLA matched BCL as targets in the Elispot assay. This can be

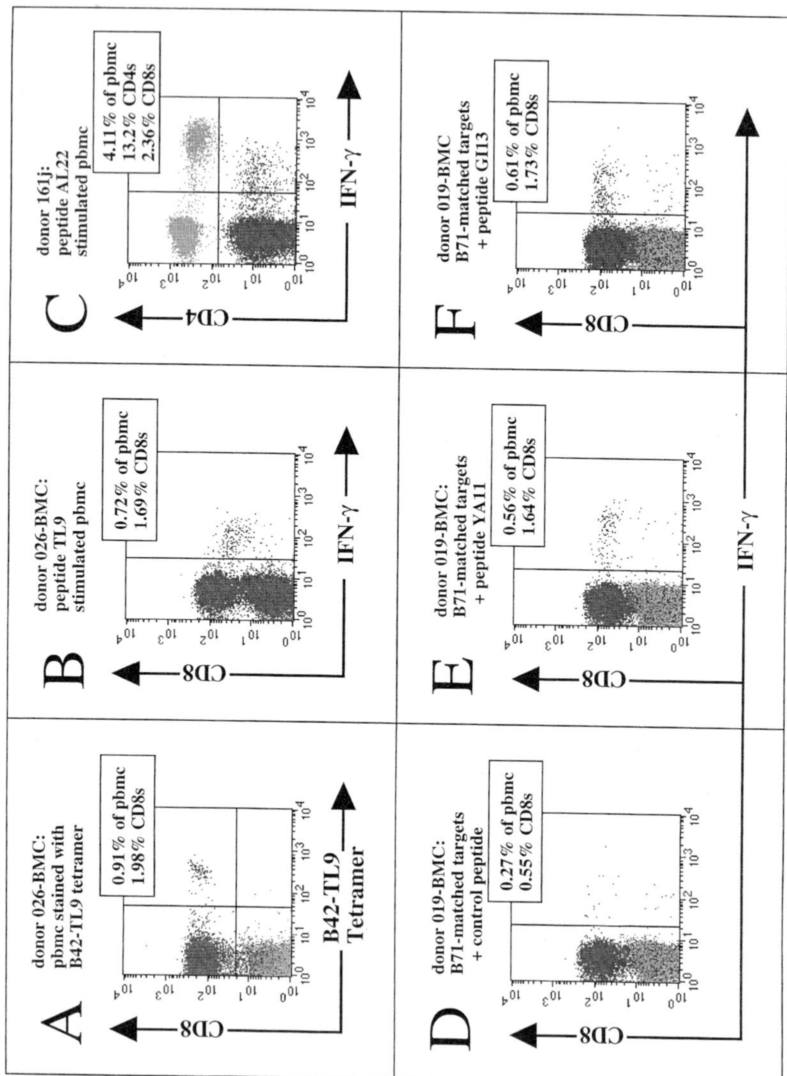

FIGURE 1. *See following page for caption.*

overcome by using either the ICS assay to determine HLA restriction (FIG. 1D and E) or T2 cells expressing particular HLA class I molecules of interest. Because T2 cells lack TAP (the transporter associated with antigen presentation),[36] EBV-processed peptides will not reach the surface of such cells.

Future additional extensions to existing flow cytometric assays of CTL function include the use of killing assays visualized by flow.[37,38] Currently, the only means of detecting cytotoxic activity is the chromium release assay, which has certainly proved a valuable tool over the last 30 years, but which is insensitive and not readily transferable to more than a small number of specialized laboratories.

In summary, the new methods now available that enable CTL and T helper cells to be detected rapidly and precisely are extremely operator-friendly and can easily be carried out in laboratories that have previously undertaken little or no studies of cellular immunity. Thus state-of-the-art assays may now be undertaken on-site in developing countries that are worst affected by the global epidemic. The single most costly item required for these studies is a flow cytometer, but taking into account the resources saved by avoiding the use of chromium release assays and the painstaking *in vitro* culture of cells required, even this piece of equipment is manifestly a most efficient use of funding.

DEFINITION OF HIV-SPECIFIC CTL RESPONSES IN C-CLADE-INFECTED AFRICANS

The principal focus of our studies has been at the University of Natal, Durban, South Africa. In many ways Durban can be seen to represent the epicenter of the current global epidemic. It is estimated that 75% of the HIV infections that have occurred to date have been in sub-Saharan Africa.[39] The epidemic in South Africa started relatively recently, with the HIV seroprevalence being <1% in antenatal mothers as recently as 1990.[40] In KwaZuluNatal, the most populated province in South Africa, reports of seroprevalence of >40% are now not uncommon.[41,42] One additional factor that makes Durban an excellent site to study HIV is that >90% of infections are clade-C,[43,44] the clade of virus that affects more infected persons worldwide than any other.[45] Finally, apart from the principal African tribal groups,

---

FIGURE. 1. (**A** and **B**) PBMC from donor 026-BMC (HLA class I type A3/-B42/ B*5703 Cw7/17), stained with the B42-TL9 peptide-MHC tetrameric complex (TL9: TPQDLNTML) in **A**, and intracellular IFN-γ staining of CD8-positive T cells following stimulation of PBMC with the same peptide, TPQDLNTML. (**C**) IFN-γ staining of CD4-positive T cells after stimulation of PBMC with the peptide, AL22 (AFSPEVIPMFSALSE-GATPQDL). CD4-positive T cells shown in light gray. IFN-γ staining of CD8-positive T cells (not shown) after stimulation of PBMC with peptide AL22 was 2.36% of CD8s. Donor 161j, HLA class I type: A*0201/3 B7/60 Cw3/7. (**D-F**) IFN-γ staining of CD8-positive T cells from donor 019-BMC following stimulation of PBMC with HLA class I-matched EBV-transformed B cells that had been pulsed with the peptides shown. HLA types of cells used: donor 019-BMC: A*0201/29 B37/71 Cw3/4. B71-matched BCL targets: 033-BMC: A34/68 B57/71 Cw3/7. (**D**) Control peptide AW11 (AEQASQEVKNW), not B71-restricted. (**E**) Peptide YA11 (YVDRFYKTLRA), B71-restricted. (**F**) Peptide GI13 (GHQAAMQMLKE-TI), B71-restricted also.

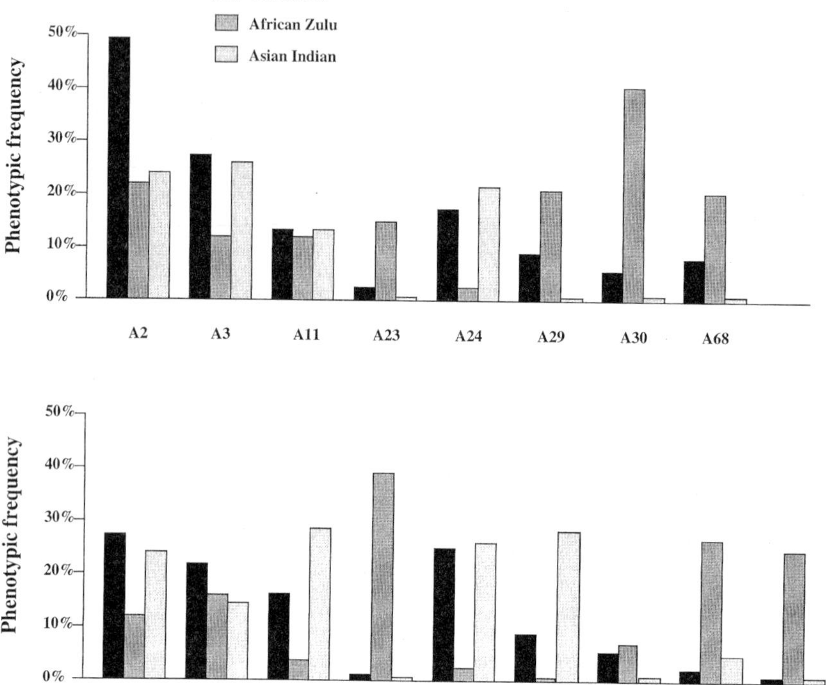

FIGURE 2. HLA class I phenotypic frequencies of selected HLA-A and B alleles, comparing North American Caucasoids with African Zulu and Asian Indians. For simplicity, class I subtypes are not included in the figure.

Zulu and Xhosa, that constitute the majority of infected persons in South Africa, Durban also has a large Asian Indian population of almost 1 million persons. Since clade-C virus is also driving the emerging epidemic in India, HIV-infected Asian Indians in Durban provide an opportunity to define the important clade-C specific epitopes that are presented to CTL and T helper cells by the HLA class I molecules prevalent in Asian Indians.

The reason that characteristic and distinct regions of HIV proteins — epitopes — are recognized by CTL and T helper cells in infected persons of different ethnic groups is that HLA class I molecules are presented at very different frequencies in each population (FIG. 2).[46,47] The best-studied HLA class I molecules so far have been those expressed in a high frequency of Caucasoid populations, such as HLA-A*0201. Unfortunately, these investigations are not always useful for two reasons. First, HLA molecules such as A*0201 are expressed in very low proportion in some populations. In Zulu, for example, the phenotypic frequency of A*0201 is <1%[48] compared with 45% in Caucasoid populations. A second reason that particular class I molecules may not be of assistance in understanding the virus-specific CTL response is that they may not feature prominently in the CTL response as a whole. For example, HLA-A1, which is expressed in approximately one-third of Caucasoids, does not appear to present HIV-specific CTL epitopes in any significant numbers.[49] Why certain HLA class I molecules, such as HLA-B27 or HLA-B57,[18,50,51] tend to dominate the CTL response and others make virtually no contribution is unclear.

In our studies of the clade-C Gag-specific CTL responses dominating the infected Zulu and Xhosa populations of Durban, South Africa, it was clear that certain regions of Gag are distinctively targeted by infected Africans compared to infected Caucasoids.[52] We confirmed that these differences principally do reflect differences in frequencies of HLA-A2, HLA-A3, and HLA-B42 in the respective populations. Caucasoid subjects, who frequently have HLA-A2 or HLA-A3, tend to target epitopes in p17 Gag (SLYNTVATL, A2 restricted; RLRPGGKKK, A3 restricted[49]), whereas African subjects, in whom similar class I molecules B42 and B81 are common, were more likely to target an epitope in p24 Gag (TPQDLNTML [TL9], B42-, or B81-restricted). This work is illustrative of the studies currently being undertaken in order first to determine the identity of the CTL and T helper epitopes that constitute the anti-HIV cellular immune response. An example of B42-TL9 tetramer staining of CTL and an ICS assay showing IFN-gamma production following stimulation of an identical aliquot of the same PBMC from a subject in Durban is shown in FIGURE 1. At the same time as this preliminary work is being completed, focus is also being placed on qualitative differences in the different CTL responses, in order to define which immune responses should ideally be induced by candidate vaccine constructs.

NOVEL APPROACHES TO DEFINING CTL EPITOPES PRESENTED BY UNSTUDIED HLA CLASS I MOLECULES

The methods for defining novel HIV-specific CTL epitopes are twofold. The first method, so-called "reverse immunogenetics,"[53] starts with an analysis of the peptides eluted from single class I molecules. By consideration of the frequency of individual amino acid residues occurring at each position in the peptide, it is possible to obtain a picture of the characteristic peptides that best bind to the class I molecule in question. For example, HLA-B7, one of the commonest HLA-B molecules, best binds peptides carrying Pro (proline) at position 2 (P2), and a medium-sized hydrophobic residue, Leu, Ile, or Met (leucine, isoleucine, or methionine), at the C-terminal position (PC) which is usually P9 in the peptide.[54] Having established this peptide-binding 'motif', it is then possible to use this to screen HIV proteins to identify candidate epitope peptides.

The second method makes no assumptions about peptide binding and simply screens for CTL epitopes by use of long peptides, 15–20 amino acids in length, that overlap by 10 amino acids and that span full-length HIV proteins (for example, ref. 55 and 56). This latter method is less directed towards understanding epitopes presented by particular class I molecules of interest, but it is less likely to miss important immunodominant epitopes that may not conform precisely to the designated peptide-binding motif. One likely explanation for the occurrence of dominant epitopes that do not bind to restriction elements as well as peptides that do not in fact induce CTL responses may be the effect of processing; peptides that are processed efficiently and reach the surface of the cell at high frequency may induce CTL responses better than peptides processed inefficiently.

A third approach to identifying novel epitopes can utilize both of these established methods. Having identified the long 15–20-mer peptide in which a response is present, often it may be possible to predict the optimal epitope once the HLA-restriction of the response is known. In the case of many of the class I molecules dominating the CTL responses in the studies of African Zulu and Xhosa being undertaken, the peptide-binding motif is not established. However, X-ray crystallographic studies have identified the MHC residues that are principally instrumental in determining the peptide-binding motif of each HLA class I molecule.[57–59] By comparing these critical residues between different class I molecules, it is possible to predict with some accuracy the peptide-binding motif of any described class I molecule.

For example, in 1996 we described a novel HLA-B*5801-restricted CTL epitope[51] in p24 Gag (TSTLQEQIGW) that was detected when studying peripheral blood mononuclear cells (PBMC) from an infected Zimbabwean. We identified this same epitope in CTL from HIV-infected subjects with HLA-B*5701. Comparison of the amino acid sequences of HLA-B*5701 and HLA-B*5801 showed close similarity in the critical residues forming the B and F pockets[60] that contribute most importantly to peptide binding. Since the peptide-binding motif for B*5801 had been established,[61] we therefore predicted that the motif for B*5701 would be very similar. HLA-B*5802, on the other hand, based solely on the linear amino acid sequence (ref. 62), did not appear likely to have the space in the F pocket to accommodate so comfortably a large residue the size of Trp (tryptophan). HLA-B*5701 and B*5801 both carry the small Ser at MHC position 116, which largely would explain the capacity of these class I molecules, as well as of HLA-B35, HLA-B53, and HLA-B62 (B*1501) for example, to accommodate large hydrophobic residues such as Trp, Phe, or Tyr into the respective F pockets (TABLE 1). Whereas B*5802 shares this Ser-116, the Trp-97 in B*5802 is likely to account for a reduced space in the F pocket. Hence, it could be predicted that although Trp might just fit into the F pocket of B*5802, optimally binding peptides would have smaller hydrophobic residues at the C-terminal position. These predictions were confirmed when the binding motif of B*5701 and B*5802 was established subsequently by analysis of peptides eluted from these class I molecules.[63] The B57 and B58-binding peptides all preferentially bound peptides with Ser, Thr, or Ala at the P2 anchor position. However, whereas individually sequenced peptides eluted from B57 and B*5801 carried the large hydrophobic residues Trp or Phe in the C-terminal anchor position (in 16/17 peptides sequenced), 4 of 7 peptides eluted from B*5802 carried much smaller hydrophobic residues at the C-terminal position, such as Val, Leu, and Ile.

Thus, based simply on knowledge of the critical contact residues likely to form the B and F pockets of HLA class I molecules and based on comparison with other class I molecules for which the binding motifs have already been established, it may be possible to predict what are the most likely optimal epitope sequences within a 15- to 20-mer peptide known to contain an epitope. This method will significantly reduce the considerable costs of synthesizing unnecessary peptides. However, the success of the method will only be partial, and for unequivocal definition of each novel epitope it remains necessary to show that peptides respectively one amino acid longer or one amino acid shorter at the N- and C-termini of the optimal epitope peptide are less well recognized in peptide titration experiments.

TABLE 1A. Critical MHC residues within the B pocket of selected HLA-B molecules and peptide-binding anchor residues at position 2 in the peptide, defined by peptide elution studies[54,76] or by prediction (see text)

HLA-	(7)	9	24	(34)	45	63	66	67	70	99	Anchor
B*0702 (B7)	Y	Y	S	V	E	N	I	Y	Q	Y	P
B*0801 (B8)	-	D	S	-	E	N	I	F	N	Y	PLI
B*1301 (B13)	-	Y	T	-	M	E	I	S	N	Y	QLM[a]
B*1401 (B64)	-	Y	S	-	E	N	I	S	N	Y	RH[a]
B*1402 (B65)	-	Y	S	-	E	N	I	C	N	Y	RH[a]
B*1501 (B62)	-	Y	A	-	M	E	I	S	N	Y	QLM
B*1503 (B72)	-	Y	S	-	E	E	I	S	N	Y	RH[a]
B*1509 (B71)	-	Y	S	-	E	N	I	C	N	Y	H
B*1510 (B71)	-	Y	S	-	E	N	I	C	N	Y	H[a]
B*1516 (B63)	-	Y	A	-	M	E	N	M	S	Y	TAS
B*1801 (B18)	-	H	S	-	T	N	I	S	N	Y	
B*2705 (B27)	-	H	T	-	E	E	I	C	K	Y	R
B*3501 (B35)	-	Y	A	-	T	N	I	F	N	Y	P
B*3701 (B37)	-	H	S	-	T	E	I	S	N	S	DE
B*3801 (B38)	-	Y	S	-	E	N	I	C	N	Y	RH[a]
B*3901 (B39)	-	Y	S	-	E	N	I	C	N	Y	RH[a]
B*4001 (B60)	-	H	T	-	K	E	I	S	N	Y	E
B*4006 (B61)	-	H	T	-	K	E	I	S	N	Y	E
B*4101 (B41)	-	H	T	-	K	E	I	S	N	Y	E[a]
B*4201 (B42)	-	Y	S	-	E	N	I	Y	Q	Y	PS[a]
B*4402 (B44)	-	Y	T	-	K	E	I	N	N	Y	DE
B*4403 (B44)	-	Y	T	-	K	E	I	N	N	Y	DE
B*4501 (B45)	-	H	T	-	K	E	I	S	N	Y	E[a]
B*5101 (B51)	-	Y	A	-	T	N	I	F	Y	Y	P
B*5201 (B52)	-	Y	A	-	T	N	I	S	Y	Y	Q
B*5301 (B53)	-	Y	A	-	T	N	I	F	Y	Y	PS
B*5401 (B54)	-	Y	A	-	G	N	I	Y	Q	Y	PLI
B*5501 (B55)	-	Y	A	-	E	N	I	Y	Q	Y	P[a]
B*5601 (B56)	-	Y	A	-	E	N	I	Y	Q	Y	P[a]
B*5701 (B57)	-	Y	A	-	M	E	N	M	S	Y	ATS
B*5702 (B57)	-	Y	A	-	M	E	N	M	S	Y	ATS
B*5801 (B58)	-	Y	A	-	T	E	N	M	S	Y	ATS
B*5802 (B58)	-	Y	A	-	T	E	N	M	S	Y	STA
B*8101 (1381)	-	Y	S	-	E	N	I	Y	Y	Y	PS[a]

[a]Anchor predicted by analogy with anchors defined by sequence of eluted peptides (no asterisk).

TABLE 1B. Critical MHC residues at the C-terminal position in the peptide, defined by peptide elution studies[54,76] or by prediction (see text)

HLA-	77	80	81	95	97	116	(123)	143	(146)	147	Anchor[a]
B*0702 (B7)	S	N	L	L	S	Y	Y	T	K	W	LM(FY)
B*0801 (B8)	S	N	L	L	S	Y	-	T	-	W	LI
B*1301 (B13)	N	T	A	I	R	L	-	T	-	W	FYLI[a]
B*1401 (B64)	S	N	L	L	W	F	-	T	-	W	LV
B*1402 (B65)	S	N	L	L	W	F	-	T	-	W	LV
B*1501 (B62)	S	N	L	L	R	S	-	T	-	W	YF
B*1503 (B72)	S	N	L	L	R	S	-	T	-	W	YF
B*1509 (B71)	S	N	L	L	R	Y	-	T	-	W	VL
B*1510 (B71)	S	N	L	L	R	Y	-	T	-	W	VL
B*1801 (B18)	S	N	L	L	R	S	-	T	-	W	LMIYF[a]
B*2705 (B27)	D	T	L	L	N	D	-	T	-	W	KLI
B*3501 (B35)	S	N	L	I	R	S	-	T	-	W	YF
B*3701 (B37)	D	T	L	I	R	F	-	T	-	W	VLI[a]
B*3801 (B38)	N	I	A	L	R	F	-	T	-	W	VLI[a]
B*3901 (B39)	S	N	L	L	R	F	-	T	-	W	VLI[a]
B*4001 (B60)	S	N	L	L	R	Y	-	S	-	L	E
B*4006 (B61)	S	N	L	W	T	Y	-	T	-	W	E
B*4101 (B41)	S	N	L	W	R	Y	-	T	-	W	VL[a]
B*4201 (B42)	S	N	L	L	S	Y	-	T	-	W	LM(FY)[a]
B*4402 (B44)	N	T	A	I	R	D	-	T	-	W	YF
B*4403 (B44)	N	T	A	I	R	D	-	T	-	W	YF
B*4501 (B45)	S	N	L	W	R	L	-	T	-	W	LIM[a]
B*5101 (B51)	N	I	A	W	T	Y	-	T	-	W	VI(F)
B*5201 (B52)	N	I	A	W	T	Y	-	T	-	W	IV
B*5301 (B53)	N	I	A	I	R	S	-	T	-	W	FL
B*5401 (B54)	S	N	L	W	T	L	-	T	-	W	LIM[a]
B*5501 (B55)	S	N	L	W	T	L	-	T	-	W	LIM[a]
B*5601 (B56)	S	N	L	W	T	L	-	T	-	W	LIM[a]
B*5701 (B57)	N	I	A	I	v	S	-	T	-	W	WFY
B*5801 (B58)	N	I	A	I	R	S	-	T	-	W	FYW
B*5802 (B58)	N	I	A	L	W	S	-	T	-	W	VILM
B*8101 (B81)	S	N	L	L	S	Y	-	T	-	W	LM(FY)[a]

[a]Anchor predicted by analogy with anchors defined by sequence of eluted peptides (no asterisk).

FUTURE DIRECTIONS IN THE CHARACTERIZATION OF
NOVEL CTL RESPONSES

As already indicated herein, definition of the epitopes targeted by CTL in the populations worst affected by the global epidemic is only a starting point. Increasingly, it is becoming clear that whilst CTL are viral in achieving control of HIV, not all CTL are created equal. Certain HLA class I molecules, notably B27, B57, have been associated with slow progression and others with rapid progression to disease in HIV infection,[64–67] associations that are presumably related to the CTL response directed through these class I molecules. Studies in LCMV-infected mice have demonstrated that subdominant CTL responses may be 100-fold more effective in clearing virus.[68] The CTL escape studies in HIV and SIV have shown that some epitopes "escape" early, whereas others escape late. Does this mean that the epitopes that allow escape early are less effective or are they more effective? Currently, we can only speculate. Perhaps the best hope to elucidate which are the most effective epitopes will come from vaccination of macaques to induce CTL responses towards particular epitopes followed by SIV challenge.

Our recent studies of CTL responses in acute HIV infection have highlighted the differences between epitopes targeted in acute and chronic HIV infection. Most obvious is the A2-SLYNTVATL (SL9) epitope which is recognized by approximately 70% of chronically infected adults who have A*0201.[14,69–71] Of 12 A2-positive subjects identified by Rosenberg and others at the Massachusetts General Hospital in Boston, only 1 had a detectable response towards this epitope,[71] whereas substantial CTL responses were evident towards other epitopes. In 2 of the 12 subjects, responses to the SL9 epitope developed >2 years later.[72] This very late appearance of the A2-SL9 response clearly shows that it has no part to play in the initial clearance of viremia following acute infection. The high frequency of CTL responses to this epitope in chronically infected subjects may thus be explained by the late appearance of CTL of this specificity in the response. Study of subjects who maintain high frequency responses to SL9 in the presence of high viral loads suggests that these CTL may not in many instances be instrumental in constraining viral replication. Further studies on the timing of each specific response in the anti-HIV immune response as it evolves through the course of the infection are of great importance in helping elucidate the effectiveness of these CTL. Close attention to the fine details of the CTL response in its entirety is required and now is feasible given the novel technologies currently available.

Better understanding of the role of each CTL specificity also opens up the opportunity to improve upon the natural antiviral immune response by inducing particular responses early to broaden and thereby strengthen it. For example, infusion of autologous dendritic cells pulsed with the appropriate peptides is a mode of immunotherapy that is rapidly emerging as a feasible and valuable means of inducing effective primary CTL responses.[73,74]

As just indicated, the CTL response is not effective alone, and the importance of the HIV-specific T helper response is only just becoming fully appreciated. Much further work if needed to define the importance of T helper epitopes and to understand the mechanism by which these cells interact with CTL to enable them to control viremia successfully. The same methods that were just described and have been applied to the study of CTL can also be applied equally to T helper responses. The fact that T helper cells can act directly as cytotoxic cells[75] in addition to facilitating CD8+ CTL function has only recently been highlighted.

CONCLUSIONS

The advent of the Elispot assay and flow-based methods of enumerating and studying CTL and T helper cells have transformed the field of HIV-specific cellular immunity. The prerequisite to understanding these responses in the populations worst affected by the global epidemic is to define the HIV-specific epitopes that constitute the targets of the antiviral immune response. Despite the previous focus of research upon Caucasoid populations infected with B-clade virus, rapid progress is now being made towards achieving this first goal. Important future steps will focus on the identification of responses that are most effective in controlling viremia and on the most efficient induction of these responses by prophylactic or therapeutic vaccination strategies.

ACKNOWLEDGMENTS

This work was supported by grants from the Elizabeth Glaser Pediatric AIDS Foundation (EGPAF Scientist Award) and the Medical Research Foundation (UK) (grant G108/274).

REFERENCES

1. WALKER, B.D., S. CHAKRABATI, B. MOSS et al. 1987. HIV-specific T lymphocytes in seropositive individuals. Nature **328:** 345–348.
2. KLEIN, M.R., C.A. VAN BAALEN, A.M. HOLWERDA et al. 1995. Kinetics of Gag-specific CTL responses during the clinical course of HIV-1 infection: a longitudinal analysis of rapid progressors and long-term, asymptomatics. J. Exp. Med. **181:** 1365–1372.
3. BEVAN, M.J. & T.J. BRACIALE. 1995. Why can't cytotoxic T cells handle HIV? Proc. Natl. Acad. Sci. USA **92:** 5765–5767.
4. FEINBERG M.B. & A.R. MCLEAN. 1997. AIDS: Decline and fall of immune surveillance? Curr. Biol. **7:** 136–140.
5. WEI, X., S.K. GHOSH, M.E. TAYLOR et al. 1995. Viral dynamics in human immunodeficiency virus type 1 infection. Nature **373:** 117–122.
6. HO, D.D., A.U. NEUMANN, A.S. PERELSON et al. 1995. Rapid turnover of plasma virions and CD4 lymphocytes in HIV-1 infection. Nature **373:** 123–126.
7. BORROW, P., H. LEWICKI, B.H. HAHN et al. 1994. Virus-specific CD8+ CTL activity associated with control of viemia in primary HIV infection. J. Virol. **68:** 6103–6110.
8. KOUP, R.A., J.T. SAFRIT, Y. CAO et al. 1994. Temporal association of cellular immune responses with the initial control of viremia in primary HIV infection. J. Virol. **68:** 4650–4655.
9. YASUTOMI, Y., K.A. REIMANN, C.I. LORD et al. 1993. Simian immunodeficiency virus-specific CD8+ lymphocyte response in acutely infected rhesus monkeys. J. Virol. **67:** 1707–11.59.
10. PHILLIPS, A.N. 1996. Reduction of HIV concentration during acute infection: independence from a specific immune response. Science **271:** 497–499.

11. SCHMITZ, J.E., M. KURODA, S. SANTRA *et al.* 1999. Control of viremia in simian immunodeficiency virus infection by CD8+ lymphocytes. Science **283:** 857–860.
12. JIN, X., D.E. BAUER, S.E. TUTTLETON *et al.* 1999. Dramatic rise in plasma viremia after CD8+ T cell depletion in SIV-infected macaques. J. Exp. Med. **189:** 991–998.
13. MELLORS, J.W., C.R. RINALDO, P. GUPTA *et al.* 1996. Prognosis in HIV-1 infection predicted by the quantity of virus in plasma. Science **272:** 1167–1170.
14. OGG, G.S., X. JIN, S. BONHOEFFER *et al.* 1998. Quantitation of HIV-1-specific cytotoxic T lymphocytes and plasma load of viral RNA. Science **279:** 2103–2106.
15. BORROW P., H. LEWICKI, X. WEI *et al.* 1997. Antiviral pressure exerted by HIV-1-specific cytotoxic T lymphocytes (CTLs) during primary infection demonstrated by rapid selection of CTL escape virus. Nature Med. **3:** 205–211.
16. PRICE, D.A., P.J.R. GOULDER, P. KLENERMAN *et al.* 1997. Positive selection of HIV-1 cytotoxic T lymphocyte escape variants during primary infection. Proc. Natl. Acad. Sci. USA **94:** 1890–1895.
17. KOENIG, S., A.J. CONLEY, Y.A. BREWAH *et al.* 1995. Transfer of HIV-1-specific cytotoxic T lymphocytes to an AIDS patient leads to selection for mutant HIV variants and subsequent disease progression. Nature Med. **1:** 330–336.
18. GOULDER, P.J.R., R.E. PHILLIPS, R.A. COLBERT *et al.* 1997. Late escape from an immunodominant cytotoxic T-lymphocyte response associated with progression to AIDS. Nature Med. **3:** 212–217.
19. GOULDER, P.J.R., D.A. PRICE, M. NOWAK *et al.* 1997. Coevolution of human immunodeficiency virus and cytotoxic T lymphocyte responses. Immunol. Rev. **159:** 17–29.
20. GOULDER, P.J.R. & B.D. WALKER. 1999. The great escape: AIDS viruses and immune control. Nat. Med. **5:** 1233–1235.
21. EVANS, D.T., D.H. O'CONNOR, P. JING *et al.* 2000. Virus-specific cytotoxic T-lymphocyte responses select for amino acid variation in simian immunodeficiency virus Env and Nef. Nat. Med. **5:** 1270–1276.
22. ALLEN, T., D.H. O'CONNOR, P. JING *et al.* 2000. Tat-specific T lymphocytes select for SIV escape variants during resolution of primary viraemia. Nature **407:** 388–390.
23. ROSENBERG, E.S., J.M. BILLINGSLEY, A. CALIENDO *et al.* 1997. Vigorous HIV-1-specific CD4+ T-cell responses associated with control of viraemia. Science **278:** 1447–1450.
24. PITCHER, C.J., C. QUITTNER, D.M. PETERSON *et al.* 1999. HIV-1 specific CD4+ T cells are detectable in most individuals with active HIV-1 infection, but decline with prolonged viral suppression. Nat. Med. **5:** 518–525.
25. KALAMS, S.A., S.P. BUCHBINDER, E.S. ROSENBERG *et al.* 1999. Association between virus-specific CTL and helper responses in HIV-1 infection. J. Virol. **73:** 6715–6720.
26. MATLOUBIAN, M., R.J. CONCEPCION & R. AHMED. 1994. CD4+ T cells are required to sustain CD8+ cytotoxic T-cell responses during chronic viral infection. J. Virol. **68:** 8056–8063.
27. BATTEGAY, M., D. MOSKOPHIDIS, A. RAHEMTULLA *et al.* 1994. Enhanced establishment of a virus carrier state in adult CD4+ T-cell-deficient mice. J. Virol. **68:** 4700–4704.
28. KALAMS, S.A. & B.D. WALKER. 1998. The critical need for CD4 help in maintaining effective cytotoxic T lymphocyte responses. J. Exp. Med. **188:** 2199–2204.
29. LALVANI, A., R. BROOKES, S. HAMBLETON *et al.* 1997. Rapid effector function in CD8+ memory T cells. J. Exp. Med. **186:** 859–865.
30. ALTMAN, J., P.A.H. MOSS, P.J.R. GOULDER *et al.* 1996. Direct visualization and phenotypic analysis of virus-specific T lymphocytes in HIV-infected individuals. Science **274:** 94–96.
31. GOULDER, P.J.R., T. TANG, C. BRANDER *et al.* 2000. Functionally inert HIV-specific cytotoxic T lymphocyte do not play a major role in chronically infected adults and children. J. Exp. Med. In press.
32. BETTS, M.R., J.P. CASSAZA, B.A. PATTERSON *et al.* 2000. Immunodominant HIV-specific CD8+ T-cell responses cannot be predicted by MHC class I haplotype. J. Virol. In press.
33. JOHNSON, R.P. Unpublished data.
34. GOULDER, P.J.R. Unpublished data.
35. ALTFELD, M., A. TROCJA, R.L. ELDRIDGE *et al.* 2000. Overrepresentation of HLA-B60 and –B61-restricted CTL activity within the total HIV-1-specific CTL response.

Rapid characterization of CTL responses and definition of multiple novel epitopes using the enzyme-linked immunospot (Elispot) assay. Manuscript submitted.

36. ANDROLEWICZ, M.J. & P. CRESSWELL. 1996. How selective is the transporter associated with antigen processing? Immunity **5:** 1–5.

37. BARCHET, W. *et al.* 2000. Eur. J. Immunol. **30:** 1356–1363.

38. SHEEY, M. *et al.* 2000. Manuscript in preparation.

39. ANONYMOUS. 1997. The current global situation of the HIV/AIDS pandemic. Wkly Epidem. Rec. **72:** 359–360.

40. ANONYMOUS. 1999. Department of Health 1998: Ninth Annual National HIV Sero-Prevalence Survey of Women attending antenatal clinics in South Africa. Health Systems Research and Epidemiology, Department of Health, South Africa, 1999.

41. WILKINSON, D., C. CONNOLLY & K. ROTCHFORD. 1999. Continued explosive rise in HIV prevalence among pregnant women in rural South Africa. AIDS **13:** 740.

42. WILKINSON, D. 1999. HIV infection among pregnant women in the South African private medical sector. AIDS **13:** 1783.

43. MOODLEY, D., T.-L. SMITH, E.J. VAN RENSBURG *et al.* 1998. HIV type 1 V3 region subtyping in KwaZulu-Natal, a high-seroprevalence South African Region. AIDS Res. Hum. Retr. **14:** 1015–1018.

44. VAN HARMELEN, J.H., E. VAN DER RYST, A.S. LOUBSER *et al.* 1999. A predominantly HIV type 1 subtype C-restricted epidemic in South African urban populations. AIDS Res. Hum. Retr. **15:** 395–398.

45. Anonymous. 1997. HIV-1 subtypes: implications for epidemiology, pathogenicity, vaccines and diagnostics. Workshop report from the European Commission and the Joint United Nations Programme on HIV/AIDS. AIDS **11:** 17–36.

46. CLAYTON, J., C. LONJOU & D. WHITTLE. 1997. Allele and haplotype frequencies for HLA loci in various ethnic groups. *In* Proceedings of XIIth International Histocompatibility Workshop. Vol 1. Dominique Charron. Ed. :665–820.

47. IMANISHI, T., T. AKAZA, A. KIMURA *et al.* 1992. Allele and haplotype frequencies for HLA and complement loci in various ethnic groups. *In* HLA 1991 – Proceedings of the XIth International Histocompatibility Workshop and Conference. Vol **1:** 1065–1220. K. Tsuji, M .Aizawa & T. Sasaszuki, Eds.

48. HAMMOND, M.G., E.D. DU TOIT, A. SANCHEZ-MAZAS *et al.* 1997. HLA in sub-Saharan Africa: 12th International Histocompatibility Workshop SSAF report. *In* Proceedings of the Twelfth International Histocompatibility Workshiop and Conference. Dominique Charron, Ed.: 345–353. EDK. Paris, France.

49. BRANDER, C. & P.J.R. GOULDER. 1999. Recent advances in the optimization of HIV-specific CTL epitopes. *In* HIV Molecular Immunology Database. 1999. B.T.M. Korber, C. Brander, B.D. Walker, R.A. Koup, J. Moore, B. Haynes & G. Meyers, Eds. Los Alamos National Laboratory: Theoretical Biology and Biophysics. Los Alamos, NM.

50. GOULDER, P.J.R. Unpublished data.

51. GOULDER, P.J.R., S. CROWLEY, P. KRAUSA *et al.* 1996. Novel, cross-restricted, conserved and immunodominant CTL epitopes in long-term slow progresssors in HIV-1 infection. AIDS Res. Hum. Retro. **12:** 1691–1698.

52. GOULDER, P.J.R., C. BRANDER, K. ANNAMALAI *et al.* 2000. Differential narrow focusing of immunodominant HIV Gag-specific CTL responses in infected African and Caucasoid adults and children. J. Virol. **74:** 5679–5690.

53. HILL, A.V.S. 1998. The immunogenetics of human infectious diseases. Ann. Rev. Immunol. **16:** 593–617.

54. RAMMENSEE, H.G., T. FRIEDE & S. STEVANOVIC. 1995. MHC ligands and peptide motifs: first listing. Immunogenetics **41:** 178–228.

55. NIXON, D.F., A.R. TOWNSEND, J.G. ELVIN *et al.* 1988. HIV-1 gag-specific cytotoxic T lymphocytes defined with recombinant vaccinia virus and synthetic peptides. Nature **336:** 484–487.

56. MADDEN, D.R., J.C. GORGA, J.L. STROMINGER & D.C. WILEY. 1992. The three-dimensional structure of HLA-B27 at 2.1A resolution suggests a general mechanism for tight binding to MHC. Cell **70:** 1035–1048.

57. GARBOCZI, D.N., D.T. HUNG & D.C. WILEY. 1992. HLA-A2-peptide complexes: refolding and crystallization of molecules expressed in *Escherichia coli* and complexed with single antigenic peptides. Proc. Natl. Acad. Sci. USA **89:** 3429–3433.

58. GUO, H.-C., D.R. MADDEN, M.L. SILVER *et al.* 1993. Comparison of the P2 specificity pocket in three human histocompatibility antigens, HLA-A*6801, HLA-A*0201, and HLA-B*2705. Proc. Natl. Acad. Soc. USA **90:** 8053–8057.

59. JARDETZKY, T.S., W.S. LANE, R.A. ROBINSON *et al.* 1991. Identification of self-peptides bound to purified HLA-B27. Nature **353:** 326–329.

60. SAPER, M.A., P.J. BJORKMAN & D.C. WILEY. 1991. Refined structure of the human histocompatibility antigen HLA-A2 at 2.6 A resolution. J. Mol. Biol. **219:** 277–319.

61. FALK, K., O. ROTZSCHKE, M. TAKIGUCHI *et al.* 1995. Peptide motifs of HLA-B58, B60, B61, and B62 molecules. Immunogenetics **41:** 165–168.

62. ARNETT, K.L. & P. PARHAM. 1995. HLA class I nucleotide sequences. Tissue Antigens **46:** 217–257.

63. BARBER, L.D., L. PERCIVAL, K.L. ARNETT *et al.* 1997. Polymorphism in the a1 helix of the HLA-B heavy chain can have an overriding influence on peptide-binding specificity. J. Immunol. **158:** 1660–1669.

64. KASLOW, R.A., M. CARRINGTON, R. APPLE *et al.* 1996. Influence of human MHC genes on the course of HIV infection. Nature Med. **2:** 405–411.

65. CARRINGTON, M., G.W. NELSON, M.P. MARTIN *et al.* 1999. HLA and HIV-1: heterozygote advantage and B*35-Cw*04 disadvantage. Science **283:** 1748–1752.

66. KEET, I.P., J. TANG, M.R. KLEIN *et al.* 1999. Consistent associations of HLA class I and II and transporter gene products with progression of human immunodeficiency virus type 1 infection in homosexual men. J. Infect. Dis. **180:** 299–309.

67. MIGUELES, S.A., M.S. SABBAGHIAN, W.L. SHUPERT *et al.* 2000. HLA-B*5701 is highly associated with restriction of virus replication in a subgroup of HIV-infected long-term nonprogressors. Proc. Natl. Acad. Sci. USA **97:** 2709–2714.

68. GALLIMORE, A., T. DUMRESE, H. HENGARTNER *et al.* 1998. Protective immunity does not correlate with the hierarchy of virus-specific CTL responses to naturally processed peptides. J. Exp. Med. **187:** 1647–1657.

69. GOULDER, P.J.R., A.K. SEWELL, D.G. LALLOO *et al.* 1997. Patterns of immunodominance in HIV-1-specific cytotoxic T lymphocyte responses in two HLA-identical siblings with HLA-A*0201 are influenced by epitope mutation. J. Exp. Med. **185:** 1423–1433.

70. BRANDER, C., K.E. HARTMAN, A.K. TROCHA *et al.* 1998. Lack of strong immune selection pressure by the immunodominant HLA-A*0201 restricted CTL response in chronic HIV-1 infection. J. Clin. Invest. **101:** 2559–2566.

71. GRAY, C., J. LAWRENCE, J.M. SCHAPIRO *et al.* 1999. Frequency of class I restricted anti-HIV CD8+ T cells in individuals receiving highly active antiretroviral therapy. J. Immunol. **162:** 1780–1788.

72. GOULDER, P.J.R., M.A. ALTFELD, E.S. ROSENBERG *et al.* 2000. HLA-A*0201-restricted cytotoxic T lymphocyte epitopes targeted differ markedly between acute and chronic HIV infection. Manuscript submitted.

73. DHODAPKAR, M.V., R.M. STEINMAN, M. SAPP *et al.* 1999. Rapid generation of broad T-cell immunity in humans after a single injection of mature dendritic cells. J. Clin. Invest. **104:** 173–180.

74. DHODAPKAR, M.V., J.R. KRASOVSKY, M. STEINMAN & N. BHARDWAJ. 2000. Mature dendritic cells boost functionally superior CD8(+) T-cell in humans without foreign helper epitopes. J. Clin. Invest. **105:** R9–R14.

75. NORRIS, P. Unpublished data.

76. RAMMENSEE, H.-G. *et al.* SYFPEITHI web site: http://1342.96.221/Scripts/hlaserver.dll/open.html

Factors Impacting on Drug Choices

Issues for Developing Countries

STEPHEN A. SPECTOR[a]

University of California, San Diego, Department of Pediatrics, Center for Molecular Genetics and Center for AIDS Research, La Jolla, California 92093-0672, USA

ABSTRACT: In considering factors that impact on drug choices for children in developing countries, it is important to learn from the advances in antiretroviral therapy that have been made in the United States and other developed countries. Abundant clinical data indicate that monotherapy with antiretroviral agents, no matter how potent, is inadequate and that children should be treated with three or more drugs. When treatment regimens are changed, at least two new drugs should be started simultaneouly to avoid the rapid development of resistance. Understanding the impact of host and viral genotypes may provide information as to how best to treat the individual child. However, at present, I believe that with limited resources, the best use of antiretrovirals for children is in disease prevention. Thus, antiretrovirals to prevent mother-to-infant transmission should be given the highest priority. Second, children in the first year of life are at highest risk of progression and should be treated with trimethoprim-sulfamethoxazole to prevent *Pneumocystis carinii* pneumonia, and targeted for receiving antiretrovirals. Moreover, treating children without an overall plan is unacceptable. Treatment with drugs because they are available will have little impact on the quality of life or disease progression unless they are used in combination. There should be no reason for children, no matter where they might live, to receive suboptimal antiretroviral therapy. For this reason, I call upon industrialized countries and the World Bank to help provide resources for the care and treatment of HIV-infected children. Additionally, I would propose that pharmaceutical companies provide support for the care and treatment of HIV-infected children. The drugs and financial support provided by pharmaceutical companies should go to a central foundation or group that will optimize the use of these resources for children in developing countries. I would also propose that in the United States, Europe, and other industrialized countries the patents on antiretroviral drugs be extended according to a formula based on the donation of a pharmaceutical company. It is only through a unified effort that we will be able to adequately treat all children infected with HIV regardless of where they might live.

INTRODUCTION

In considering factors that impact on drug choices for children in developing countries, I believe it is important that we examine what has been learned in the United States and other developed countries so that we can apply this knowledge to

[a]Address for correspondence: Dr. Stephen A. Spector, University of California, San Diego, Stein Clinical Research Building, 9500 Gilman Drive, La Jolla, CA 92093-0672. Voice: 858-534-7170; fax: 858-534-7411.

saspector@ucsd.edu

improve treatment for HIV-infected children globally. In April 1998, "Guidelines for the use of antiretrovirals in pediatric HIV infection," was published in the *Morbidity and Mortality Weekly Report*. These guidelines were the product of numerous pediatric HIV specialists coming to consensus on how best to treat HIV-infected children.

CURRENT RECOMMENDATIONS FOR TREATMENT OF THE HIV-INFECTED CHILD

The guidelines outline several basic principles for the treatment of pediatric HIV disease. The guidelines are reviewed monthly and modified when appropriate in an attempt to keep pace with new information and advances in treatment. For most asymptomatic children infected with HIV, the guidelines recommend that antiretroviral therapy be initiated, whereas a small minority of experts would withhold treatment until virologic, immunologic, or clinical signs of progressing HIV disease were present. All experts agree, however, that for any child identified before 12 months of age, with immunologic impairment or clinical symptoms associated with HIV infection, antiretroviral therapy should be instituted. All experts agree that when antiretroviral therapy is begun, initiating treatment with three or more drugs is most appropriate. Recommended antiretroviral regimens for children include: a protease inhibitor plus two nucleoside reverse transcriptase inhibitors (NRTIs), efavirenz plus two NRTIs, or efavirenz plus nelfinavir plus one NRTI. Alternative regimens include: nevirapine plus two NRTIs or abacavir plus zidovudine/lamivudine (3TC). Specific regimens are not recommended including the use of any monotherapy, stavudine (d4T) plus zidovudine (ZDV) (because of demonstrated antagonism both *in vitro* and *in vivo*), and ddC combined with ddI, d4T, or 3TC because of potential additive toxicity (particularly peripheral neuropathy). Children who have signs of virologic, immunologic, or clinical failure are recommended to have their treatment regimens modified with the reinstitution of treatment with at least two new drugs.

IMPACT OF HIGHLY ACTIVE ANTIRETROVIRAL THERAPY (HAART)

A recent study that evaluates the pharmacokinetics, safety, tolerability, and antiviral effects of efavirenz and nelfinavir combined with one or two NRTIs demonstrates the ability of antiretrovirals to significantly suppress HIV plasma RNA and increase CD4+ lymphocyte counts. In this study, 50 (88%) of 57 children achieved plasma RNA levels below 400 copies/ml after a median of 8 weeks, whereas 36 (63%) of 57 achieved plasma RNA levels below 50 copies/ml a median of 20 weeks after initiation of therapy. The treatment has had excellent durability of response and tolerance with sustained elevations in CD4+ lymphocyte counts. Thus, initiation of potent combination therapy in these antiretroviral experienced children with a non-nucleoside reverse transcriptase inhibitor (NNRTI) and protease inhibitor (PI) led to an excellent virologic, immunologic, and clinical response.

A child for whom we have provided care in San Diego, I believe exemplifies some of the pitfalls of early therapies and the advances that have been made over the last several years with the availability of HAART. This child was born in 1989 and at 3 months of age was diagnosed with *Pneumocystis carinii* pneumonia and HIV infection. Zidovudine (ZDV) therapy was initiated, and she had a brief response before having a significant decline in the CD4+ lymphocyte count. At 32 months of age she had ddC added to the ZDV therapy and again had a modest but short-lived response to therapy. By 50 months of age her CD4+ lymphocyte count was 47/μL, and the antiretroviral therapy was switched to ZDV/ddI/Nevirapine. After a modest response, she again failed therapy, and soon the CD4+ lymphocyte count was below 10 cells/μL. Her growth fell below the third percentile; she was cognitively impaired and spent most of her day in bed. It was now 1995 and protease inhibitors were available. The administration of d4T/3TC/Ritonavir was begun through a gastrostomy tube. The response was dramatic. Her weight increased from below the third percentile to the fiftieth percentile. The HIV RNA load was undetectable, and the CD4+ lymphocyte count rose to over 800 cells/μL. She responded to recall antigens on skin testing and in LPA assays to a number of different antigens. Her neurocognitive impairment was reversed clinically and improvement was demonstrated on magnetic resonance imaging. We started three new drugs including a new class of drugs, protease inhibitors, and the patient dramatically responded. However, another lesson can be learned from this patient, one that I believe is relevant to our consideration of antiretrovirals in developing countries. That is, although done unintentionally, we treated this patient with the antiretrovirals that we had available to us at the time. The treatment was, in fact, inadequate and today would be considered substandard. Much has been learned about how not to use antiretrovirals. We must learn from these lessons and not let ourselves be forced into making the same mistakes.

Increasingly antiretroviral therapy in the U.S. and other developed countries has converted HIV from an invariably fatal infection to a chronic illness. We often argue as to what is undetectable virus. Are less than 400 copies of HIV RNA/ml undetectable? How about less than 50 copies/ml? Isn't there still virus in lymph nodes or the bone marrow or other remote sites? The answer is yes, virus is always present somewhere in the body. Treatments significantly do decrease the overall viral burden. Moreover, overall survival and quality of life have been greatly improved. As an example, in 1995, 49 (25%) of 199 children participating in antiretroviral studies within the PACTG died compared to 20 (4%) of 474 in 1998. Thus, a dramatic improvement in survival has been observed over the last several years in children participating in PACTG studies.

IMPACT OF CHEMOKINE RECEPTOR AND CHEMOKINE GENOTYPE ON HIV-RELATED DISEASE

With the identification of specific chemokine receptors as co-receptors with CD4 for HIV attachment and entry into cells, considerable research has examined the association of genetic polymorphisms in adults of chemokines and chemokine receptors.[3,4] These data indicate that the CCR5Δ32 polymorphism impacts on both HIV transmission as well as disease progression. Persons homozygous for Δ32 rarely become infected with HIV (fewer than 10 persons worldwide have been identified as HIV-infected with this genotype). Although the CCR5wt/Δ32 does not prevent infection, it significantly delays disease progression. Similarly, in adults the CCR264I variant is associated with delayed disease progression as well as the chemokine genotype SDF1-3'A/3'A.[5,6] In children, little data are available regarding these genotypes. To my knowledge, no infant has been infected perinatally with the CCR5Δ32/Δ32 genotype.

To further identify the impact of chemokine receptor genotypes on disease progression, we examined the genotypes of children who participated in the PACTG 152 protocol. Children who participated in this study were randomized to receive either zidovudine, didanosine, or zidovudine/didanosine. Patients were followed for clinical endpoints. The results of the study demonstrated that ddI and ZDV/ddI provided superior efficacy when compared to the ZDV alone group.[7] However, no difference in clinical endpoints was observed for ddI compared to the ZDV/ddI groups. Of the 152 participants, we identified 8 with the CCR5wt/Δ32 genotype; 11 received ZDV, 9 ddI, and 8 ZDV/ddI.[8] Children with the wt/Δ32 genotype progressed more slowly than did other children regardless of the treatment regimen to which they were randomized. Moreover, children with the CCR5wt/Δ32 genotype entered the study with lower HIV-1 plasma RNA levels, higher CD+ lymphocyte counts, and better weight for age Z-scores than did children with the wt/wt genotype and at completion of the study maintained these differences. We have also examined the impact of the CCR2 and SDF1 genotypes on disease progression. In these cases, our findings in children differ from those in adults. Children with the CCR264I variant showed no difference in disease progression from those with the wt/wt genotype. In further variance with findings in adults, children with the SDF1-3'A/3'A genotype progressed more rapidly than do those with the wt/wt or heterozygote. In fact, 6 (75%) of 8 children with the 3'A/3'A variant demonstrated disease progression during the course of the study (p <0.001) (Barroga *et al.*, manuscript in preparation). Thus, it may be possible to identify certain children who are at increased risk for disease progression and target antiretroviral therapy for these high-risk children.

APPROACH TO TREATMENT OF THE HIV-INFECTED CHILD IN THE DEVELOPING WORLD

A critical question for developing countries is whether we can target treatment for those children who are most likely to progress and would therefore benefit most from therapy. The first group that would clearly benefit from antiretrovirals is those children identified as infected who are below 12 months of age. In one study performed in Uganda, 34% of HIV-infected children died within the first year of.[1] Similarly, in San Diego, 21% of children identified as HIV-infected within the first year of life died prior to the availability of antiretrovirals.[2] Thus, targeting children identified within the first year of life for antiretroviral therapy is a high priority.

What can and should be done for HIV-infected children in developing countries? First, with limited resources, the best use of antiretrovirals for children is in disease prevention. Thus, antiretrovirals to prevent mother-to-infant transmission should be given the highest priority. Second, children in the first year of life are at highest risk of progression and should be treated with trimethoprim-sulfamethoxazole to prevent *P. carinii* pneumonia and be targeted for receiving antiretrovirals. We have learned in the U.S. and other industrialized countries that monotherapy is suboptimal treatment. Moreover, treating children without an overall plan is unacceptable. Treatment with drugs because they are available will have little impact on the quality of life or disease progression unless they are used in combination.

A GLOBAL PARTNERSHIP IS NEEDED

There should be no reason for children, no matter where they might live, to receive suboptimal antiretroviral therapy. For this reason, I call upon industrialized countries and the World Bank to help provide resources for the care and treatment of HIV-infected children. Additionally, I would propose that pharmaceutical companies provide support for the care and treatment of HIV-infected children. The drugs and financial support provided by pharmaceutical companies should go to a central foundation or group that will optimize the use of these resources for children in developing countries. I would also propose that in the U.S., Europe, and other industrialized countries the patents on antiretroviral drugs be extended according to a formula based on the donation of a pharmaceutical company. It is only through a unified effort that we will be able to make an impact on this critical situation.

Although in many ways we in industrialized countries are a world apart from people in developing countries, we are one world. We must take advantage of this historic opportunity to prevent HIV transmission from any infected mother to her infant and provide the resources necessary to provide care, education, and treatment for HIV-infected children.

ACKNOWLEDGMENTS

This research is supported by Grants AI39004, AI27563, and the UCSD Center for AIDS Research (AI36214).

REFERENCES

1. MARUM, L.H., D. TINDYEBWA & D. GIBB. 1997. Care of children with HIV infection and AIDS in Africa. Aids **11**(Suppl. B): S125–134.
2. SPENCER, L.T., M.T. OGINO, W.M. DANKNER & S.A. SPECTOR. 1994. Clinical significance of human immunodeficiency virus type 1 phenotypes in infected children. J. Infect. Dis. **169**: 491–495.
3. LITTMAN, D.R. 1998. Chemokine receptors: keys to AIDS pathogenesis? Cell **93**: 677–680.
4. LUSTER, A.D. 1998. Chemokines: chemotactic cytokines that mediate inflammation. N. Engl. J. Med. **338**: 436–445.
5. MANGANO, A., J. KOPKA, M. BATALLA et al. 1999. Influence of CCR5, CCR2, and SDF-1 genetic polymorphisms on HIV-1 disease progression in childhood. 6th Conference on Retroviruses and Opportunistic Infections. Foundation for Retrovirology and Human Health. Chicago, IL.
6. SMITH, M.W., M. DEAN, M. CARRINGTON et al. 1997. Contrasting genetic influence of CCR2 and CCR5 variants on HIV-1 infection and disease progression. Science **277**: 959–965.
7. ENGLUND, J.A., C.J. BAKER, C. RASKINO et al. 1997. Zidovudine, didanosine, or both as the initial treatment for symptomatic HIV-infected children. AIDS Clinical Trials Group (ACTG) Study 152 Team. N. Engl. J. Med. **336**: 1704–1712.
8. BARROGA, C.F., C. RASKINO, M.C. FARGON et al. 2000. The CCR5Δ 32 allele slows disease progression of human immunodeficiency virus-1-infected children receiving antiretroviral treatment. J. Infect. Dis. **182**: 413–419.

Factors with a Negative Influence on Compliance to Antiretroviral Therapies

AUGUSTIN CUPSA,[a] CRISTIAN GHEONEA, DUMITRU BULUCEA, AND SORIN DINESCU

University of Medicine and Pharmacy of Craiova, 1100 Craiova, Romania

A key element in the management of the HIV patient, adherence to antiretroviral therapy (ART), is influenced by a broad spectrum of factors.[1] Of utmost importance in pediatric HIV, especially where younger children are concerned, is the role of the family in the correct administration of the prescribed medication. When dealing with the worldwide problem of nonadherence to ART,[2,3] the management of HIV-infected children involves specific factors pertaining to the family. These factors require adequate monitoring and amelioration by targeted strategies.[4,5]

OBJECTIVES

It was our objective to evaluate long-term compliance with ART by the parents or those acting *in loco parentis* of horizontally HIV-infected children; to determine the incidence, motivation, and risk factors associated with discontinuing/abandoning (D/A) ART in the families with HIV-infected children in an administrative unit in southern Romania, a region with distinctive ethnic, socioeconomic, and cultural features.

METHODS

From the total number of 325 pediatric patients managed at the Active Surveillance Center for the HIV-Infected Children and Their Families (ASCHIV) of Craiova, Dolj County, Romania, we followed up prospectively, starting in 1996, over a period of 18 months, 150 patients (52.6%), aged 8.5 ± 2.5 (5.7–11) years. The children, raised in their own families or in family-type structures, were started on mono or dual ART.

The definition of compliance was accepted as adherence to ≥85% of the prescribed ART. Compliance assessment was performed by obtaining self-reports of D/A ART from children and/or their families and identification of their reasons; interviews on the modes of administration and the medication taken one day before their monthly appointments at ASCHIV; establishing the punctuality of presentation for

[a]Address for correspondence: Cupsa Augustin, M.D., Ph.D., University of Medicine and Pharmacy of Craiova, 4 Petru Rares Str., 1100 Craiova, Romania. Voice: (+4)-051-145603; fax (+4)-051-413838.

cupsa@medinf.comp-craiova.ro

scheduled appointments; and ad-hoc visits of ASCHIV teams to the patients' houses and checking the existing provisions of drugs.

The following characteristics were considered in the analysis presented here: those of patients (gender, level of education, clinical and immunological categories as defined by the 1994 CDC Classification, the ART regimen) and those of the families (place of residence, ethnic group, distance from home to ASCHIV, family structure and size, socioeconomic status, mother's education). *In loco parentis* arrangements consisted of foster parents or extended family members who had custody of the HIV-infected children abandoned by their families. ART medication was distributed at the ASCHIV according to a monthly schedule. The statistical analyses were performed using STATISTICA 7.0 software. (The p value was calculated by chi square comparison of proportions.)

RESULTS

Forty cases (26.67%) in which patients discontinued or abandoned ART were studied. The structure of the group studied is detailed in TABLE 1. The primary reason for suspending ART (see TABLE 2) was an inability to comprehend the disease and the treatment (12 cases, 30%), with the second most frequent reason given being mistrust of the therapy or fear of side effects (8 cases, 20%). Irregular ART supply by ASCHIV was responsible for D/A in 4 cases (10%). Two families preferred naturalistic and homeopathic therapies. Six respondents (15%) associated two or more reasons for discontinuing/abandoning ART.

Study of the factors with a negative influence on compliance (see TABLE 1) showed an increased incidence of D/A in patients with minor clinical and immunological manifestations (4/8 vs. 36/142, $p = 0.045$). Their reasons were related to a lack of comprehension of the disease and the treatment. D/A was more frequent among families from rural communities (26/74 vs. 14/76, $p = 0.02$). A negative association with compliance was presented by disorganized natural families and in loco parentis arrangements (23/65 vs. 17/85, $p = 0.03$), families with very low income (21/57 vs. 19/93, $p = 0.03$), and low educational level of the mother/caregiver (26/75 vs. 14/75, $p = 0.026$). There was no significant statistical correlation between D/A of the ART and medication, ethnic group, or distance from ASCHIV.

CONCLUSIONS AND LESSONS LEARNED

Nonadherence to ART among the families of the children infected with HIV in Dolj County is present in a significant number of cases. Certain factors with a negative influence on compliance can be positively influenced by the health care personnel (adapting the type and rhythm of counseling, especially for disorganized families and those with a low educational level). Nevertheless, other factors require complex interventions on the community level (i.e., improving the socioeconomic status of families with difficulties and providing financial support for a constant supply of ART medication).

TABLE 1. Correlation of cases discontinuing/abandoning ART with patient and family characteristics

| Characteristics | Study group | | D/A group | | |
	$n = 150$	Percent	$n = 40$	Percent	p value
Gender					
Male	82	54,7	22	26,8	
Female	68	45,3	18	26.4	
Level of education for the children					
Organized educational program	96	64	31	32.3	
Sporadic, at home	54	36	9	16.7	
Distribution by clinical categories					
A	8	5.3	4	50	0.04
B	64	42.7	14	21.9	
C	78	52	22	28.2	
Distribution by immunological categories					
1	8	5.3	4	50	0.04
2	53	35.3	12	22.6	
3	89	59.3	24	30.8	
ART					
Monotherapy	55	36.6	14	25.5	
Dual therapy	95	63.4	26	27.4	
Residence					
Urban	76	50.6	14	18.4	0.02
Rural areas	74	49.4	26	35.1	
Ethnic group					
Romanians	83	55.3	21	25.3	
Gypsies	64	42.7	19	29.7	
Other	3	2	-		
Distance from home to ASCHIV					
< 30 km	74	49.4	14	18.9	
≥ 30 km	76	50.6	26	34.2	
Family structure					
Natural, organized	85	56.6	17	20	
Natural, disorganized[a]	48	32	18	37.5	0.03
Loco parentis	17	11.3	5	29.4	
Economic status[b]					
Low	57	38	21	36.8	0.03
Good	71	47.3	14	19.7	
Very good	22	14.6	5	22.7	
Level of education for the mother					
None	21	14	7	33.3	
Eight grades	54	36	19	35.2	0.02
High school	39	26	6	15.4	
College or more	36	24	8	22.2	
Number of children in the family					
1–2	76	50.6	19	25	
≥ 3	74	49.4	21	28.4	

[a]Single parent, extended family.
[b]Family monthly income lower than one monthly minimum wage.

TABLE 2. Reasons for discontinuing/abandoning antiretroviral therapy

Reasons	No. of cases	Percent
No comprehension of the treatment	7	17.5
No comprehension of the disease	5	12.5
Fear of side effects	5	12.5
Side effects	4	10
Temporary availability of medication	4	10
Mistrust of the therapy	3	7.5
Changing to alternative therapies	2	5
Multiple reasons	6	15
Lost of ASCHIV evidence	4	10

On the basis of the data gathered from this study, a complex program (including viral load determinations) for monitoring cases and preventing nonadherence was implemented at ASCHIV, to face the new challenges[6] raised by the introduction of HAART for pediatric cases in 1999.

REFERENCE

1. CHESNEY, M. 1999. The challenge of adherence. BETA (Bulletin of Experimental Treatment for AIDS) January 1999 issue.
2. MEHTA, S., R.D. MOORE & N.M.H. GRAHAM. 1997. Potential factors affecting adherence with HIV therapy. AIDS **11**: 1665–1670.
3. WILLIAMS, A. & G. FRIEDLAND. 1997. Adherence, compliance, and HAART. AIDS Clin. Care **9(7)**: 51–58.
4. DUNN, A-M., J.P. NAVARRA & J. CERVIA. 1998. Adherence to antiretroviral medications in HIV-infected children: a collaborative approach with guidelines for care. Abstract No. 32378. 12th World AIDS Conference, Geneva.
5. GROSS, E., C.K. BURR, D. STORM, *et al.* 1998. Monitoring treatment adherence in pediatric HIV: identifying the issues from providers and families. Abstract No. 32438. 12th World AIDS Conference, Geneva.
6. BASSETTI, S., M. BATTEGAY, H. FURRER, *et al.* 1999. Why is highly active antiretroviral therapy (HAART) not prescribed or discontinued? JAIDS **21**: 114–1192.

Immunologic and Virologic Outcome of a Multitreated Cohort of 78 HIV-Infected Children

CATHERINE DOLLFUS, M. DESUQUE, G. VAUDRE, AND C. COURPOTIN
Hôpital Armand-Trousseau, AP-HP, Paris, France

INTRODUCTION

Recent years have witnessed successive advances in HIV therapeutic management. Here, we present an evaluation of longitudinal therapeutic changes in the population of a large French pediatric center and their virologic and immunologic outcomes. Our center's policy has always been to initiate treatment in all HIV-infected children, regardless of their immunologic status, upon ascertaining the diagnosis. Therapeutic strategies were drawn from the adult experience and pediatric protocols and, since 1996, have been aimed toward maintaining an undetectable viral load, while taking into account quality of life, including school schedules.

POPULATION AND METHODS

Hôpital Armand Trousseau HIV Pediatric Clinic was started in 1987. A computerized data management system became available in 1993. Of the 118 HIV-infected children enrolled in the database between January of 1993 and December of 1998, 18 children died and 22 moved to a different place or were lost to follow-up; 78 children are included in this study.

The standard of care comprises monthly routine outpatient visits and blood tests including measurement of viral load and CD4 cell count every 3 months, or more frequently depending on medical judgment.

The description of the patient population is based on the 1994 revised classification system for HIV infection in children (Centers for Disease Control).[1] It reflects the worst stage ever reached by the children on the basis of clinical and immunologic parameters, not the current status. Treatment data refer to current and previously used treatments and therapeutic history (number and duration of single or combination antiretroviral drug treatments).

Immunologic and virologic outcome, derived from the results of the last two consecutive blood tests available up to December 31, 1998, is defined by means of the following criteria:

- Immunologic success: no evidence of immunosuppression (CD4 $\geq$ 25%), improvement from previous moderate (CD4 = 15 to 24%) to no evidence of immunosuppression, or from previous severe (CD4 < 15%) to moderate or no evidence of immunosuppression.

- Virologic success: plasma HIV-1 viral load maintained $\leq$500 copies/ml.

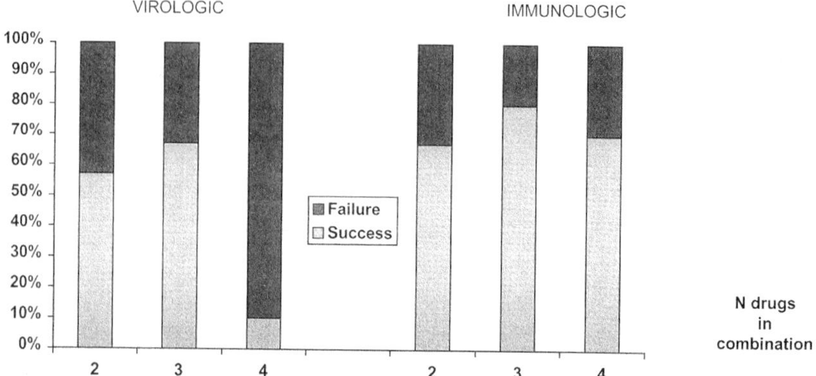

FIGURE 1. Virologic and immunologic success and failure rates according to current treatment at last follow-up.

Any other condition in this analysis is considered to be a failure of the treatment.

RESULTS

The population consists of 78 children age 1 to 21 years old with a median age of 8 years (mean 8.5 years). Of these, 94% have been vertically infected, 3% acquired the virus through blood transfusion, and 3% acquired the virus from an unknown source. According to the CDC classifications, 44% were at clinical stage A, 40% at B, 16% at C; immunologic status was at stage 1 in 28% of the patients, stage 2 in 37%, and stage 3 in 35%.

Seventy-seven children were treated: 21 received dual therapy, 45 received a combination regimen of three drugs (42 including a protease inhibitor), 10 children received a four-drug combination, and one child was on a five-drug combination including two protease inhibitors.

Treatment history reflects medical decisions based on evolving scientific knowledge and drug availability. Eighty-three percent of our population, whose treatment was initiated before 1995, started with a single NRTI with a majority receiving zidovudine; 11% of the children started with two combined NRTIs. For only 6% (first treated in 1997 or 1998) was highly active antiretroviral therapy (HAART) with three drugs the first treatment choice. The maximum duration of zidovudine monotherapy was 95 months (mean 30 months). With the increasing availability of various treatment options and the development of viral quantification, we have observed a tendency toward more frequent treatment change. The mean duration of the first two NRTI combinations was 12 months and, for the first triple combination therapy, was 7 months.

Virologic success according to our definition was observed in 56% of the patients (57% of those receiving the two-drug treatment, 67% of those receiving the three-drug treatment, and 10% of those receiving the four-drug .treatment); 70% of chil-

TABLE 1. Immunologic and virologic results in our population compared to French national adult data[a]

	Immunologic success	Immunologic failure	Total
Virologic success	45% (37%)	11% (12%)	56% (49%)
Virologic failure	31% (29%)	13% (22%)	44% (51%)
Total	76% (66%)	24% (34%)	100% (100%)

[a]Données DM12.

dren had a viral load of less than 5000 copies/ml. Immunologic success was observed in 76% of patients overall, which breaks down to 67% of those with the two-drug combinations, 80% of those with the three-drug combinations, and 70% of those with the four-drug combinations (FIG. 1).

DISCUSSION

These results are superior to those of the French national adult data (données DMI2) using the same stringent criteria and demonstrate that good results can be achieved in a pediatric population when motivated staff can support children and families (TABLE 1).

In developed countries the HIV pediatric population is experiencing an improved immunologic status with an obvious impact on morbidity and mortality.[2] Yet, with a tendency to accelerate treatment changes and the mean duration of unchanged HAART combination being 7 months, the number of new combinations is not infinite.

REFERENCES

1. CALDWELL, M.B. *et al.* 1994. Revised classification system for human immunodeficiency virus infection in children less than 13 years of age. Morbid. Mortal. Wkly. Rep. **43:** 1–10.
2. RÉSEAU NATIONAL DE SANTÉ PUBLIQUE. 1998. Surveillance du SIDA en France. Situation au 30 juin 1998. Bull. Epidemiol. Hebd. **37:** 157–163.

Lymphoid Interstitial Pneumonitis in Pediatric AIDS

Natural History of the Disease

CORINA E. GONZALEZ,[a,b] RUDI SAMAKOSES,[c] ANNE MARIE BOLER,[b] SUVIMOL HILL,[d] AND LAUREN V. WOOD[b]

[b]HIV/AIDS Malignancy Branch, National Cancer Institute, National Institutes of Health, Bethesda, Maryland 20892, USA

[c]Pramongkutklao College of Medicine, Bangkok, Thailand

[d]Diagnostic Radiology Department, National Institutes of Health, Bethesda, Maryland 20892, USA

INTRODUCTION

Lymphoid interstitial pneumonitis (LIP), as well as other conditions characterized by abnormal lymphoid proliferation, has been described with increased frequency in patients with HIV infection. Lymphoid interstitial pneumonitis is particularly common in pediatric AIDS and has been reported in up to 40% of vertically infected infants and children with pulmonary disease.[1–4] Although it is known that LIP can cause significant morbidity, the natural history and pathogenesis of this condition are not well understood. Recent advances in the understanding of the pathogenesis of interstitial lung disease suggest that it may be a cytokine-mediated process, the initiation and perpetuation of which is dependent on immune responses to HIV antigens and direct effects of HIV and/or other pathogens such as Epstein-Barr virus (EBV).[5,6] The natural history of pediatric HIV infection is that of a progressive disease leading to profound immunosuppression with continuous viral replication.[7,8] This process entails changes in the host immunity that can definitely affect the course of lymphoid proliferations. Similarly, antiretroviral therapy, particularly highly active antiretroviral therapy (HAART), can also affect the course of these conditions. Because HIV-infected patients survive longer as a result of improved antiretroviral therapy and supportive care, long-term studies on the course of LIP and other lymphoid interstitial disorders (LPDs) are now possible.

NATURAL HISTORY OF LYMPHOID INTERSTITIAL PNEUMONITIS

Early prospective studies in HIV-infected children identified LIP as a favorable prognostic factor associated with intermediate HIV disease progression.[7,8] Other studies associated severe CD4[+] T-lymphocyte depletion with complete resolution of

[a]Address for correspondence: Corina E. Gonzalez, M.D., Children's National Medical Center, Pediatric Medicine Suite 3.5-600, 111 Michigan Ave., N.W., Washington, DC 20010.
cgonzale@cnmc.org

TABLE 1. Presence of other lymphoproliferative disorders in HIV-infected children with lymphoid interstitial pneumonitis evaluated at the National Cancer Institute

Lymphoproliferative disorders	LIP positive ($n = 22$)	LIP negative ($n = 535$)	p value (Fisher's exact test)
Lymphadenopathy + hypergammaglobulinemia	9	47	<0.0001
Salivary gland enlargement	6	26	0.0009
Diffuse infiltrative lymphocytosis syndrome (DILS)	2	7	0.045
Mucosa-associated lymphoid tumor (MALT-lung)	2	1	0.004
Non-Hodgkin's lymphoma (NHL) (excluding MALT)	2	15	Not significant
All NHLs (including MALT)	4	16	0.008

radiological findings of LIP in chest x-rays.[9] These reports did not, however, address the clinical course of the disease. A retrospective study from the National Cancer Institute (NCI) evaluated the clinical and radiological manifestations as well as pulmonary function tests, EBV serology, treatment variables, and course of HIV infection in 22 HIV-infected children with biopsy-proven LIP for a median period of 4 years (range 0.5–10).[10] The study found that LIP-related clinical and radiological manifestations as well as abnormal pulmonary function tests resolved or significantly improved over time independent of disease severity or HIV disease status (see FIG. 1). Three (14%) patients developed radiological sequelae including bronchiectasis, emphysema, and bulla formation. One patient developed pulmonary hypertension secondary to chronic hypoxemia. LIP did not cause mortality in this study. HIV infection in these patients had an intermediate to slow progressive course. The variable most strongly associated with survival was the use of HAART.

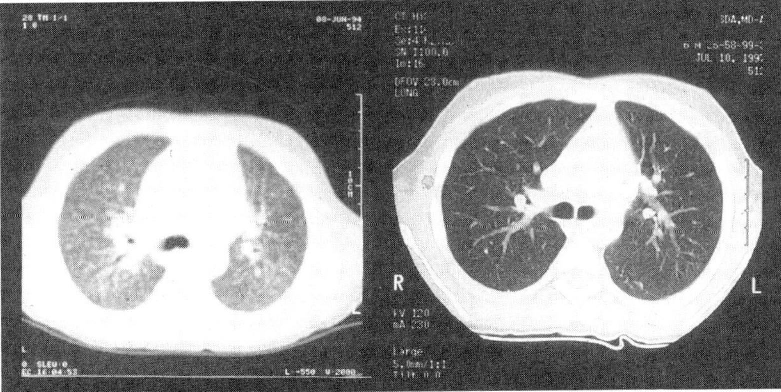

FIGURE 1. Two computerized tomography scans of the chest of an HIV-infected child with biopsy-proven lymphoid interstitial pneumonitis. Pulmonary interstitial infiltrates improved or resolved over time in most of the patients evaluated in the NCI study; this is a representative case. *Left panel*: CT scan of the chest, 1994. *Right panel*: CT scan of the chest, 1997.

CONCOMITANT LYMPHOPROLIFERATIVE DISORDERS

Little is known about the association of LIP or other LPDs and lymphoid malignancies in pediatric AIDS. Certainly, the borderline between these conditions is not well defined. There have been reports in adult AIDS patients of associations between LPD and non-Hodgkin's lymphoma (NHL).[11] The NCI study reported that the incidence of other LPDs, including NHL, was significantly higher ($p < 0.05$) in HIV-infected children with LIP than in those who did not have LIP (see TABLE 1). Of note is that two (50%) of the four NHLs were mucosa-associated lymphoid tissue lymphoma (MALT) of the lung. These observations underscore a possible association between benign lymphoproliferations and lymphomas. In this study, the presence of NHL was not associated with severity of the LIP disease. In fact, half of the patients were asymptomatic but had radiological evidence of LIP and underwent lung biopsies as part of the workup for pulmonary nodules. The role of EBV in the pathogenesis of these conditions is still under investigation. In the same study from NCI, EBV serology was positive in approximately 80% of HIV-infected children with and without LIP diagnosis. In addition, EBV was found in about half of the NHLs by *in-situ* hybridization using a EBV-encoded small RNA-1 riboprobe.

IMPACT OF ANTIRETROVIRAL THERAPY ON THE NATURAL HISTORY OF LIP

The recovery of $CD4^+$ T lymphocytes seen in HIV-infected children treated with HAART has raised the concern about potential LIP exacerbation.[12] In the study from NCI, 13 (59%) of 22 patients received HAART (7 expired before HAART became available for pediatric use and 2 received only nucleoside analogues), and none of them experienced an exacerbation of the LIP disease. Moreover, all patients, regardless their immunological and/or virological response to HAART, improved their respiratory status over time.

CONCLUSIONS

LIP-related clinical manifestations, radiological findings, and abnormal pulmonary function tests gradually improved or resolved over time independent of the severity of the disease or the HIV disease status. LIP long-term morbidity is less frequent but certainly possible and is generally associated with severe disease. There is evidence of a possible association between LIP and NHLs, particularly MALT of the lung, which warrants close clinical follow-up of HIV-infected children with a LIP diagnosis. Recovery of $CD4^+$ T-lymphocyte cells after HAART was not associated with exacerbation of LIP.

REFERENCES

1. ANDIMAN, W.A. & W.T. SHEARER. 1998. Lymphoid interstitial pneumonitis. *In* Pediatric AIDS: The Challenge of HIV Infection in Infants, Children, and Adolescents. P.A. Pizzo & C.M. Wilfert, Eds.: 323–334. Williams & Wilkins. Baltimore, MD.

2. RUBINSTEIN, A., R. MORECKI, B. SILVERMAN, *et al.* 1986. Pulmonary disease in children with acquired immune deficiency syndrome and AIDS-related complex. J. Pediatr. **108:** 498–503.

3. SAID, J. 1997. Human immunodeficiency virus-related lymphoid proliferations. Sem. Diagn. Pathol. **14:** 48–53.

4. JOSHI, V.V., J.M. OLESKE, A.B. MINNEFOR, *et al.* 1985. Pathologic pulmonary findings in children with the acquired immunodeficiency syndrome. Hum. Pathol. **16:** 241–246.

5. AGOSTINI, C., R. ZAMBELO, L. TRENTIN, *et al.* 1996. HIV and pulmonary immune responses. Immunol. Today **17:** 359–364.

6. COHEN, C.A., E.A. FITZPATRICK, C. HARTSFIELD, *et al.* 1997. Pulmonary lymphoid cell activation and cytokine expression in murine AIDS-associated interstitial pneumonitis. Am. J. Resp. Cell. Mol. Biol. **16:** 153–161.

7. THE EUROPEAN COLLABORATIVE STUDY. 1994. Natural history of vertically acquired human immunodeficiency virus-1 infection. Pediatrics **94:** 815–816.

8. SCOTT, G.B., C. HUTTO, R.W. MAKUCH, *et al.* 1989. Survival in children with perinatally acquired human immunodeficiency virus type 1 infection. N. Engl. J. Med. **321:** 1791–1796.

9. PROSPER, M., J.A. OMENE, S. LEDLIE, *et al.* 1995. Clinical significance of resolution of chest x-ray findings in HIV-infected children with lymphocytic interstitial pneumonitis (LIP). Pediatr. Radiol. **25:** S243–S246.

10. GONZALEZ, C.E., R. SAMAKOSES, A.M. BOLER, *et al.* 1999. Collected abstracts of the Advances in Pediatric AIDS meeting (Montreal, Canada): No. 283. New York Academy of Sciences. New York.

11. OKSENHENDLER, E., M. DUARTE, J. SOULIER, *et al.* 1995. Multicentric Castleman's disease in HIV infection: a clinical and pathological study of 20 patients. AIDS **10:** 61–67.

12. PALELLA, F.J., JR., K.M. DELANEY, A.C. MOORMAN, *et al.* 1998. Declining morbidity and mortality among patients with advanced human immunodeficiency virus infection. N. Engl. J. Med. **338:** 853–860.

Impact of Chemotherapy for AIDS-Related Malignancies in Pediatric HIV Disease

CORINA E. GONZALEZ,[a,b] MELISSA ADDE,[c] PERDITA TAYLOR,[b] LAUREN V. WOOD,[b] AND IAN MAGRATH[c]

[b]HIV/AIDS Malignancy Branch, National Cancer Institute, National Institutes of Health, Bethesda, Maryland 20892, USA

[c]Pediatric Oncology Branch, National Cancer Institute, National Institutes of Health, Bethesda, Maryland 20892, USA

INTRODUCTION

Children with the acquired immunodeficiency syndrome (AIDS) are at increased risk of developing a malignancy. Non-Hodgkin's lymphoma (NHL) and Kaposi's sarcoma are the most common malignancies associated with AIDS. Treatment of these conditions requires chemotherapy to effect disease control or cure. Chemotherapy, however, has been associated with profound and repetitive periods of myelosuppression as well as with infectious complications, which may be poorly tolerated by patients with AIDS. There is a paucity of information regarding the impact of chemotherapy on HIV disease, particularly on viral replication and immunity. The literature in pediatric AIDS is limited to case reports or short case series. In general, these studies show poor response rates to chemotherapy and short survival times, which may indicate that chemotherapy has a profound deleterious effect on HIV disease.[1–4]

USE OF CHEMOTHERAPY IN AIDS-RELATED MALIGNANCIES

The decision to treat a malignancy in a child with HIV infection must be guided by the stage and type of the cancer as well as the overall performance status of the patient. If treatment is initiated, it should be with the intention to cure the malignancy. Chemotherapy in AIDS patients can be a double-edged sword since its antitumor effects must be balanced against its possible deleterious effect on the underlying condition. Potential problems include increased risk of infections, worsening of pre-existent hematological deficits, and development of more severe chemotherapy-related toxicity because of the underlying HIV disease or its treatment. Comprehensive supportive care including addition of hematopoietic growth factors, intravenous immunoglobulin, adequate nutritional support, and prophylaxis of selected infections such as *Pneumocystis carinii* pneumonia, herpetic, or fungal infections, as well as carefully selected antiretroviral therapy, may improve the treatment-associated morbidity and mortality in pediatric AIDS patients.

[a]Address for correspondence: Corina E. Gonzalez, M.D., Children's National Medical Center, Pediatric Medicine, Suite 3.5-600, 111 Michigan Ave., N.W., Washington, DC 20010.
cgonzalez@cnmc.org

CLINICAL MANIFESTATIONS DURING AND AFTER CHEMOTHERAPY

Most of the reported study series of children with AIDS and malignancies, predominantly NHLs, show a short median survival time of about 6 months following initiation of chemotherapy treatment.[1–4] The majority of patients who received multiagent chemotherapy suffered early mortality at 2 to 3 months, either because of progression of the malignancy or because of the development of major treatment-related toxicity. Opportunistic (OI) and/or serious infections generally occurred after 2–3 months on therapy. As shown in TABLE 1, in a series of 11 patients from the National Cancer Institute (NCI) who received 3 to 5 cycles of two systemic drugs in combination with antiretroviral therapy consisting of two nucleoside reverse transcriptase inhibitors, the main complications during chemotherapy included myelotoxicity and infections.[5] Interestingly, neither reactivation nor development of new opportunistic infections occurred during chemotherapy. Consistent with prior reports, OIs occurred within a median time of 6 months (range 2–9 months) during the follow-up period after chemotherapy. Only one patient died as a result of an OI. Aplastic anemia was observed in two patients after receiving chemotherapy. These patients presented with neutropenia and mild thrombocytopenia before starting chemotherapy, probably due to several factors including disseminated *Mycobacterium avium complex* infection.

ABSOLUTE CD4$^+$ T-LYMPHOCYTE COUNTS DURING AND AFTER COMPLETION OF CHEMOTHERAPY

CD4$^+$ T lymphocytes exhibit a profound decrease after chemotherapy in immunocompetent children with malignancies. It has been reported, however, that these patients develop a rapid thymus-dependent regeneration of CD4$^+$ T lymphocytes that occurs within a median of 10 months after chemotherapy.[6] In the same series of HIV-infected children with malignancies from NCI, patients reached their nadirs of CD4$^+$ percentage and absolute counts at or near the completion of chemotherapy. Three (33%) of the nine patients evaluated recovered CD4$^+$ cells to baseline levels within a median of 9 months after chemotherapy. All of them had baseline absolute CD4$^+$ counts >100 cell/µl. Given the limited number of patients, it is not clear whether the baseline level of immunosuppression associated with AIDS influenced the capacity for immunological recovery following chemotherapy or whether the use of chemotherapy influenced the response of these patients to HAART.

VIRAL REPLICATION DYNAMICS DURING AND AFTER COMPLETION OF CHEMOTHERAPY

The effect of chemotherapy on viral dynamics is unclear and is a frequent source of concern. Limited reports on adult AIDS patients have shown that viral load (VL) levels do not significantly increase and may even decrease during chemotherapy.[7–9] In the NCI study of HIV-infected children with malignancies, VL levels showed an

TABLE 1. Summary of the National Cancer Institute Study on HIV-Infected Children with Malignancies Treated with Chemotherapy

Demographic features	
Number of patients	11
Males (%)	8 (73)
Females (%)	3 (27)
Median age (years) (range)	7 (1–14)
HIV infection features at tumor diagnosis	
CDC classification B-1 (%)	1 (9)
B-3 (%)	3 (27)
C-3 (%)	7 (64)
Median absolute CD4+ T lymphocyte count	
(cells/µl) (range)	113 (92–1989)
Median HIV-1 RNA level	
($\log_{10}$ copies/ml) (range)	5 (3.1–5.9)
Tumor characteristics	
Non-Hodgkin's lymphoma (NHL)	
Number of patients (%)	10 (91)
Stage[a] I: 2, II: 3, III: 5	
Neuroendocrine carcinoma (NEC)	
Number of patients (%)	1 (9)
Stage: metastatic	
Chemotherapy regimens[b]	
NHL: Primary regimen: CYP + MTX	3 cycles
Relapse regimen: IFM + Ara-C	3 cycles
NEC: Primary regimen: CIS + VP-16	5 cycles
Total number of cycles	41
Antiretroviral therapy during chemotherapy	
AZT + DDI (No.) (%)	9 (82)
3TC + D4T (No.) (%)	2 (18)
Complications during chemotherapy	
Infectious (number of episodes) (%)	14 (10 cycles)
Fever and neutropenia	6 (55%)
Documented serious infections[c]	8 (73%)
(Gram + cocci Bacteremia 3, Periorbital cellulitis 2,	
RSV pneumonia 1, *Clostridium difficile* diarrhea 2)	
Noninfectious (number of episodes) (%)	
Severe myelotoxicity	41 (91%)
(<500 neutrophils/µl and/or <25,000 platelets/µl)	
Complications postchemotherapy	
Infectious (number of patients) (%)[c,d]	8 (73%)
PCP	2
CMV retinitis	1
CMV colitis1	1
Esophageal candidiasis	1
Pulmonary aspergillosis	2
Bacterial sepsis	1
Noninfectious (number of patients) (%)	2
Aplastic anemia	2 (18%)

ABBREVIATIONS: CDC, Centers for Disease Control and Prevention; CYP, cyclophosphamide; MTX, methotrexate; CIS, cisplatin; PCP, *Pneumocystis carinii* pneumonia; CMV, cytomegalovirus.

[a]St. Jude's staging system for lymphomas.

[b]Systemic regimen. Patients with NHLs also received intrathecal chemotherapy consisting of cytarabine (AraC) and MTX.

[c]Serious infections were defined as any infection listed as C condition in the CDC AIDS case definition, or disseminated infection, or infection to the lung, meninges, bone or joint, or abscess of an internal organ or body cavity.

[d]Developed with a median time of 6 months after completion of chemotherapy (range 2–9 months).

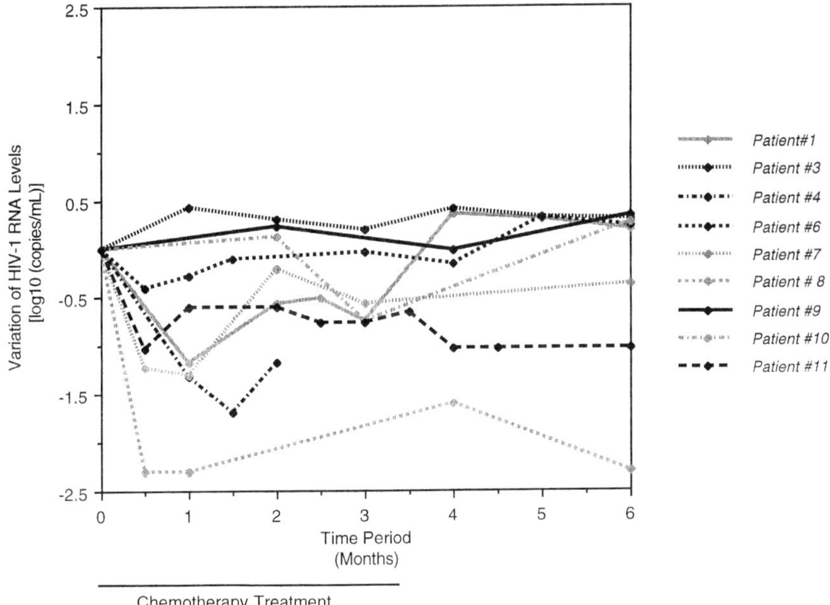

FIGURE 1. HIV-1 RNA levels during and after 6 months of starting chemotherapy for AIDS-related malignancies in HIV-infected children. HIV-1 RNA levels showed a decrease associated with chemotherapy in seven of nine patients ($R_2 = 0.88$ by least squares regression analysis). The other two patients had minor increases in HIV-1 RNA levels that fell within the range of biological variation.

overall downward trend during chemotherapy (see FIG. 1). Only two of nine patients had a minimal increase (0.4 and 0.2 $\log_{10}$) in VL levels that fell within the range of biologic variation, whereas the other seven demonstrated a significant downward trend with a median VL reduction of 0.87 $\log_{10}$ (0.14–2.1). After completion of chemotherapy, VL increased and reached or surpassed baseline levels by the end of the first year of follow-up in seven (78%) of nine patients.

CONCLUSIONS

Patients with AIDS are less tolerant of chemotherapy. Adequate and comprehensive supportive care is necessary in order to decrease morbidity and mortality in these patients. Chemotherapy does not induce viral replication. Further, in the only study reported in children, there was an overall decrease of VL levels during chemotherapy. This observation may be relevant for designing the antiretroviral and chemotherapy regimens for AIDS children with malignancies. Once the decision to treat is made, sparing drugs with potentially serious interactions, such as protease inhibitors and nonnucleoside reverse transcriptase inhibitors, may be a strategy that should be considered. Recovery of CD4 counts in HIV-infected children after chemotherapy is possible.

REFERENCES

1. ARICO, M., D. CASELLI, P. DíARGENIO, *et al.* 1991. Malignancies in children with human immunodeficiency virus type 1 infection. Cancer **68:** 2473–2477.
2. EVANS, J.A., D.M. GIBB, F.J. HOLLAND, *et al.* 1997. Malignancies in UK children with HIV-infection acquired from mother to child transmission. Arch. Dis. Child. **76:** 330–333.
3. TIRELLI, U., M. SPINA, E. VACCHER, *et al.* 1995. Clinical evaluation of 451 patients with HIV-related non-Hodgkin's lymphoma: experience of the Italian cooperative group on AIDS and tumors (GICAT). Leuk. Lymphoma **20:** 91–96.
4. MONTALVO, F.W., R. CASANOVA & L.A. CLAVEL. 1990. Treatment outcome in children with malignancies associated with human immunodeficiency virus infection. J. Pediatr. **116:** 735–737.
5. GONZALEZ, C.E., M. ADDE, P. TAYLOR, *et al.* 1999. Collected abstracts of the Advances in Pediatric AIDS meeting, Montreal, Canada, No. 282. New York Academy of Sciences. New York.
6. MACKALL, C.L., T.A. FLEISHER, M.R. BROWN, *et al.* 1995. Age, thymopoiesis, and $CD4^+$ T-lymphocyte regeneration after intensive chemotherapy. N. Engl. J. Med. **332:** 143–149.
7. RUTSCHMAN, O.T., M. PECHÈRE, J. KRISCHER, *et al.* 1997. Chemotherapy for AIDS-related malignancies does not increase HIV viraemia. AIDS **11:** 944–945.
8. LITTLE, R., G. FRANCHINI, D. PEARSON, *et al.* 1997. HIV viral burden during EPOCH chemotherapy for HIV-related lymphomas. J. Acquir. Immun. Def. Syndr. Hum. Retrovir. **14:** A42 (Abstr.).
9. LEE, F.C., A. LEIBLIN, J. CARDEN, *et al.* 1997. Viral load changes in patients undergoing chemotherapy for AIDS-KS. J. Acquir. Immun. Def. Syndr. Hum. Retrov. **14:** A42.

Maternal Mortality Associated with Tuberculosis–HIV Coinfection in Durban, South Africa

M. KHAN, T. PILLAY,[a,c] J. MOODLEY,[b] AND C. CONNOLLY

Medical Research Council South Africa, [a]Department of Paediatrics and Child Health and [b]Obstetrics and Gynaecology, University of Natal, Durban, South Africa

INTRODUCTION

With the combined escalation of tuberculosis (TB) and HIV-1 infection in our region, we document the impact of both diseases on maternal mortality at King Edward VIII, Durban, South Africa, between January 1996 and December 1998. A prospective case controlled study was performed in 1997 and 1998 and a retrospective analysis in 1996.

METHODS

Known maternal deaths during the study period were studied. HIV-1 status, the presence of TB, maternal clinical features, and perinatal outcome were documented. The overall maternal mortality rate for the hospital was calculated, as were the specific rates for HIV-1 infection and TB. The attributable fraction of deaths due to HIV-1 was calculated in the overall group as well as in the group with TB coinfection.

RESULTS

A total of 50,518 maternities and 101 known maternal deaths were recorded. The overall hospital-based mortality rate was 200/100,000; for HIV-1–infected women, this was calculated as 323/100,000 and HIV-1–negative mothers, 148.6/100,000. The attributable fraction of deaths due to HIV-1 at the hospital was 16%. Fourteen of the 15 mothers who had TB were HIV-1 coinfected. The hospital-based mortality rate for TB and HIV-1 coinfection was 121.7/1,000; for TB without HIV-1 coinfection, this was 38.5/1,000. Of all maternal deaths due to TB, 54% were attributable to HIV-1 infection. TB was the third commonest cause of death following pregnancy-induced hypertension/eclampsia and sepsis. Of maternal deaths, 34.6% were associated with stillbirths, but perinatal outcomes were no different between groups of mothers with TB, HIV-1, or no infection.

[c]Address for correspondence: Dr T. Pillay, Nuffield Department of Medicine, c/o Wolfson College, OX2 6UD, Oxford, UK.
tpillay@gwmail.jr2.ox.ac.uk

TABLE 1. Description of maternal deaths associated with TB

Age	Peripartum and labor problems	TB defined	Pregnancy outcome
25	Sepsis, shock, diarrhea, congenital TB in neonate	Disseminated TB	1.8 kg, 38 weeks SGA congenital TB
16	Bilateral pleural effusion, pneumonia, pyrexia, preterm labor	Pulmonary TB (PTB)	1.3 kg 32 weeks SGA congenital TB
23	Cavitating TB pneumonia, varicella, pyrexia, preterm labor	PTB	26 weeks SGA
34	Wasting syndrome, reactivation TB-smear microscopy and culture positive for M tuberculosis	PTB	Intrauterine death
39	Meningioma, PTB, smear microscopy and culture positive for M tuberculosis, HIV negative[a]	PTB	Intrauterine death, 30 weeks
34	Miliary TB, confusion, tuberculoma brain, smear microscopy and culture positive for M tuberculosis	Miliary TB Tuberculoma brain	Intrauterine death, 24 weeks
26	Miliary TB, disseminated intravascular coagulopathy	Miliary TB	Intrauterine death, 28 weeks
23	Cavitating pneumonia, smear microscopy and culture positive for M tuberculosis, preterm labor	PTB	Intrauterine death, 29 weeks
30	Pneumonia, pyrexia, diarrhea, smear microscopy and culture positive for M tuberculosis, preterm labor	PTB	Intrauterine death, 24 weeks
25	Paraparesis, kypho-scoliosis	TB spine	3.5 kg, 38 weeks
	TB pneumonia	PTB	Intrauterine death, 22 weeks
39	TB pneumonia, pericardial effusion	PTB, ?cardiac TB	Intrauterine death, 32 weeks
29	Pleural effusion	PTB	Intrauterine death, 19 weeks
23	Basal meningitis	TB meningitis	3.25 kg, 3 5weeks
24	Perineal abscess, pneumonia, sputum smear microscopy positive for M tuberculosis	PTB	2.45 kg, 34 weeks

[a]All mothers except case 5 were HIV-1 coinfected.

CONCLUSION

TB and HIV-1 are emerging as significant contributors to maternal mortality in KwaZuluNatal. Any attempt to improve maternal health must include careful screening and investigation for TB in high-risk pregnant women.

TABLE 2. Characteristics of maternal deaths associated with TB

	TB positive ($n = 15$)	TB negative ($n = 86$)	$p =$
HIV-1 infected	14 (93.3%)	16 (18.6%)	< 0.01
Age (median, range)	27.5 (16–39) yr	27.3 (15–45) yr	0.9
Parity (median, range)	2 (1–5)	2 (1–14)	0.8
Abortion	2	10	0.8
Booking status	10 (66.6%)	58 (67.4%)	0.8
Days to death (median, range)	1 (1–120)	5 (0–33)	0.5
Ventilatory support	2 (13.3)	47 (54.6%)	0.01
Days on ventilator (median, range)	3.5 (2–5)	6 (1–30)	
Neonatal outcome Alive	5 (33.3%)	37 (43.0%)	0.5

ACKNOWLEDGMENT

This study was supported in part by the MRC and the University of Natal, Durban, South Africa.

Counseling in Children with HIV/AIDS

JESSICA KISA LUKANDWA,[a] R.M. NASABA, AND I. KALYESUBULA

Makerere University, Kampala, Uganda

INTRODUCTION

The Mother-Child Clinic (Ward II) Mulago Hospital was established in 1988 as a Research Collaboration between Makerere University (MU) and Case Western Reserve University (CWRU) in response to the HIV/AIDS epidemic. In 1996, Johns Hopkins University (JHU) replaced (CWRU). Since 1988, the clinic has had 153 HIV-1–positive children whose mothers participated in the HIV/AIDS research projects of Natural History of HIV Transmission from mother to child and the Neurodevelopment of children born to HIV-positive mothers. Of the 153, 119 have died and 34 of these still living are 5-11 years of age. These together with three children from the Infectious Disease Clinic (IDC) run by the Department of Paediatrics have benefitted from the services.

NEED FOR COUNSELING

These HIV-infected children, who are becoming sexually active, need to be aware of their sero status to prevent them from infecting their peer group members. (Many children have their first sex encounter at the age of 9 years, according to the 1998 Lakai study in Uganda.) Infected children experience high levels of stress, as they are often very sick and most of the interventions required are traumatic. They require invensive treatments and investigations, and they begin to question why this is so. To explain their continued ill health, an HIV/AIDS counselor has to break the sad news. They are fearful and feel insecure, as they have seen their parents in agony when they fall sick and eventually die; therefore, they need to be communicated with and be prepared to accept and go through the same experience as their parents. Also, they need help in regaining trust in adults, which they lost when their sick parents never revealed their HIV status to them. Communities still stigmatize HIV-infected people, children included; therefore, these children face isolation and unkind comments against them in school, by adopting families, and at health care centers. As a result, they need counseling to cope with these situations.

[a]Address for correspondence: Box 663, Kampala, Uganda. Voice: 256-41-534262; fax: 256-41-533531.
cwru@imul.com

OBJECTIVES

HIV/AIDS counselors need to inform older HIV-1 infected children of their sero-status. Moreover, there is the need to improve the well being of HIV-I–infected children by social support through continuous counseling.

Of the 153 HIV-positive children whose mothers participated in the HIV/AIDS research projects, 119 died and 34 of them are 5–11 years of age. Of these 34, 8 of them know their sero-status through counseling services: (i) They are referred to an HIV/AIDS counselor by doctors whenever they see a need, and therefore are given follow-up appointments. For instance, if an HIV-positive child is brought in by a caregiver with a medical problem, such as herpes zoster, a counselor is responsible for giving full information on what might have brought about her/his illness. (ii) Sometimes they are brought in by their caregivers when behavioral problems occur after unkind remarks by people in the community, health workers, peer group members, or teachers, and they refuse to go back to school or come to the clinic for treatment. In either case, HIV/AIDS counselors seek consent from the caregiver to talk to the child alone, so that he/she can feel free to express himself/herself, because counseling communication skills for adults and children differ. Children can be communicated with through either drawing or writing their likes and dislikes and thereafter discussing why he/she drew or wrote the things he/she did. Finally, the caregiver and the child are counseled together, and eventually children make the decision to learn of their sero-status. They are then given appointments for support through continuous counseling. Caregivers are also offered counseling in starting income generating projects (IGPs) to support these children economically and socially. (One child's grandmother is raising chickens to support the child economically and socially.)

To illustrate the value of counseling HIV-1–infected children, we present here two case histories.

CASE 1. The child, a 9 1/2 year old girl, was born in March 1990 and was HIV-1 infected at birth. Her mother participated in the Natural History of HIV-1 Transmission from Mother to Child project. Her maternal grandparents took care of her after the death of her parents at 2 years and continued to bring her to the clinic for follow-up visits. Because of chronic ear problems, she was referred to an ENT surgeon who remarked to the grandmother in the child's presence that, "AIDS patients are expected to have the symptoms the child was having." This was when she first heard that she had AIDS. She began to lose interest in school. When the grandmother asked her why she did not want to study, she told her that all AIDS persons die and she too was going to die. After counseling, she returned to school. She enjoys playing with friends and likes Sunday school.

CASE 2. The child, a 14-year-old boy, was born in 1985. His mother died in 1996. In addition to a chest problem that he had had since the age of 1 month, he developed herpes zoster in 1997, when he was 12 years old. He was taken to a health center by his eldest sister. The clinical officer referred him to IDC Mulago Hospital. After medical treatment the doctor referred him to an HIV/AIDS counselor to discuss his frequent ill health, which had been affecting his performance at school and was responsible for his absences. Pre-test counseling was provided, and an HIV-1 test proved him to be HIV-1 infected. Post-test counseling helped him to accept his condition and to understand why he was behind his age mates at school. He continues to attend school and follow-up visits at the clinic. He has been referred to Mildmay Centre, Uganda, for socialization with other HIV-infected children. He loves playing football with friends and helps with housework when he is well.

CONCLUSION

HIV-infected children are being helped to accept their state of life. They are learning to cope with sickness. They are gaining the freedom to express their feelings and to socialize with peer group members in support groups of other children with HIV/AIDS and in the community.

In the future, we want to establish counseling centers for HIV-1 infected children so that they can be made aware of their HIV status by professionals with experience in communicating with children. We must educate communities, health care workers, and schoolteachers by organizing seminars so as to prepare them to receive and accept HIV-positive children amongst them. Health care workers and schoolteachers must be made aware of places where these HIV-positive children can be referred for support, such as, support groups of other children with HIV/AIDS for socialization and continuous counseling support.

T-Helper Cell Responses among HIV-Infected Children in Soweto, South Africa

T.M. MEYERS,[a,e] L. KUHN,[d] S. MEDDOWS-TAYLOR,[c] K. SIMMANK,[a] G.G. SHERMAN,[b] AND C.T. TIEMESSEN[c]

[a]Department of Paediatrics, Chris Hani Baragwanath Hospital, University of the Witwatersrand, Johannesburg, South Africa

[b]Department of Haematology, University of the Witwatersrand, Johannesburg, South Africa

[c]National Institute of Virology, University of the Witwatersrand, Johannesburg, South Africa

[d]School of Public Health, Columbia University, New York, New York, USA

INTRODUCTION

The prognosis of HIV-infected children is highly variable. Some infected children remain clinically healthy for many years, even in the absence of antiretroviral treatment. The dynamics of viral replication, particularly in the first few months of life, are strongly associated with this observed variability,[1] but host immunologic factors are less clearly defined. Typically, HIV infection results in early and progressive defects in T-cell function, and these deficits have been observed in children.[2] Less well understood is the role of HIV-specific T-cell function. In one report of HIV-infected adults, HIV-specific CD4+ T-helper cell responses were strongly associated with long-term nonprogression,[3] but this has not been replicated and these responses have not been investigated in children. In this study, we measured CD4+ helper cell responses in HIV-infected South African children who had not been exposed to antiretroviral therapy and investigated whether these responses were correlated with markers of clinical disease progression.

MATERIALS AND METHODS

Confirmed HIV-infected children (all vertical transmission) aged between 3 months and 11 years and a control group of confirmed uninfected children were recruited from outpatient and inpatient services at Chris Hani Baragwanath Hospital, Soweto, South Africa. HIV-infected children who manifested a severe clinical course were age-matched to an equal number of HIV-infected children who manifested a mild clinical course and to uninfected control children. After obtaining parental consent, a relevant clinical history was obtained and physical examination was performed in each child. A blood sample was drawn for HIV RNA quantification, CD4/CD8 subset analysis, and helper cell function assays.

[e]Address for correspondence: Dr. T. Meyers, Department of Paediatrics, Chris Hani Baragwanath Hospital, P O Bertsham, 2013, Johannesburg, South Africa. Voice: +27 11 933 8488; +27 82 330 0822; fax: +27 11 938 9074.

tammymeyers@hotmail.com

TABLE 1. Age distribution, CD4$^+$ T-lymphocyte counts, and HIV RNA quantity among 32 HIV-infected children with a mild and a severe clinical course and 10 uninfected controls recruited from Chris Hani Baragwanath Hospital, Soweto, South Africa

Age (years)		Uninfected controls	HIV-infected "mild" clinical course	HIV-infected "severe" clinical course
0–2	n	6	4	6
	Mean CD4 count (SD)	3138 (1342)	2927 (743)	1042 (547)
	Mean $\log_{10}$ HIV RNA (SD)	—	5.34 (0.87)	5.55 (0.5)
2–5	n	2	10	5
	Mean CD4 count (SD)	1910 (1303)	1042 (683)	407 (287)
	Mean $\log_{10}$ HIV RNA (SD)	—	4.54 (0.61)	5.46 (0.32)
5–11	n	2	2	5
	Mean CD4 count (SD)	1215 (103)	597 (71)	262 (169)
	Mean $\log_{10}$ HIV RNA (SD)	—	4.72 (1.28)	5.04 (0.43)
Total	n	10	16	16
	Mean CD4 count (SD)	2508 (1381)	1458 (1086)	600 (508)
	Mean $\log_{10}$ HIV RNA (SD)	—	4.77 (0.78)	5.36 (0.61)

T-helper cell function was measured using a previously described bioassay.[4] Freshly separated peripheral blood mononuclear cells (PBMC) were either unstimulated or stimulated with phytohemagglutinin (PHA), tetanus (TET), and a cocktail of synthetic HIV-1 envelope peptides (*env*). After 7 days' incubation, culture supernatants were tested for interleukin (IL)-2 induced proliferation using an IL-2–dependent continuous T-lymphocyte cell line. Results were expressed as stimulation indices (ratios of counts of stimulated to unstimulated cultures), and stimulation indices >3 were considered positive.

At the time of analysis, data were available for 16 HIV-infected children with a severe and 16 with a mild clinical course and for 10 uninfected control children. The clinical categories were strongly associated with CD4+ T-lymphocyte counts and with HIV RNA quantities (TABLE 1).

RESULTS AND DISCUSSION

All 10 uninfected controls and 31 of 32 HIV-infected children had positive T-helper cell responses to PHA. HIV-infected children were less likely to have a detectable T-helper cell response to TET than were uninfected children (9 of 32 [28%] HIV-

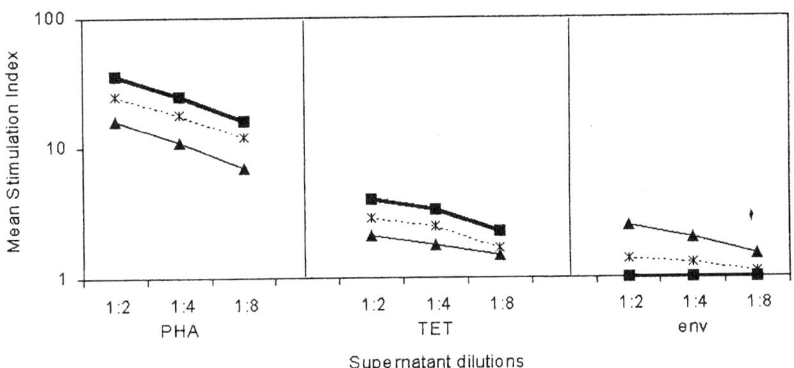

FIGURE 1. Strength of *in vitro* T-helper cell responses (mean stimulation indices) to phytohemagglutinin (PHA), tetanus (TET), and a cocktail of synthetic HIV-1 envelope peptides (*env*) measured using a previously described bioassay[4] among 16 HIV-infected children with a mild and 16 with a severe clinical course and 10 uninfected controls recruited from Chris Hani Baragwanath Hospital, Soweto, South Africa. Symbols: ▬■▬ uninfected; ···✳··· HIV-infected mild, ▬▲▬ HIV-infected severe.

infected vs 5 of 10 [50%] uninfected), but this difference did not reach significance ($p = 0.20$). No positive responses to *env* were detectable in any of the 10 uninfected children, but they were detected in 7 of 32 (22%) HIV-infected children.

The strength of T-helper cell responses to PHA was significantly higher among uninfected (mean SI = 36) than among HIV-infected children (mean SI = 20, $p = 0.001$) and was lower in HIV-infected children with a severe clinical course (mean SI = 16) than among those with a mild clinical course (mean SI = 25, $p = 0.005$). A similar proportion of HIV-infected children with a mild (25%, 4 of 16) or severe (31%, 5 of 16) clinical course responded to tetanus, but mean stimulation indices to tetanus tended to be higher in children with a milder disease course. By contrast, T-helper cell responses to HIV peptides were in the opposite direction: 2 of 16 (13%) children with a mild clinical course and 5 of 16 (31%) with a severe clinical course had positive responses to *env* (FIG. 1).

We observed defects in generalized T-cell function in HIV-infected children, even among those with a clinically mild disease course. However, HIV-specific T-cell function was not correlated with a milder clinical profile; rather, HIV-specific T-helper cell responses were somewhat stronger in children with a more severe clinical profile. Strong HIV-specific T-helper cell responses initiated at the time of infection may protect against subsequent disease progression, but these responses measured some time after infection may not have the same prognostic significance. In addition, viral replication above a certain threshold may be necessary to maintain T-helper cell responses in an infected child. In the context of pediatric HIV infection, the development and role of HIV-specific T-helper cell responses appear to be more complex than previously recognized. We are extending this research to a larger number of children and will continue with clinical follow-up to investigate these relationships further.

REFERENCES

1. SHEARER, W.T., T.C. QUINN, P. LaRUSSA *et al.* 1997. Viral load and disease progression in infants infected with human immunodeficiency virus type 1. Women and Infants Transmission Study Group. N. Engl. J. Med. **336:** 1337–1342.
2. ROILIDES, E., M. CLERICI, L. DePALMA *et al.* 1991. Helper T-cell responses in children infected with human immunodeficiency virus type 1. J. Pediatr. **118:** 724–730.
3. ROSENBERG, E.S., J.M. BILLINGSLEY, A.M. CALIENDO *et al.* 1997. Vigorous HIV-1-specific CD4+ T cell responses associated with control of viremia. Science **278:** 1447–1450.
4. CLERICI, M., A.V. SISON, J.A. BERZOFSKY *et al.* 1993. Cellular immune factors associated with mother-to-infant transmission of HIV. AIDS **7:** 1427–1433.

Measles Infection in HIV-Infected African Infants

ROBERT T. PERRY,[a,d] FRANCIS MMIRO,[b] CHRISTOPHER NDUGWA,[c] AND RICHARD D. SEMBA[a]

[a]Department of Ophthalmology, The Johns Hopkins University School of Medicine, Baltimore, Maryland 21205, USA

[b]Department of Obstetrics and Gynaecology, Makerere University Medical School, Kampala, Uganda

[c]Department of Paediatrics and Child Health, Makerere University Medical School, Kampala, Uganda

ABSTRACT: Measles infection remains a serious threat to child survival in the developing world despite vaccination and treatment with vitamin A. This report reviews the epidemiology of measles in HIV-infected children in Africa. In hospitalized infants, the rate of malnutrition before measles and the rate of death after measles are both higher in HIV-positive than in HIV-negative infants. However, the rates of pneumonia and diarrhea in infants hospitalized with measles are the same in HIV-positive as in HIV-negative infants. In an autopsy study, measles was associated with death in HIV-positive children, only for those over 15 months of age. A cohort study found that infants of HIV-positive women were more likely than infants of HIV-negative women to have measles before 9 months of age, although the rates of complications did not differ between the two groups. The HIV status of the infants and the measles serology were too incomplete to draw firm conclusions, though only 1 of 54 infants tested was seropositive for measles at 6 months of age. In the context of the HIV epidemic, further work is needed to determine the risk of measles and its complications in HIV-positive infants and the optimal age of measles immunization.

INTRODUCTION

Measles infection remains a major cause of morbidity and mortality in children despite the use of an effective vaccine, treatment with vitamin A, and clinical management of complications. In Africa and Asia, it was estimated in 1997 that 29 million children had measles and 928,000 of them died.[1] The risks of acquiring measles and its associated complications are both affected by the host's immune status. The HIV pandemic has resulted in a large group of children with reduced immune function in areas where measles are endemic. This article reviews the available informa-

[d]Address for correspondence: Robert Perry, MD, MPH, Ocular Immunology Division, 550 N Broadway, Suite 700, Baltimore, MD 21205, USA. Voice: +1-410-955-3572; fax: +1-410-955-0629.

rperry@welchlink.welch.jhu.edu

tion on the interaction of HIV infection and the acquisition and complications of measles, focusing on Africa.

HIV AND MEASLES IN THE UNITED STATES AND EUROPE

In children with impaired immunity, the manifestations, complications, and case fatality rate from measles are more severe. Case reports and reviews from centers caring for childhood cancer in the United States and Britain have shown that children may present without the typical rash, have a higher rate of pneumonitis and encephalitis, shed measles virus for prolonged periods, and, if complications develop, are more likely to die despite intensive care.[2] With the advent of the HIV epidemic, reports from the United States suggested that HIV-infected infants may also present without rash, develop complications more frequently, and have case fatality rates approaching 50%.[3]

HIV AND MEASLES IN AFRICA

The experience in Africa is less clear. The rates of complications and death are higher in HIV-negative (HIV−) children in Africa than in the United States, in part from higher rates of malnutrition,[4] from children living in more crowded conditions,[5] and from a greater proportion of young infants contracting measles.[6]

Sension and colleagues[7] found 16 HIV-seropositive (HIV+) and 298 HIV− children with measles among hospitalized infants in Kinshasa, and 91% had IgM antibodies against measles virus to confirm the clinical diagnosis. The case fatality rate (CFR) was higher, but not significantly so, in HIV+ (31.3%) versus HIV− (28.1%) children. In children over 9 months of age, the CFR was higher in HIV+ (50%) than HIV− (28.8%) children, although the difference did not reach statistical significance. In unvaccinated infants, the CFR was 80% in HIV+ compared to 32% in HIV− infants, with a RR of 2.5 (95% CI [0.9, 3.9]). In Lusaka, Zambia, Oshitani and colleagues[8] calculated the CFRs for 68 HIV+ and 288 HIV- hospitalized children with clinically diagnosed measles. The CFR was lower for HIV+ vaccinated boys than for those not vaccinated (24% vs. 31%, $p < 0.05$), but it was the same for HIV− children regardless of gender or vaccination status. However, for HIV+ girls, the CFR was higher for those vaccinated than for those unvaccinated (42% vs. 17%, OR 3.57, $p = 0.18$).

In a study of the causes of death of HIV+ children, Lucas and colleagues[9] in Abidjan, Cote d'Ivoire, performed autopsies on HIV+ and HIV− children of similar age and height.[9] They found 18 children who died of measles, most with pneumonitis and 1 with encephalitis. Under 15 months, the odds of dying with measles were the same for HIV+ as for HIV−. Children 15 months and older dying from measles were more likely to be HIV+, with 8 cases among 42 HIV+ deaths compared to 2 cases among 48 HIV− deaths (OR = 5.4, 95% CI [1.1, 27.2]).

The foregoing studies are hospital based and may reflect the characteristics of children ill enough to be admitted rather than the general experience with measles. Embree and colleagues[10] looked for measles in infants born to women followed for a study of mother-child transmission of HIV in Nairobi. Before 9 months of age, 10 of 109 (9%) infants of HIV+ women and 5 of 194 (3%) infants of HIV− women had measles, with 1 death in each group, both from pneumonia. However, half the children born to HIV+ women were not tested for HIV because of death (1) or age <15 months (4), and only 2 of the others were confirmed HIV+. After measles, 6 of 10 infants born to HIV+ women and 4 of 5 infants born to HIV− women had pneumonia, 2 born to HIV+ and 1 to HIV− had diarrhea, and 7 born to HIV+ and 2 to HIV− had growth failure. An additional 11 cases of measles occurred in infants >9 months old with no increase in children of HIV+ women. Measurement of measles antibody titers in women prepartum and in their infants who had measles early showed that all mothers were immune, whereas among the infants, 5 of 8 cord blood samples had protective titers, and at 6 months, only 4 of 24 had detectable antibodies to measles, 1 who went on to have clinical measles.

CONCLUSIONS

The effect of HIV infection on the experience of measles in children with HIV infection in Africa is not as clear as in the United States and Britain. As with HIV− children,[11] HIV+ children have a lower CFR with measles after vaccination, although in Zambia it appears that with normal-titer vaccine, females with HIV may be at higher risk of death. Overall, however, the CFRs are not consistently higher in HIV+ children. One reason may be reliance on HIV serology. Earlier experience in Africa is that the CFR is higher for infants than older children,[12] and these infants would be overlooked when looking for those >15 months and eligible for HIV serologic testing. In Africa, infants lose maternal antibodies to measles at a faster rate than do infants in the developed world,[6] placing the child at risk of measles at an earlier age. In studies from Africa, 25% of HIV-related mortality occurs in children <1 year.[13] However, autopsy study found an association between HIV infection and measles mortality only in children >15 months.

Further studies are therefore needed to examine the risks of complications and mortality in HIV-infected children with measles and to examine its relationship to the level of maternal antibodies present in infants of various ages. This would guide recommendations for an earlier age of measles immunization in HIV-infected infants, weighing poor response from remaining maternal antibodies and immaturity of the infant's immune system against lower levels of maternal antibodies in infants of HIV-infected women and the deterioration of immune status that affects HIV-infected infants with age.

ACKNOWLEDGMENT

R.T.P. is also a fellow in Pediatric Infectious Diseases at the University of Maryland, Baltimore, Maryland.

REFERENCES

1. ANONYMOUS. 1998. Measles: progress towards global control and regional elimination, 1990–1998. Wkly. Epidemiol. Rec. **73:** 389–394.
2. KERNAHAN, J., J. MCQUILLIN & A.W. CRAFT. 1987. Measles in children who have malignant disease. Br. Med. J. (Clin. Res. Ed.) **295:** 15–18.
3. KAPLAN, L.J., R.S. DAUM, M. SMARON & C.A. MCCARTHY. 1992. Severe measles in immunocompromised patients. JAMA **267:** 1237–1241.
4. DOSSETOR, J., H.C. WHITTLE & B.M. GREENWOOD. 1977. Persistent measles infection in malnourished children. Br. Med. J. **1:** 1633–1635.
5. AABY, P. 1988. Malnutrition and overcrowding/intensive exposure in severe measles infection: review of community studies. Rev. Infect. Dis. **10:** 478–491.
6. BURSTROM, B., P. AABY & D.M. MUTIE. 1995. Measles in infants: a review of studies on incidence, vaccine efficacy and mortality in east Africa. East Afr. Med. J. **72:** 155–161.
7. SENSION, M.G., T.C. QUINN, L.E. MARKOWITZ *et al.* 1988. Measles in hospitalized African children with human immunodeficiency virus. Am. J. Dis. Child. **142:** 1271–1272.
8. OSHITANI, H., H. SUZUKI, M.E. MPABALWANI *et al.* 1996. Measles case fatality by sex, vaccination status, and HIV-1 antibody in Zambian children. Lancet **348:** 415.
9. LUCAS, S.B., C.S. PEACOCK, A. HOUNNOU *et al.* 1996. Disease in children infected with HIV in Abidjan, Cote d'Ivoire. Br. Med. J. **312:** 335–338.
10. EMBREE, J.E., P. DATTA, W. STACKIW *et al.* 1992. Increased risk of early measles in infants of human immunodeficiency virus type 1-seropositive mothers. J. Infect. Dis. **165:** 262–267.
11. AABY, P., K. KNUDSEN, T.G. JENSEN *et al.* 1990. Measles incidence, vaccine efficacy, and mortality in two urban African areas with high vaccination coverage. J. Infect. Dis. **162:** 1043–1048.
12. BURSTROM, B, P. AABY & D.M. MUTIE. 1993. Child mortality impact of a measles outbreak in a partially vaccinated rural African community. Scand. J. Infect. Dis. **25:** 763–769.
13. RYDER, R.W., M. NSUAMI, W. NSA *et al.* 1994. Mortality in HIV-1-seropositive women, their spouses and their newly born children during 36 months of follow-up in Kinshasa, Zaire. AIDS **8:** 667–672.

Virologic Response of Nine Therapy-Experienced Children Receiving 64 Weeks of Nelfinavir Salvage Therapy

C.L. VAVRO,[a,c] A.M. ZIMMERMANN,[a] D.R. McCLERNON,[a] S.L. KEHNE,[a] L.A. MARTEL,[b] M.E. VALENTINE,[b] AND R.E. McKINNEY[b]

[a]Department of Virology, Glaxo Wellcome, Inc., Research Triangle Park, North Carolina 27709, USA

[b]Pediatrics, Duke University Medical Center, Durham, North Carolina 27710, USA

INTRODUCTION

While protease inhibitor (PI) use in adults has been studied extensively,[1,2] little is currently known about the efficacy of PIs in children.[3] This study examines long-term exposure to nelfinavir (NFV) salvage therapy in reverse transcriptase inhibitor (RTI)-experienced children. The goals of this study were (1) to examine virologic and immunologic responses of RTI-experienced, PI-naïve children to triple salvage therapy with NFV, and (2) to determine whether the genotype of the HIV-1 reverse transcriptase and protease coding regions or the biologic phenotype of HIV-1 at baseline is predictive of the response to NFV therapy in this population.

MATERIALS AND METHODS

Study Population. The study population consisted of nine RTI-experienced, PI-naïve, HIV-1–infected children who received triple (8 children) or quadruple (1 child) therapy with NFV for 64 weeks. At study onset, all subjects added NFV and switched at least one of their current RTIs. The study was conducted at Duke University Pediatric Infectious Disease Center with Institutional Review Board approval. Parents or legal guardians of the children provided written informed consent prior to enrollment.

Lymphocyte Subset Analysis. At the specified clinic visits, whole blood was collected from each subject in EDTA-containing Vacutainer tubes. Lymphocyte subsets were obtained using standard whole blood cytometric methods. Absolute values were calculated using total lymphocyte numbers obtained from a complete blood count using a Coulter Counter.

Clinical Sample Culture. Blood samples (3 ml) were collected every 4 weeks from the subjects. Ten million (10^7) donor peripheral blood mononuclear cells (PMBCs) were co-cultivated with 5×10^6 subject PBMCs.[4] To monitor viral replication, reverse transcriptase levels were measured twice weekly using ^{3}H-deoxythymidine incorporation, as previously described, and cell pellets and aliquots of cell-free supernatant were frozen at peak reverse transcriptase levels.[5]

[c]To whom all correspondence should be addressed.

Viral Phenotype Determinations. Subject peripheral blood mononuclear cells were co-cultivated with an equal number of MT2 cells for approximately 23 days. Every 2–3 days each well was monitored for reverse transcriptase levels and syncitia formation by an examiner blinded to the specific subject and culture history.[6] Cultures were scored as syncitium-inducing or non-syncitium–inducing cultures.

Plasma HIV-1 RNA Quantitation. Plasma HIV-1 RNA levels were determined for each subject using the Roche Amplicor Monitor (v. 1.0) method (Roche Diagnostic Systems, Branchburg, NJ), with a lower limit of detection of 400 copies/ml. Virologic response was defined as a $>1 \log_{10}$ decrease in viral load from baseline (pre-study), which was sustained over the 64-week study period. Responders were defined as subjects who experienced by week 4 a $>1 \log_{10}$ decrease in viral load from baseline, which was sustained throughout the 64-week period. Transient responders were defined as subjects who experienced a $>1 \log_{10}$ decrease in viral load from baseline, which was sustained at the end of the first 28-week period but which had returned to baseline levels or higher at the end of the 64-week study period. Nonresponders were defined as subjects who failed to experience or sustain a $>1 \log_{10}$ decrease in viral load from baseline.

Viral Amplification and Sequencing. Nucleic acid isolation was performed using NucliSens HIV-1 QT Isolation kits (Organon Teknika, Durham, NC) which employ silica-based technology.[7] The first 240 codons of the reverse transcriptase region and the 99 codons of the protease region were amplified using reverse transcriptase-polymerase chain reaction. DNA sequence analysis was performed using dye terminator chemistry and the Perkin-Elmer ABI 373 (Perkin-Elmer, Foster City, CA).

RESULTS

Virologic Response. Of the nine RTI-experienced children in this 64-week study, there were two responders, one transient responder, and six nonresponders. The two responders had a mean decrease in viral load of $2.91 \log_{10}$ copies/ml, which contributed to the mean decrease of $0.72 \log_{10}$ copies/ml for the entire study population of nine subjects. The six nonresponders and one transient responder together had a mean decrease in viral load of $0.09 \log_{10}$ copies/ml. Plasma HIV-1 RNA levels for each subject throughout the study period are presented in TABLE 1.

Immunologic Response. All subjects had an increase in CD4 cell levels, with an average increase from baseline of 328 CD4 cells. The transient responder and five of the six nonresponders had a >200 absolute CD4 cell increase at or near 64 weeks. By contrast, the two responders had a dramatic and sustained increase in absolute CD4 cells, with a mean increase of 1,847 cells/mm^3 at 64 weeks. Absolute CD4 cell counts for each subject throughout the study period are presented in TABLE 1.

Viral Biological Phenotype Analysis. Eight of nine subjects had biological phenotype determinations performed at baseline. Six of eight subjects (subjects 1, 3, 4, 5, 7, and 8), including two responders, had viral isolates expressing the syncitium-inducing phenotype at baseline. The remaining two of eight subjects (subjects 6 and 9) had viral isolates expressing the non-syncitium–inducing phenotype at baseline, and both were nonresponders.

Genotypic Analysis. For seven of nine subjects, genotypic analysis of the protease coding region was performed on samples on or near week 64 of therapy. Five of these

TABLE 1. HIV-1 RNA levels ($\log_{10}$ copies/ml) and absolute CD4 cells (cells/mm^3) throughout the study[a]

PID	Pre	Week 4	Week 16	Week 28	Week 36	Week 44	Week 60	Week 64	Week 68
1	4.89/32	5.40/208	5.06/112	5.41/206	5.19/149	4.70/139	4.77/98	nd	nd
2	5.13/208	4.58/285	4.28/304	4.61/340	3.89/474	nd	4.41/467	nd	nd
3	5.09/10	2.37/102	2.30/nd	2.30/893	2.38/891	2.17/1571	nd	2.78/2019	nd
4	5.39/0	5.37/16	nd	5.43/557	5.88/651	5.81/456	nd	5.80/227	nd
5	5.13/0	2.82/17	4.98/nd	5.68/nd	5.88/198	5.53/248	nd	nd	4.99/208
6	5.86/83	4.58/165	5.73/207	5.88/314	6.20/328	nd	nd/186	5.88/164	5.59/135
7	4.94/0	2.65/27	3.44/239	3.40/355	4.51/466	4.87/663	4.93/nd	5.11/786	nd/751
8	5.87/60	3.50/200	3.34/725	nd	2.30 /1304	nd/1794	2.34/1421	nd	2.36/1745
9	5.26/4	2.70/12	2.30/52	2.20/nd	4.48/100	5.15/nd	nd/120	4.98/216	nd

[a]Abbreviations: nd = not done.

TABLE 2. Genetic analysis of the reverse transcriptase and protease coding regions[a]

PID	Study Visit	Reverse Transcriptase Coding Region	Protease Coding Region
1	Pre	M41L, T69T/A, M184V, T215Y	M36I
	Wk 16	M41L, M184V, T215Y	nd
	Wk 20	M41L, M184V, T215Y	D30N, M36M/I, N88N/D
	Wk 60	M41L, L210W, T215Y	K20R, D30N, M36I, L63P, N88D
2	Pre	D67N, T69D, K70R, T215Y	nd
	Wk 24	D67N, T69D, K70R, T215Y	M46I, L63P
	Wk 62	D67N, T69D, T215Y	L10I, M46I, A71T, V77I, L90M
3	Pre	M41L, D67N, T69D, V75M, T215Y	nd
	Wk 12	Y181C	nd
	Wk 28	nd	K20M, M36I, L90M
4	Pre	M41L, D67N, M184V, T215Y	V77I
	Wk 24	M41L, D67N, M184I, T215Y, K219R	nd
	Wk 28	M41L, D67N, M184I, L210W, T215Y, K219R	D30N, V77I, N88D
	Wk 62	M41L, D67N, M184I, L210W, T215Y	L10V, D30N, M36I, M46I, D60E, L63P, A71T, V77I, N88D
5	Pre	M41L, D67N, T69D, M184I/M, T215Y, K219R	nd
	Wk 28	M41L, D67N, T69D,K101N, Y181C, M184I, T215Y, K219R	D30N, M36I
	Wk 69	M41L, D67N, T69D, K101N, Y181C, M184I, T215Y, K219R	K20R, D30N, M36I, L63P, A71T, N88D
6	Pre	M41M/L, D67A, Y181C	K20M, M36I, L90M
	Wk 28	D67N, K70R, K103N, M184V, T215Y, K219E	nd
	Wk 64	M41L, D67N,K70R, V75I, M184V, T215Y, K219E	L10V, K20M, L63P, A71V, V77I, L90M
7	Pre	M41L, D67N, M184V, T215Y, K219R	nd
	Wk 48	M41L, M184V, L210W, T215Y	M36I, A71V,
	Wk 64	M41L, M184V, L210W, T215Y	D30N, M36I, L63P, A71V, N88D, L90M
8	Pre	M41L, K101Q, Y181C/Y, T215Y, K219N	nd
	Wk 16	nd	M36I, A71V, L90M
	Wk 24	M41L, Y181C, T215Y, K219N	nd
9	Pre	M41L, M184V, T215Y	nd
	Wk 24	nd	L20M, M36I, L90M
	Wk 63	nd	D30N, N88D

[a]Abbreviations: nd = not done; pre = pre-study (baseline).

seven subjects had mutations at codons 30 and 88 (TABLE 2); mutations D30N and N88D are associated with NFV resistance.[8] All seven subjects were nonresponders to NFV triple therapy. The remaining two of nine subjects, both responders, had plasma HIV-1 RNA values below the level of detection; as a result, sequence analysis could not be performed.

CONCLUSIONS

With this group of therapy-experienced subjects, only two children experienced sustained virologic response on NFV triple or quadruple therapy. However, all subjects experienced an increase in absolute CD4 cell count, regardless of the virologic response. Virologic response to NFV could not be predicted by the presence of the syncitium-inducing phenotype at baseline. The presence of mutations at both codons 30 and 88 was associated with virologic failure.

ACKNOWLEDGMENTS

This work was supported by Glaxo Wellcome, Inc. The authors thank Barbara Rutledge for manuscript preparation.

REFERENCES

1. JARVIS, B. & D. FAULDS. 1998. Nelfinavir: a review of its therapeutic efficacy in HIV infection. Drugs **56:** 147–167.
2. MOYLE, G.J. *et al.* 1998. Safety, pharmacokinetics, and antiretroviral activity of the potent, specific human immunodeficiency virus protease inhibitor nelfinavir: results of a phase I/II trial and extended follow-up in patients infected with human immunodeficiency virus. J. Clin. Pharmacol. **38:** 736–743.
3. SHARLAND, M. *et al.* 1998. Immune reconstitution in HAART-treated children with AIDS [lett.]. Lancet **352:** 577–578.
4. JACKSON, J.B. *et al.* 1988. Rapid and sensitive viral culture method for human immunodeficiency virus type 1. J. Clin. Microbiol. **26:** 1416–1418.
5. SCHWARTZ, O. *et al.* 1988. A rapid and simple colorimetric test for the study of anti-HIV agents. AIDS Res. Hum. Retroviruses **4:** 441–448.
6. HARADA, S. *et al.* 1985. Infection of HTLV-III/LAV in HTLV-1 carrying cells MT-2 and MT-4 and application in a plaque assay. Science **229:** 563–566.
7. BOOM, R. *et al.* 1990. Rapid and simple method for purification of nucleic acids. J. Clin. Microbiol. **28:** 495–503.
8. PATRICK, A.K. *et al.* 1998. Genotypic and phenotypic characterization of human immunodeficiency virus type 1 variants isolated from patients treated with the protease inhibitor nelfinavir. Antimicrob. Agents Chemother. **42:** 2637–2644.

Prevention of Ill Health in Children Born to HIV-Positive Women

MEDIATRIX BIHIIRA, J. KEITH, E. KISEKKA, T. KAYONGO, H. BACHOU,
E. OKECH, AND E. NAKIGUDDE

Morning Star Babies Home, Kampala, Uganda

INTRODUCTION

Morning Star Babies Home was established as a nongovernmental organization
in September 1998 in Kampala, Uganda. It was created to provide comprehensive
health care for some of the abandoned and orphaned AIDS children of Uganda and
the growing demand for specialized homes, specifically targeted at the needs of HIV-
infected and HIV-affected infants.

The four existing babies' homes in Kampala (Sanyu, Nsambya, Watoto, and
Naguru) were full to capacity and were unable to provide the specialized and individualized care needed by infants under 5 years of age. From January to March 1998,
the Kampala Police recorded 132 abandoned children, 15 of whom were infants under 2 years of age.

RATIONALE

A large percentage of abandoned babies are born to HIV-infected mothers. Some
of these women abandon the infants in hospitals immediately after delivery. Others
abandon them after they realize that they are either too sick or too poor to look after
the infants. Recently widowed fathers who are unable to balance the responsibilities
of a job and the care of a newborn at the same time bring some of the infants to the
Home. In the latter case, the Home takes over the care of the infant up to the age of
6 months, when the father or other relatives can take over. While the child is in the
Home, the relatives receive training on the nutritional, health, and nurturing needs
of the infant. Relatives also receive counseling on how to handle the social and emotional needs of an infected infant.

OBJECTIVES

The main objective of the Home is to provide a safe, healthy, and nurturing environment for abandoned and orphaned infants, some of whom are born to HIV-infected women. The Home achieves this by having two nurses, one social worker, one
doctor, and three caregivers on call. The combined effort of this team takes care of
all the infant's needs.

Many of the infants arrive at the Home malnourished, wasted, underfed, and sickly. The Home provides nutrition appropriate to the promotion of proper physical

growth and development. It also provides health care services including the required immunizations and treatment of illnesses.

When an infant first arrives at the Home, he is washed, weighed, fed, and examined by a doctor within 48 hours of arrival. If a medical record is available, it is reviewed and updated. If one is not available, the nurse obtains a history from the relative or most recent caregiver. The Home provides counseling to relatives having difficulty accommodating a child whose parents have died of AIDS. As well as training on how to care for newborn or sickly infants, they counsel relatives on the importance of integrating the infected infant into the family's normal day-to-day activities. All of these services are provided free of charge.

METHODOLOGY

The Home receives the following types of babies from the probation and child welfare office: (a) abandoned infants, (b) orphaned infants, (c) infants with parents who are too sick or too poor to support them properly, and (d) the infants of recently widowed fathers. All of these babies are received between the ages of 0 and 2 years and are kept until they are 5 years old. If the child is eligible but older than 2 years, he/she is referred to foster centers elsewhere. During this period, the Home identifies foster parents or foster homes that can take the infants permanently. The resident nurse registers the infants and takes a detailed medical and social history from the infant's last caregiver. Anthropometric measurements and vital signs are taken and the required vaccinations given. The physician examines each baby within 48 hours. Detailed medical records of each infant are maintained and kept separate from the infant's legal file. The Home currently (August 1999) has nine children, six boys and three girls ranging in age from 2 weeks to 2.5 years.

OBSERVATIONS

Information acquired from the last caregivers suggests that most of these children's parents do not have strong relationships. Most parents are unemployed. The poverty levels often found in HIV-affected homes can limit the chances for adequate care of the ill children. The lack of financial security in a home causes some mothers to leave their homes and desert their children while they look for a new partner who can provide for them.

FUTURE PLANS

The Home will liaise with medical centers, which offer palliative care and antiretroviral drug therapy to HIV-infected persons. The Babies Home intends to reach out and educate the people in the community about child care, children's rights, and alternative treatment centers. The Home also plans to identify income-generating projects to enable it to take care of children who by the age of 5 years have not been placed with foster parents or centers. The Home has and will continue to create awareness in the community that not all children born to HIV-infected mothers will contract HIV/AIDS. It will also create awareness about HIV transmission, risk reduction, and prevention.

REFERENCE

1. KEITH, J. 1998. Morning Star Babies Home Information Bulletin. Morning Star Babies Home. Kampala, Uganda.

Index of Contributors